LECTURES,

CLINICAL AND DIDACTIC,

ON THE

DISEASES OF WOMEN.

BY

R. LUDLAM, M.D.,

PROFESSOR OF OBSTETRICS AND THE DISEASES OF WOMEN AND CHILDREN IN THE HAHNEMANN MEDICAL COLLEGE, OF CHICAGO;

LATE PRESIDENT OF THE AMERICAN INSTITUTE OF HOMŒOPATHY;

PRESIDENT OF THE CHICAGO ACADEMY OF MEDICINE; GYNÆCOLOGIST TO THE SCAMMON HOSPITAL;

OBSTETRICAL EDITOR OF THE UNITED STATES MEDICAL AND SURGICAL JOURNAL;

AUTHOR OF A VOLUME OF CLINICAL LECTURES ON DIPHTHERIA; ETC., ETC.

"Artists are few,
"Teachers are thousands, and the world is large."
DR. HOLLAND.

CHICAGO: C. S. HALSEY.

PHILADELPHIA: F. E. BŒRICKE. LONDON: HOMŒOPATHIC PUB. CO.

1872.

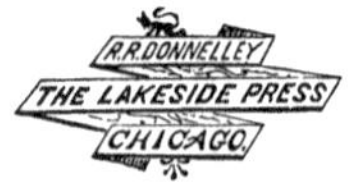
R.R. DONNELLEY
THE LAKESIDE PRESS
CHICAGO

TO

I. TISDALE TALBOT, M.D.,

OF BOSTON,

PRESIDENT OF THE AMERICAN INSTITUTE OF HOMŒOPATHY AND EDITOR OF THE NEW ENGLAND MEDICAL GAZETTE,

IN APPRECIATION OF HIS ABILITY AS A PHYSICIAN, HIS ATTAINMENTS AS A SCHOLAR, AND OF HIS HIGH PERSONAL CHARACTER; —

ALSO,

TO THE ALUMNI AND STUDENTS OF THE

HAHNEMANN MEDICAL COLLEGE,

OF CHICAGO,

IN ACKNOWLEDGMENT OF THEIR KIND ATTENTION TO THESE LECTURES, AND OF THE MANY EXPRESSIONS OF THEIR REGARD WHICH HAVE STIMULATED AND ENCOURAGED THE PREPARATION OF THE WORK;

THIS VOLUME IS RESPECTFULLY DEDICATED BY THEIR FRIEND AND FELLOW-LABORER,

THE AUTHOR.

PREFACE.

The following lectures are the substance of those delivered by the author in the college and hospital in which he has served in the capacity of a teacher for many years. Most of them were condensed by careful hands in the lecture-room; others were written at home; all are based upon actual experience. The text illustrates a series of cases which were selected because they were typical, and not because they were anomalous. They, therefore, constitute what naturalists style a type-collection. Each of these cases is genuine, the report thereof being from notes which were taken upon the spot, and not trusted to the *tabula rasa* of professional memory. The great majority of them were obtained from the College Dispensary and the Hospital; others were derived from a large consulting field, and a few (to add to the variety and force of the illustration) from the author's private case-book.

These cases have not been given in all their tedious detail, especially after the treatment was begun, but they have been analyzed and prescribed for in accordance with the author's best skill and judgment. Whenever it has seemed especially important, the result has been noted. They are not offered as models of excellent and accurate prescribing, which are complete in themselves and perfect of their kind; but are designed to be suggestive of the scope of practical medicine, surgery and hygiene, as applied to this specialty.

Clinical lectures permit the practical recognition of many minor points that are likely to be passed over in more stately treatises; and hence, if faithfully reported, approximate the more nearly to actual bed-side experience. The old maxim which holds that "History repeats itself" is true in Medicine. The clinical history of the various diseases to which attention has been called in these lectures will repeat itself in the experience of those who first heard them in the amphitheatre, and who may hereafter consult them in the printed form. That the lessons drawn may be suggestive, valuable and trustworthy in every particular, has been the chief object in their preparation.

The author herewith returns thanks to his professional brethren for their practical suggestions and the complimentary reception and recognition of his services in years that are past. This relation has not only been most grateful to him, but it has also served greatly to extend the field of his observation and experience in this specialty.

The lectures were reported by Drs. A. W. Woodward, H. T. F. Gatchell, E. Mussina, and the lamented W. Brendemuehl. The fidelity with which this work was done merits the thanks of the reader as well as of the author. And so likewise does the careful supervision of the press by my friend and colleague Prof. R. N. Foster. With these acknowledgments and without any apology for haste in its preparation, the work is herewith submitted to the profession.

CHICAGO, AUGUST 1, 1872.

CONTENTS.

LECTURE I.

LECTURE II.

LECTURE III.

LECTURE IV.

LECTURE V.

LECTURE VI.

LECTURE VII.

LECTURE VIII.

LECTURE IX.

LECTURE X.

LECTURE XI.

LECTURE XII.

LECTURE XIII.

LECTURE XIV.

LECTURE XV.

LECTURE XVI.

LECTURE XVII.

LECTURE XVIII.

LECTURE XIX.

LECTURE XX.

LECTURE XXI.

LECTURE XXII.

LECTURE XXIII.

LECTURE XXIV.

LECTURE XXVII.

LECTURE XXVIII.

LECTURE XXIX.

LECTURE XXX.

LECTURE XXXI.

LECTURE XXXII.

LECTURE XXXIII.

LECTURE XXXIV.

LECTURES,

CLINICAL AND DIDACTIC,

ON THE

DISEASES OF WOMEN.

LECTURE I.

PROLAPSUS UTERI WITH DROPSY, DATING FROM THE CLIMACTERIC PERIOD.

GENTLEMEN:

The first case to which your attention will be directed this morning belongs to a class of which I shall doubtless have occasion to speak quite often in my clinical course on the Diseases of Women.

Case.—Mrs. ——, aged 52, has had four children, the youngest of which is now fifteen years old. She has had but one abortion, and that occurred prior to the birth of her last child. Her menstruation was first established at the age of twelve years, and it ceased at forty, that is to say, twelve years ago. She says that her mother met with her "change" at the same age. The first symptom of ill health that this woman remarked in her own case, was a bloated feeling in the abdomen, which was sometimes quite full and distended, and again would subside to almost its natural size. This enlargement, she says, was uniform in its development, and not limited to any particular portion of the abdomen. There has been no tenderness on pressure, and no soreness. The swelling is notably increased by exercise, and is accompanied by bloating and puffiness of the limbs, the feet, and the face.

The bowels are habitually constipated, and if she fails to take a laxative pill, she has a great deal of straining at stool, and finally passes only dry, hard scybala. By reason of this urging at stool, she is quite positive that the womb is sometimes very much prolapsed, so much so, indeed, as to threaten protrusion from the vulva. She is also certain that at these times she has felt it lying between the labia majora. When she lies with the head low and the hips raised, the "tumor" disappears. The Dispensary Physician, Dr. Streeter, has made a careful vaginal examination of this case, and diagnosticates it as one of confirmed prolapsus uteri. The swelling of the integument is evidently dropsical, as is proved by its "pitting" under the pressure of my finger. The urine is scanty and high colored; the appetite capricious.

Parturition a cause of uterine deviations, and the climacteric period predisposes thereto.

Uterine displacements are so frequently related, either directly or indirectly, to abortion and to labor at term, that it will be well for you, in every case, to inquire whether the patient has recently passed through the process of parturition. This woman's last labor occurred fifteen years ago, and the probability that the uterine deviation dates from that event is very much lessened by the fact that it was not noticed until three years later. The prolapsus came on with the "change," or the advent of the grand climacteric, which, in her case, occurred at the early age of forty years. It is, therefore, possible for the uterus to become displaced at the end of the child-bearing period, and from other causes than a defect in its proper involution, or folding upon itself, after labor.

Dropsy at the climacteric, and constipation, causes of prolapsus.

Now the most obvious reason why she, at her time of life, has a prolapsus so decided, and which is only remotely, if at all, related to pregnancy, is the co-existence of dropsy, to which many women are liable at the climacteric. The ascites and general anasarca are indicative of a weakened and relaxed fibre, which strongly predisposes to uterine displacements. Add to this the direct pressure imposed upon the womb, also the semi-paralyzed condition of the rectum, and of the perineum (which has lost its resiliency), and the displacement downwards, even to the extent of procidentia, is readily explained. The only support that the uterus has from below, is from the contractile wall of the vagina, which rests like a column upon the perineum; and the chief muscles of the latter are connected with the rectum and the anus. In the constipation which is incident to chronic cases of this kind, the tone and elasticity of these tissues is partially or wholly lost. The straining at stool may therefore not only serve to perpetuate the luxation, but also to change its degree, and even its variety. It may convert a case of retroflexion into one of retroversion, or of simple prolapsus into procidentia. This relaxed or weakened condition of the muscular floor of the pelvis is, as I have already said, much more likely to follow upon the heels of labor, either premature or at term; but it also occurs in those who, like this patient, have borne numerous children, and who become subsequently afflicted with protracted and debilitating disease.

Treatment. — The relief afforded by the horizontal position, with the hips elevated, is significant. Many cases of prolapsus need but little beside appropriate postural treatment. It often happens that the displaced uterus will gravitate into its proper position, if the patient can keep off her feet. But it is not always possible, nor would it be best, for women with this infirmity to go to bed and remain there. Those of the poorer classes must work, and they all need exercise. And thus it may become necessary to supply a means of support which shall supplement the relaxed muscular fibre of the vagina and of the perineum. It is in just such examples of prolapsus as this, occurring in women somewhat advanced in life, who are ill in other respects, and constitutionally weak, and withal obliged to walk and to work daily, that I am accustomed to recommend the wearing of the perineal pad, as a means of temporary relief. It will accomplish more, and is more available in most instances, than any other form of supporter. In conjunction with the proper internal remedies, its effect is to tone up the parts which afford the natural support for the uterus, and at the same time to allow the patient to move about with impunity. I shall speak, in a subsequent lecture, of the proper indications for pessaries, and the value of them in this and other forms of uterine displacement, as they occur under different circumstances.

Postural treatment, and the perineal pad.

It is important that this patient should refrain from all violent exercise, more especially from lifting heavy weights, and from scrubbing, sweeping, and ironing. She should not permit herself to strain at stool, neither sit in a constrained position for any considerable time. Her food should consist largely of albuminous matters, designed to improve the quality of the blood; and of vegetable

Hygienic precautions, and remedies.

substances, particularly of such as are somewhat laxative, as fruits, and bread made of unbolted flour.

The remedies that are most prominently indicated for this particular case are nux vomica and apis mellifica. And, since neither of them will cover the two sets of symptoms which are present, I recommend them to be given in alternation, the former at evening, and the latter in the morning and at noon of each day. The nux vomica is especially indicated on account of the constipation, the straining at stool, the passage of scybala, and the threatened escape of the uterus from the pelvic cavity. There are the best possible pathogenetic and physiological reasons for its employment, although, in chronic cases like this, I think it should not be given more than once or twice daily. In similar cases, lycopodium, or sepia, will sometimes prove of the greatest utility.

Internal remedies.

The manifest relation between the commencement of the dropsical symptoms, and the arrest or cessation of the menstrual function furnishes us with a characteristic indication for the apis mellifica. In using this remedy, my own preference is for the second or third decimal triturations.

LEUCORRHŒA WITH CHRONIC OVARITIS.

Case.—Mrs. ——, aged 30, was married seven years ago, but has had no children, and has never suffered a miscarriage. She has had leucorrhœa for the last ten years. The discharge is of a yellowish white color, sometimes thick and creamy, and again thin, copious, and quite fluid. After having been upon her feet for a long time, the flow becomes more profuse. She is certain that the quantity discharged frequently amounts to three or four ounces in a day. When the matter which is most liquid escapes, she feels most exhausted. She complains, at such times especially, of a sense of weariness, and of dragging pains in the loins and hips. For a long time, she remarked, the leucorrhœal discharge was most profuse either immediately before, or directly after, her menstrual "returns;" but for some time past she could discern no especial increase at this or any other period of the month.

She menstruates regularly every four weeks, but the proper flow is gradually lessening in quantity, so that at present she is "sick" but two days instead of three, or three and a half, as heretofore. The only suffering experienced during menstruation is a severe burning pain, which is located just within the anterior superior spinous process of the left ilium and above the groin, or in other words, in the region of the left ovary. This pain, which is sometimes very severe, always extends down the corresponding thigh to the knee. She has never had it upon the right side. She is quite confident that she has not menstruated a single time, during the last ten or twelve years, without experiencing this peculiar, burning, cramp-like, neuralgic pain. When the catamenia cease, it immediately declines, and she has never had it in the inter-menstrual period. Riding and walking increase its severity.

Examination by the speculum discloses a scrofulous suppurating ulcer at the os externum, extending into the canal of the cervix. The mucous membrane, investing the vaginal portion of the uterine neck, is considerably swollen and congested. The left ovarian region is exceedingly sensitive to external and internal palpation. She has been treated by four physicians, three of whom cauterized the cervix severely, but without any benefit to the patient. Indeed, she steadily continued to grow worse, and, as you see, her general health is now very much impaired.

Burning pain in ovaritis. Ovulation sometimes a constant cause of ovaritis.

A chief point of interest in this case is the lesion of the left ovary and its consequences. For, the local symptoms which occur so regularly, are so characteristic and so constant that we are forced to conclude that the ovarian disease is the primary one. There is, indeed, something quite distinctive about this "burning" pain in the inguinal region, which extends down the limb of the same side. When it comes on with the return of the catamenia, and ceases during the inter-menstrual period, you may be certain that the corresponding ovary is inflamed. This inflammation may exist for years, with a brief, sub-acute and self-limited attack each month. The cause of this fresh and painful recurrence of inflammation is the physiological afflux of blood to the organ; without this afflux the proper function of the ovary can not be performed, any more than the gastric juice can be secreted if the delicate capillaries of the gastric mucous membrane are not injected with blood. It is the periodical repletion of the vessels of an inflamed ovary that gives rise to the peculiar, burning, cramp-like, neuralgic pains of which our patient has just made complaint, and that has literally been the thorn in her side for these many years.

Reflex relations of the ovary.

The reflex relations of the ovaries are numerous, varied, and important. They are in sympathy with the lungs, the mammary glands, the uterine mucous membrane, the nerve centers of animal life, and especially with the uterine cervix and its secretory apparatus. The neck of the uterus is not more intimately associated with the womb itself, of which it is the natural outlet, than it is with the ovaries. These little organs, although remotely located, have really as much to do with the active dilatation of the os uteri, and the escape of the menstrual flow through it, as they have with its first formation in the uterine cavity. They not only serve as time-keepers for the menstrual organism, but they also open the gateway of the generative intestine for the escape of its periodical discharge.

Sympathy between the uterine cervix and the ovaries.

This peculiar sympathetic function is exceedingly liable to derangement. In a state of health, both of the ovaries and of the cervix, it is intact. But suppose that either of these parts becomes the seat of serious and protracted disease — nothing is more certain than the consequent, although indirect, implication of the other. It would be almost, or quite impossible for our patient to have had this form of sub-acute ovaritis for so long a period without the cervical leucorrhœa also. Protracted and persistent leucorrhœal discharges, whether from the uterus or the vagina, or both together, are always indicative of structural disease somewhere. The lesions which produce them may be idiopathic or secondary. They may depend upon causes which are purely local, upon those which are constitutional, or upon such as are reflex. In the case before us there is little doubt that the ulceration depends on the inflammation of the left ovary, which is the fount and origin of the disorder for the relief and cure of which we have been consulted.

Leucorrhœa may substitute menstruation.

The gradual diminution of the menses is significant and suggestive. When ovaritis is accompanied by uterine ulceration, which is not cancerous or phagedenic, there is almost always a tendency in the menstrual secretion to become more and more scanty. Under these circumstances, the leucorrhœa sometimes substitutes menstruation, when it is termed " vicarious." This result is more likely to follow the inflammation of both ovaries than of one.

Uterine and vaginal catarrh from ovaritis.

In *catarrhal* leucorrhœa, without ulceration of the cervix, and whether it comes from the uterus or the vagina, the discharge is usually increased either before or directly after the catamenial flow. Here the ovarian sympathy spends itself in giving rise to an extraordinary secretion of mucus, and menstruation is more apt to be profuse than scanty. Some of the worst forms of menorrhagia, or excessive menstruation, are engrafted upon this kind of leucorrhœa, which may also arise from ovarian irritation and inflammation.

Barrenness caused by leucorrhœa.

Sterility is a natural and almost necessary consequence of either of the forms of leucorrhœa just named, which might, without any great impropriety, be styled ovarian leucorrhœa. As our patient's disease commenced before her marriage, there are the best of reasons why she has never been pregnant.

The importance of special pathology.

Treatment. — It is possible that enough has already been said to illustrate the importance of a correct knowledge of special pathology in cases of this kind. And yet I must embrace so favorable an opportunity to say a few words upon a subject concerning which you will find so much in our books and journals. I apprehend that no man or woman ever yet made a prescription without having in his or her mind a theory of the ailment to be treated. However improperly it may have been done, the simplest domestic remedy is not given until the disease has been classified. And among the fraternity, *nolens volens*, we are as much addicted to the habit of naming diseases before we treat them, as to the naming of our babies before they are baptized. And because this theory, which represents our idea of the special pathology of the disease in question, and typifies our knowledge or our ignorance of it, is "as inevitable as one's shadow," it is vitally important that it be correctly established. If we would unravel the tangled skein, we must get hold of the proper thread. In order to be skillful and successful in the interpretation and cure of diseased states, we must begin at the right end of the series.

According to the theory that the ulceration gave rise to the leucorrhœa, and that what would heal the former would also cure the latter, this patient has been cauterized by three physicians in turn. Their applications may have patched up the case, but, for reasons which you now understand better than they seem to have done, the cure was not permanent. The lesion of the os reappeared, simply because the ovarian affection had been overlooked and neglected. And not only did the cruel expedient to which they resorted fail to cure the lesion of the os uteri; it also increased the ovarian congestion and inflammation. For the sympathy between the cervix and the ovaries is such that whatever harms one will almost certainly implicate and injure the other.

Indiscriminate cauterization of the os uteri.

Your preceptors are fully aware of the fact that a large share of the ovarian affections which they are called upon to treat have been caused in this manner. And your own future experience will one day confirm the observation, that the *indiscriminate* employment of escharotics in uterine ulceration is mischievous to the last degree. If those three doctors had been more competent diagnosticians, they would have been less likely to commit such an unpardonable error in practice.

Let us endeavor to improve upon this treatment. We must study this case most carefully, not for the purpose of naming the disease, and afterwards treating it by name, for that plan has already been tested; but to analyze the symptoms presented, and to remove them in the most rational and sensible manner. In a case of this kind the ovarian symptoms are a thousand times more significant than those which pertain to the leucorrhœal discharge. The proper plan is, therefore, first to treat the disease of the left ovary, and afterwards, if anything remains of the uterine ulceration and its consequent discharge, to address our remedies specifically to them.

The prominent symptoms for which we must select a remedy in this case are, therefore, severe pain in the *left* ovary, which is of a burning character, extending down the corresponding limb, which recurs with every return of the catamenial period, and is aggravated by riding or walking; the menses become more scanty, and are accompanied and followed by leucorrhœa. The appropriate remedy is thuja oc., of which she will take a dose every evening during the month.

Inter-menstrual treatment.

The most proper and effective treatment in cases of this kind is one that is brought to bear during the inter-menstrual period. Palliatives and kindred expedients, only designed to relieve suffering while menstruation continues, are in no sense curative. The persistency of the symptoms just named, and the unequivocal indication presented for the thuja, warrant us in promising a great, although it must be a gradual, improvement in our patient's health. In addition to the internal remedy, she should syringe out the vagina twice daily with tepid castile suds. In some cases of this kind I add a few drops of the crude tincture of thuja, and in others of calendula, to the water injected into the vagina. But it should be an indictable offense, for the physician to prescribe or apply astringent washes and escharotics, for the relief of such a case of leucorrhœa as that to which your attention has now been called.

You will not understand me to recommend this prescription for all cases of ovarian inflammation indiscriminately. Before the session has closed, I shall doubtless have occasion to advise the employment of various other remedies in the treatment of this disease.

MORNING SICKNESS OF PREGNANCY, AND RETROVERSION.

Case. — Mrs. G., aged 35, has reached the third month of her fifth pregnancy. Her first two children, a son and a daughter, were carried to term and are now living. She has aborted twice at about three and a half months, in consequence, as her physician told her, of retroversion of the womb. The chief peculiarity of the case is that the nausea and vomiting which are incident to the early months of gestation are experienced by her at night only. It commences each evening at ten, and continues, with occasional interruptions, until after midnight, and sometimes until two o'clock in the morning. She enjoys her breakfast and dinner, but has no appetite for tea.

She is very confident that when she was pregnant with her two living children, the gastric symptoms came on as with most women, in the morning and not at night. And also that, in case of the two which she lost prematurely, the nausea and vomiting occurred, as in the present instance, during the evening and night. For this reason she dreads an impending abortion, and is fully persuaded in her own mind that it is quite impossible for her to go to "term." This conviction is also confirmed by the dictum of her former physician, who declared positively that it would be out of the question for her to carry her offspring beyond the fourth month.

Upon careful digital examination, I found an evident deviation or displacement of the uterus. The os uteri was nearer the symphysis pubis than natural, and at the Douglas' cul-de-sac there was a hard, globular tumor, which yielded to steady pressure in the direction of the sacral promontory, and finally passed upwards out of reach. This little manipulation afforded her great relief. She insists that the replacement of the womb has always palliated the gastric distress, and sometimes stopped it entirely for days together.

This is an exceptional case. It is seldom indeed that the reflex gastric symptoms in the early months of pregnancy are so pronounced. I have, accordingly, chosen it as the theme for a few practical remarks. The case is a typical one, which illustrates the intimate relationship through indirect nervous communication, between the uterus and the stomach. This peculiar sympathy is shown in various ways. I have known a patient to vomit within five or ten minutes after, and in consequence of the application of the nitrate of silver to the uterine cervix. A sudden dropping down of the womb in some cases of prolapsus produces the same effect. In many cases of tardy labor dependent upon rigidity of the os uteri, emesis removes the cause of the delay by relaxing the cervix. For it often happens that, when delivery has been delayed for some hours, the sudden relaxation of the os is announced by retching, and a desire to vomit. Ulceration of the cervix may indirectly occasion the most intractable vomiting. Bennet and others are of opinion that the worst cases of "morning sickness" are referable to this cause. Uterine displacements are known to produce it, and it is more than possible that the slight prolapse of the womb, which is incident to the first months of gestations, may help to account for this very distressing symptom.

Reflex gastric symptoms in early pregnancy.

In the example before you, the retroversion, which is temporarily induced by more or less of exercise upon her feet during the day, and which is relieved when the patient rests at night, is evidently the chief cause of the retching and vomiting. When the fundus and body of the uterus topple over backwards, they not only press upon the anterior sacral or sciatic plexus of nerves, which is situated at the side of the rectum, but also upon the sacral ganglia of the great sympathetic. The hypogastric plexus is also implicated in the displacement. The ease with which the organ can be replaced, and the manifest relief afforded, are not only useful in the matter of diagnosis, but suggestive as to the postural treatment proper for our patient. For, the mere prescription of a remedy, or remedies, to be given internally for the relief of the gastric symptoms, is but a fractional part of the physician's duty

Retroversion a possible cause of morning sickness.

in a case of this kind. It will often happen, that by placing such a patient in a proper posture, and regulating her diet, as well as the time of eating her meals, and the amount and quality of exercise taken, we can accomplish more than by the most appropriate constitutional means. The cause of the suffering is purely local, and the treatment should be partly, if not exclusively, local also.

Abortion a contingent of retroversion of the gravid uterus.

In less than a month, if the excessive vomiting and the displacement do not cause abortion, this woman's womb will pass out of the pelvic basin into the abdominal cavity, in order that it may undergo the proper development. If we can succeed in averting the contingency of miscarriage, (which is, perhaps, doubtful,) she may go on well to term. For when the womb has escaped from the lower pelvis, its liability to dislocation will be removed, and the proneness to gastric derangement cease. Provided the retroversion is not inveterate, the gastric disorder will be self-limited.

If not excessive, morning sickness is salutary. Apt to return at night in retroversion.

The idea has long been entertained and advocated by obstetrical writers that, unless a pregnant woman has "morning sickness" at some period of gestation, she will be apt to miscarry, or perhaps to have a difficult and dangerous labor at its close. Although there are frequent exceptions to this rule, many persons passing through pregnancy from first to last without any particular derangement of the stomach, and finally doing well, it nevertheless remains true, that its presence is a more favorable sign, if it be not extreme in degree or misplaced in the period of its recurrence, than its absence. From careful observation in this respect, I am led to conclude that the habitual return of this symptom at evening, or as sometimes happens, in the middle of the night, renders it a more serious and obstinate affair than when it comes in the early part of the day, whether before or after breakfast.

A prognosis of inevitable abortion unwarranted.

While it is no part of my duty or desire to reflect unkindly upon my professional brethren, I must be emphatic in warning you against perpetrating the folly and wrong which this patient's former physician committed when he declared it impossible for her ever to carry another child past the fourth month. His opinion was not properly deduced from the facts of the case, and is, therefore, fallacious. Because this poor woman had retroversion in the early stage of two successive pregnancies, and afterwards aborted, it by no means follows that a third or a fourth attempt to complete the process of gestation can not prove successful. If such a verdict were as harmless as it were unjustifiable, we would pass it by without further notice. But you are witnesses to the fact that it weighs down this patient's spirits like an incubus, and discourages her in the outset. Such dicta are inexcusable and mischievous. There are few circumstances that will warrant you in telling a woman that she cannot possibly go through with pregnancy, and give birth to a living child. Daily experience proves that even the most learned and reliable practitioners are likely to be mistaken when they pass such a sentence upon their patients. The range of physiological possibilities is a wide one, and since Nature will do as she pleases, it will be wise in us not to assume to limit her powers in this direction.

How to replace the womb.

Treatment.—The first indication presented is to restore the womb to its natural position. This may usually be accomplished by a species of vaginal taxis, pressure being made with one or more of the fingers against the body of the displaced organ in the direction of the sacro-vertebral angle. In order to be most efficient and least harmful, this operation should be performed in a slow and cautious, not in a rapid and careless manner. The desired result will be facilitated by calling gravitation to our aid. For this purpose, in most cases, it may suffice for the patient to lie upon her side, or better still, upon her abdomen. We may, however, find it best to place her in the prone position upon the knees and breast, over one or more large pillows, as recommended in the treatment of prolapse of the funis, and for the correction of presentation of the face, side and shoulder. It may also be necessary to introduce the finger, or some other instrument, into the rectum in such a manner as to aid in replacing the uterus. Gariel's air-bag may be passed into the bowel behind the displaced organ, and afterwards so inflated as to lift the fundus, and compel the womb to correspond as it should with the axis of the superior strait. Or you may employ this little instrument, devised by my friend, Prof. Guernsey,* which is admirably fitted to fill the same indication.

* Vide Guernsey's Obstetrics, etc., 1867; page 16.

In using this instrument, Dr. G. recommends that, after the bladder and rectum have been emptied, "the patient should be placed on the bed, near its edge, upon her knees and elbows, so that the force of gravity may assist in the reduction. The ball of the instrument, well lubricated, is to be brought to the anus, with the convex surface of the rod upwards, then gently pressed until within the sphincter; when the handle should be slightly elevated, so as to bring the ball against the anterior wall of the rectum. The instrument is now to be firmly and carefully pressed up the rectum, when the ball will elevate the fundus,—care being taken to raise the handle more and more as progress up the rectum is made; and presently the uterus will regain its normal position immediately posterior to the symphysis pubis.

The uterine sound as a means of reducing the dislocation.

In all cases of uterine displacement incident to pregnancy, and whether for purposes of exploration or of treatment, you should carefully abstain from the introduction of any instrument whatever through the canal of the cervix into the uterine cavity. Such an operation would be almost certain, sooner or later, to be followed by abortion. And I flatter myself that no member of this medical class would willingly commit the crime of murder, even for the sake of curing a case of prolapsus, or of retroversion of the womb! I have known a physician, however, who, through cupidity and ignorance, found it convenient to diagnosticate many examples of the latter displacement in pregnant females, and afterwards to reduce the dislocation by means of the uterine sound — a most cruel and unwarrantable expedient.

Postural treatment.

But simply to replace the organ in such a case as the one before us is not always sufficient. Unless we provide against a recurrence of the displacement, more especially when the patient assumes an upright position, the increased size and weight of the womb will bring it down again. To obviate such a result, and thus indirectly to control the gastric symptoms, she should remain in the horizontal position upon the bed or sofa, and should lie either upon the side or upon the abdomen. If she can keep off her feet altogether until such time as the uterus has ascended into the abdomen, the vomiting will be greatly relieved, and perhaps cured, and, what is still more important, the chief danger of abortion will also be averted.

It is only now and then that a pessary is of real utility in the uterine deviations contingent upon pregnancy. The watch-spring pessary, covered with rubber, will sometimes answer a good purpose temporarily, and is less objectionable than most others. Either of the stem pessaries would be more likely to cause than to prevent a miscarriage, and moreover they are not suited to cases of retroversion.

The pessary.

In two similar instances I have succeeded in keeping the womb *in situ* by the introduction of a small sized air-pessary, to be then inflated, into the posterior and superior portion of the vagina, in such a manner as to prevent the body and fundus of the organ from falling towards the coccyx. When distended with air, this rubber bag becomes a species of cushion against which the uterus may rest without injury, and indeed it can do no possible harm to the soft parts. Nor is it half so liable as instruments that are made of more solid materials, to stimulate reflex uterine contractions, and thereby to excite an abortion. Some practitioners prefer Hodge's lever pessary in this as in other cases of retroversion. If judiciously used, it very rarely happens that the means which I have indicated will not serve to replace the womb and to keep it in position. A few cases are recorded in which the displacement has persisted until the end of gestation. Where the retroversion is inveterate, and in case of emergency, it has been thought expedient sometimes to promote the evacuation of the uterine contents by rupturing the amniotic sac through the uterine cervix, or by the operation of *paracentesis uteri*, as first recommended by the celebrated Dr. William Hunter.

Retroversion may persist until term.

In a report upon the retroversion of the gravid uterus, read before the Obstetrical Society of London, by Dr. W. Tyler Smith,* you will find the following instructive case:

"I was consulted in August, 1859, by a lady, a patient of Dr. Duigan, of Gainsborough. She was the mother of two children, and, in the previous May, had a miscarriage, which left her in a very weak state. She had lost blood largely, and had since been irregular at the periods. Her chief complaint was of a distressing pain at the bottom of the back, and the least attempt at walking or exertion produced faintness. On making a digital examination, the uterus was found to be retroverted, the fundus hanging upon the lower part of the rectum, and so enlarged as to make me be-

* Trans. of the Obstetrical Society of London; Vol. II., page 297.

lieve that pregnancy existed. She remained in town about a month; and the increase in the size of the uterus in this time converted the belief into certainty. There is no other condition in which the increase of the gravid uterus in the early months can be so readily estimated as in retroversion. The globular fundus is so perfectly within reach of the finger, as to render it possible to measure its increase with a precision which cannot be obtained when the uterus is in its natural position. In this case, the fundus could be lifted from the rectum, so as to afford temporary relief, but it would soon return to the position of retroversion. Acting on this hint, I introduced an air-pessary of considerable size, which gave great relief, and enabled her to move about to an extent which had previously been impossible. With the air-pessary the uterus remained in a state of semi-retroversion. She continued to wear the instrument, with great comfort, for upwards of two months, and only left it off when quickening and the movements of the child made it certain that the uterus had risen out of the pelvis. She was delivered in April last of a living child, and carefully rested after her confinement, lying, as much as possible, in the prone position. In this case, the pelvis was of large size, and it is the only instance I have seen of persistent retroversion in the gravid state, in which there was no vesical symptom whatever. I have seen this patient twice since her delivery. The first time there was no sign of retroversion, but the second it had returned to some extent, and I advised the use of the air-pessary again."

ON WEANING A CHILD, AND THE SUBSEQUENT TREATMENT OF THE MAMMARY GLANDS — GALACTORRHŒA.

Case. — Mrs. Z——, aged 30, applies for advice concerning the propriety of weaning her child, and likewise for instructions relative to the best method of procedure if this expedient is deemed proper. The baby is eleven months old, and healthy in every respect, not having had a day's sickness from its birth. The mother's health is also excellent. The milk is furnished in good amount and quality, and although she really dreads to wean the little one, she will nevertheless do so if it is thought best. By the advice of her former physician she nursed an elder child, now four years of age, until it was eighteen months old. Her infant feeds well, and, if it were allowed, would eat almost anything. It has a mouthful of teeth. She fears that when she takes it from the breast altogether, she may have trouble with the glands themselves. For she is somewhat peculiar in this respect, that with her the milk continues to be secreted for a long time after it has ceased to be regularly drawn off. Thus when she weaned her little girl, two years and a half ago, the milk "continued to come into the breast," as she says, for four or five months longer, her menstruation being quite regular meanwhile. And following an abortion, that she once experienced at the fourth month, she had a considerable flow of milk for the space of nearly six months. For this reason she feels exceedingly anxious to know what course is the proper one.

Fashionable pretexts for the indiscriminate weaning of infants.

In the practice of your profession you will be frequently consulted in cases similar to this. You will observe that some mothers apply for professional sanction to wean their children early, and, indeed, that many of them prefer not to nurse their babies at all. These most unnatural and baneful practices are, unfortunately, becoming more frequent. In all our cities and towns—and in these days of railways and telegraphs there are no more country villages—the custom of rearing children at second-hand, or by proxy, is becoming more and more popular and prevalent. The most silly pretexts are preferred by people in fashionable life for denying the little infant the mother's breast. One such mother will decline to ruin her bodily form and figure by nursing her own child, another considers it vulgar, a third is too much of an invalid herself, while a fourth is unwilling to sacrifice the pleasures of the table, of the toilet, or of gay and fashionable society, of late hours, or of some favorite form of dissipation, for the cares and crosses of maternity. Among women of the great middle class of society there is a growing aversion to what is both natural and necessary for the welfare of their delicate offspring. For the most trivial, and even shameful reasons, too many little innocents are thus denied their most appropriate aliment. The consequence is that a large share of American mothers never experience those reflex influences that would tend to soften and sweeten their own natures; and that thousands of children are poisoned by all sorts of artificial substitutes for healthy human milk.

Another class of mothers place a premium on the luxury of nursing their own children. They are never quite ready and willing to wean them. If your future observation accords with my own, you will have reason to conclude that, with many members of this class, the pleasure derived from the performance of this very natural function constitutes the chief enjoyment of their married life.

Not unfrequently, however, there is another reason for the resolve on the part of these women to prolong the period of lactation. As a rule, menstruation is suspended until the child is taken from the breast. This they all know as well as we do. They are also aware that, while the nursing woman does not menstruate, she is not very likely to conceive again. Hence many mothers voluntarily continue to suckle their children beyond the proper time, in the hope that they may thus avoid too rapid an increase in the family. But since there are many exceptions to the rule that a nursing woman may not become pregnant, and more especially because the health of the child, and of the mother also, may be injured thereby, it will become your manifest duty, in some cases, to insist that this practice shall be relinquished.

Ill effects of too prolonged lactation.

As a rule, if both the patient and her child are well, the little one should not be weaned before it is about a year old. After this period the mother's milk becomes deficient in casein,—a physiological reason why lactation should not be prolonged. In deciding upon the most proper time for taking the children from the breast, something depends upon circumstances. If, for example, the little thing has cut its teeth freely and early, and manifests a disposition for a mixed diet, being ready and eager to eat almost anything that is offered, there will be little risk in weaning it. It will, however, be more safe for the child to cease nursing in cool or cold weather, as in the fall or winter, than in the late spring or early summer months. If a severe epidemic, more especially any alimentary disorder, such as cholera infantum or dysentery, is prevalent among young children, you should counsel the mother to wait until the epidemic has subsided before she puts her child away. The almost utter impossibility, in our larger cities, at certain seasons, of procuring good, healthy cow's milk for the infant, may afford another valid reason for prolonging lactation even beyond the twelfth month. Statistics prove that after the ninth month, weaning is more apt to be followed by mammary abscess than at any period between the second and ninth months.

The proper time for weaning.

In the case in which we have just been consulted, the child's age is favorable, it has its complement of teeth, eats well, and is thrifty in every regard; the season (November) is propitious; and there is no disease which at this time is especially prevalent among infants and young children. We therefore advise that this woman's babe be weaned.

Treatment.—And now the question is fairly before us; what course is most proper for the mother? In her case there is a manifest predisposition to a profuse and prolonged secretion of milk. Ordinarily the quantity of milk secreted is in proportion to the frequency with which the breast is drawn, or emptied; the more it is nursed, the greater the yield. But in this case a profuse flow is furnished by the gland, although none of the product is forcibly withdrawn. Here there is a danger lest the milk may accumulate and give rise to inflammation, and, ultimately, to mammary abscess. Hence we must, if possible, institute measures that will avert such a calamity. For it is a species of martyrdom for any woman to suffer from an abscess or abscesses of the mammary gland, and we should use our best endeavors to spare her such an infliction.

Prophylactic treatment.

Where, as in this instance, the flow of milk is very profuse, and especially if the child is several months old, I think the wiser course is to wean it gradually—say to nurse it only at night for a time, and to feed it during the day. This plan will prevent the accumulation of a very large quantity of milk in the breasts, and also allow the general organism to accommodate itself to the new condition of things, points which are in some cases most significant. If the mother stops nursing abruptly, there will be greater risk of local trouble, and of a general derangement of her health, than if the change is less sudden and extreme.

This rule, which has its exceptions, is also applicable in case it becomes necessary to wean the child at a very early age. In general, however, it is thought advisable to put the infant away from the breast at once, as less troublesome than gradual weaning. Afterward, if the ducts become obstructed, and the glands distended, hard and painful, a resort is to be had to some artificial means of emptying them, and of averting farther trouble.

Antigalactics.

Medicines which are believed to have the power of lessening the quantity of milk secreted are termed *Antigalactics*. They are used both internally and externally. Of those which are adapted to internal use the more prominent are belladonna, bryonia, calcarea carbonica, and phosphorus. Besides these, other remedies are suited to lessen a redundancy of this flow, when it is attended by peculiar symptoms, all of which are lacking in this case. For, Mrs. Z. is not ill at the present time, and the most diligent search might fail to disclose a single symptom of an abnormal condition. Our treatment must, therefore, be prophylactic. It should be designed so to diminish the quantity of this secretion as to insure the breasts against local disease or injury, and the general system from all contingent disorders. To fill this indication I have more confidence in the calcarea carbonica than in any other remedy. I prefer it in the third decimal trituration. Your future experience may cause you to decide in favor of some other form or potency of this remedy. This is a matter which cannot be settled for you in the lecture-room.

The age of the child a criterion of the danger of mammary abscess.

In general, the younger the child the greater the danger of mammary abscess from weaning it. There are, however, exceptions to this rule also, in which it is almost or quite impossible to take the child from the breast at any period without incurring the risk of this accident. When a physician tells you that he has always been able to avoid such a result in his practice, you may safely conclude that he has been unusually fortunate, or that his observation has been limited.

Local applications.

Local adjuvants are not only admissible, but, in certain cases, necessary also. Most practitioners prefer camphor for this purpose. Cloths may be wet with the common tincture and applied directly to the breast. Or it may be anointed with a mixture of camphor and sweet oil — the camphorated oil of the shops. A saturated solution of camphor in glycerine makes a more pleasant and equally useful preparation, which may be kept constantly applied over the gland by means of flannel compresses.

Several of my medical friends assure me that they have derived the most satisfactory results from the topical employment of cold water, as a preventive against mammitis and mammary abscess in cases of this kind. I have no experience therewith. They recommend to apply a wet compress directly over the gland, and to protect the clothing by a dry one outside. This is to be renewed from time to time, the water being at the temperature of ordinary well or hydrant water. They claim that the faithful use of this simple means will spare much subsequent trouble to all concerned. Another method consists in covering the breast with one or more layers of flannel, and then applying a bladder which is partly filled with broken ice. Persistent rigors and chilliness, however, contra-indicate the use of cold applications of all kinds.

A stimulating lotion may also be made of black pepper (*Piper nigrum*), by permitting it to stand for a considerable time in good brandy. The pepper should, however, be in the grain and not ground, or pulverized, otherwise, by insinuating itself into the delicate skin, especially in the region of the areola, it might occasion much suffering. This lotion may be applied in the same manner as recommended for the glycerole of camphor.

In inflammatory cases in which the pain and throbbing of the gland are severe, or if the pains are neuralgic, the application of the belladonna plaster will sometimes afford the greatest possible relief. It may serve not only to abort the suppurative process, but also to put a stop to the further secretion of milk. This expedient seems especially adapted to those cases in which it is advisable, directly after labor, to institute measures for the prevention of a free flow of the lacteal product. Dr. Marley recommends to smear the breast with the extract of belladonna.* He has employed this treatment for the prevention of mammary abscess with almost uniform success in 44 cases, in which a prompt arrest of the lacteal secretion was necessary.

When the breasts are large and flabby, the extra weight may be relieved by a broad handkerchief, a net-work supporter, or by strips of adhesive plaster properly applied. These plaster-strips are sometimes used to secure uniform compression of the glands, and thereby diminish their secretion. The bandage of Seutin has been extolled for the same purpose.

Means of support for the breasts.

Our patient should abstain from soups and all kinds of liquid food, and satisfy her appetite chiefly with solids. It would not be best for her to drink largely of any fluid whatever, more especially of water or malt liquors. She will take a dose of the calcarea carbonica every night, and apply the camphorated oil externally.

The proper diet.

* Transactions of the Obs. Society of London. Vol. I., p. 31.

LECTURE II.

MOLAR PREGNANCY — FALSE CONCEPTION.

GENTLEMEN:

In my obstetrical course you were told that, in forming a correct diagnosis of pregnancy, an exclusive reliance upon any of its presumptive or of its probable signs would be likely to mislead you. I will open my lecture this morning with a case in point, the counterpart of which, in some respects at least, you will surely meet with as medical practitioners.

Case. — Mrs. W——, aged 42, was married eight months ago. She was at that time a widow; but had never had any children. She says that within the eight months, or since her last marriage, she has not menstruated. Prior to that, menstruation was normal in every respect. She has had no vicarious hæmorrhage, or leucorrhœal flow. When the menses ceased she began to have morning-sickness, which continued for six weeks. She had also various caprices of the appetite, with faintness before dinner, and inordinate craving for food. There was no perceptible development of the ovum, or enlargement of the abdomen. The mammæ became swollen and sensitive.

Six days ago, after walking to church upon the icy pavement, she began to "flow." The hæmorrhage from the uterus was passive, irregular, and slight, until the third night, when, after having had a great deal of pain about the back and loins, with some headache and debility, she awakened out of sleep very much frightened by the escape of a fleshy mass from the uterus and vagina. The flowing soon ceased, and to-day she has ventured to walk to the Clinique. In addition to the details already given, she says that all her unpleasant and indescribable feelings about the hips and abdomen were greatly relieved by a bandage worn tightly about those parts.

This was an example of spurious pregnancy, sometimes styled false conception, pseudo-pregnancy, quasi-gestation, molar gestation, and should not be confounded with pseudo-cyesis. The product was a fleshy mole, which

Morbid anatomy.

the patient has preserved, and brought with her, and which we will now proceed to examine. Fortunately for us, she has kept it in water, and the examination will not be difficult. You will observe that the mass is about the size of a small lemon. On cutting through its walls, we come down to the amnion, which is intact. Slitting this open, a slight flow of its proper liquor escapes. Here is the rudimentary embryo, which, although it has been eight months in utero, is not larger than it should have been at the sixth week of pregnancy. The undeveloped funis is but a mere thread, and ragged at its free extremity. Between the outer membranes, or rather within the thickened wall outside of the amnion, blood has been effused, and small coagula are seen.

These appearances indicate an arrest of embryonic development. Conception probably took place as it should have done, and all went on well for a limited period. But, for some unknown reason, the nourishing supplies that were derived from the uterine surface, and designed for the ovum, were appropriated to the abnormal, pathological growth of the chorion. The little embryo was therefore sacrificed. It died from a lack of those elements which were necessary to the development and repair of its tissues, and the hypertrophied chorion and decidua constitute this carneous or fleshy mass which is called a mole.

Death of the embryo.

Although women of all ages are liable to this form of spurious pregnancy, yet it is a singular fact, that those who have reached their fortieth year seem more prone to it than those who are younger. As in the case before us, it is not uncommon among women who marry a second time late in life. The formation of these moles (which are the consequence, not the cause, of the death of the ovum) is intimately connected with the history of abortion. Rigby says most expressively: "When any cause has occurred to destroy the life of the embryo, during the early weeks of pregnancy, one of two results follows, either that expulsion takes place sooner or later, or the membranes of the ovum become remarkably changed, and continue to grow for some time longer, until at length they form a fleshy, fibrous mass, called a mole, or false conception."

Influence of age.

The true mole is always a product of conception. When the mass has been expelled, it is not difficult to recognize it, and to separate it from spurious formations which resemble it in some respects, by the presence of a rudimentary embryo within its cavity. If, however, the embryo died during the first month, it may have been dissolved, and we shall, therefore, fail to find it on dissection. Such a mole may be retained within the uterus for many months, or it may be cast off and expelled at or about the period at which the menses should have returned had the woman not been pregnant. It sometimes happens that the hæmorrhage attendant upon labor of this kind is profuse and long-continued. Generally, however, it ceases with the delivery of the fleshy mass. Ambrose Paré cites a case in which a mole was retained in the womb for seventeen years.

Retention of embryo.

Among the clinical points worthy of note in the case before us, you will observe that, until her last marriage, this woman's menstruation was habitually regular and healthy. It is important to take this fact into account, for it sometimes happens that menstrual disorders predispose to abnormal developments of the membranes which enclose the ovum. Membranous dysmenorrhœa may indirectly cause this form of spurious pregnancy.

Molar pregnancy and menstruation.

Following the arrest of the catamenia there was no vicarious discharge. Morning sickness set in, and our patient was supposed to be pregnant. This continued for six weeks, or most probably until the death of the embryo, and was accompanied by the capricious appetite, fainting, etc., to which so many women are liable after conception.

Probable signs of pregnancy.

For the best of reasons there was no observable change in the abdomen. The usual development of the uterine tumor was prevented. There was no necessity for the womb to ascend out of the pelvis, as it would have done had gestation gone on properly. The embryo was dead, and its growth became impossible. The uterine cavity was already large enough to contain it, and hence there was no need of its further expansion. If the case had been one of hydatids (falsely so-called), the abdominal enlargement might have taken place. For these hydatigenous growths sometimes fill the womb, and cause it to enlarge in very much the same manner as if it contained a healthy fœtus. They may also be retained even some months beyond "term" before they are finally expelled. You should not forget that these uterine hydatids are really due to a defective organization of the placenta, or, more properly speaking, to a cystic degeneration of the villi of the chorion.

We have no means of knowing the precise changes that took place in the breasts in this case. It is possible that the areolæ may have been discolored, and the follicles about the nipples developed, as in true pregnancy. These glands are liable to become swollen and sensitive from other causes, and this general symptom of pregnancy would therefore be very uncertain and unreliable. At this time there is nothing peculiar in the appearance of the mammary glands. Usually, in similar cases, the series of changes proper to these organs, and which provides for the extra-uterine needs of the infant, is arrested when, from any cause, the embryo dies. Even when the mole or the hydatid mass is carried to the ninth month, or beyond, before it is extruded, there is generally little or no secretion of milk.

These signs do not indicate the progress of pregnancy.

From these remarks you will infer that, although the suppression of the menses, the morning sickness, and the fickleness of appetite, are to be regarded as presumptive signs of conception, and may signify that the fecundated ovum has reached the uterine cavity, and commenced to develop therein, still they do not afford a certain criterion of the progress of gestation. They may have marked its commencement; but do not indicate its possible arrest or failure. This patient had the morning sickness during the first six weeks, but afterwards the only remaining symptom of pregnancy was the non-appearance of the menses. And the prolonged arrest of this flow is to be accounted for by the presence of this foreign body, or mole, within the womb.

Cause of the delivery.

Concerning the final cause of labor in this form of pseudo-pregnancy, various theories have been advanced. Perhaps the most reasonable is that which refers it to the menstrual cycle, when the physiological afflux of blood to the uterine, mucous membrane facilitates, if it does not actually insure, the entire separation of the decidua. At this particular period the cervix uteri is also more or less relaxed, as if menstruation were coming on, and some slight exciting cause, as, for example, a fall, or sudden shock, or forcible exercise, as in walking on an icy pavement, may precipitate labor. Dilating pains follow or accompany the hæmorrhage. In due time expulsive contractions set in, and the womb is emptied of its contents. The suffering may be either slight or severe, its quality and degree varying with the laxity of fibre of the uterine neck, the rapidity of the labor, the size of the mole, and the temperament of the patient. It is only in exceptional cases that the mass drops away with so little pain as this patient had. Although there are women who frequently and habitually suffer from this form of spurious pregnancy, it does not follow that one such mishap is certain to be succeeded by a second of a similar kind. Even at her age, Mrs. W. might, perhaps, pass through another pregnancy successfully.

LEUCORRHŒA THE CAUSE OF IMPAIRED LACTEAL SECRETION.

Case.— Mrs. ——, aged 30, of scrofulous diathesis, has one child, which is now two and a half months old. She has had leucorrhœa for more than two years. It showed no abatement during pregnancy, and continued through her lying-in and lactation. At birth, her infant weighed ten pounds; now it weighs only eight pounds. Its digestive system has been constantly deranged, and its little life threatened by vomiting, indigestion, and diarrhœa. The mother's breasts have not been diseased in any way, but have remained plump, soft, and natural. The quality of the milk, however, was impaired. It was thin, watery, and of a bluish cast.

A fortnight ago the child was, by my advice, taken from the breast, and ordered good cow's milk, diluted in the proportion of one-third water to two-thirds milk. Immediately it began to improve and gain flesh, and it is now nearly well. The only treatment this patient has ever had for the leucorrhœa, consisted of harsh astringent injections of alum-water, tannin, etc. These expedients have had the effect to arrest the flow temporarily. She describes the discharge as milky, and says it is accompanied by more or less of aching in the vagina and itching of the pudenda. The flow is more profuse after exercise. It has been her habit heretofore to menstruate too freely and frequently.

Leucorrhœa and scrofulosis.

Leucorrhœa is sometimes very persistent. It may be associated, either as cause or effect, with a depraved and enfeebled condition of system. The worst cases occur in scrofulous subjects. In this class of patients there is a strong predisposition to glandular disease, and leucorrhœa should properly be classed among the glandular affections. Let us inquire into the significance of the fact that it is so frequently engrafted upon the scrofulous dyscrasia.

In the lecture upon hæmatogenesis, or blood-making, which you heard only last evening, my colleague, the professor of physiology, directed your attention to the important function of the lymphatic glands, as related to that process. You were told that the chyle and lymph which are subjected to the action of these glands, are so changed thereby as afterwards to constitute a most essential part of the blood. The mesenteric glands manipulate the chyliferous fluid which is *en route* for the general circulation. Both the superficial and the deep-seated lymphatics are designed to absorb any surplus of serum that may have been poured out in excess of the needs of the different tissues. They are the original physiological economists. They stamp their impress upon this fluid, and then pass it along into the blood-current again. This is the function of lymphosis. As indicated in the lecture to which I have just referred, it concerns the assimilation of the oleo-albuminous element of the food. It is the first step in the process of histogenesis or tissue-making. If this step is not properly taken, the blood becomes impaired in quality, and all the functions are likely to be implicated.

Now this physiological knowledge is of practical application to the case before us. Scrofulous persons are unhealthy because this glandular system is predisposed to disease. Inflammation, or any of its consequences, may so impair the function of the lymphatics as to impoverish the blood, and even to render it harmful to the life-processes. Under these circumstances the albuminous principle is not available for the repair of the tissues. It circulates as a foreign element, which must, in some way, be eliminated and expelled from the organism. It may find an outlet through the kidneys, or some other excretory apparatus; but in escaping is very likely to develop a catarrhal inflammation of one or another of the mucous membranes. The mucous secretions are changed in amount and quality. They become the vehicle for carrying off those very elements which are needed in nutrition, but which have been rejected because the initiatory step in the process of their assimilation was not properly taken. In political parlance, there is so much "red-tapeism," so much respect for method and precedent, in the affairs of our bodily organization, that the other organs and textures will neither recognize nor appropriate this class of proximate principles, unless they have been identified and stamped, or acted upon beforehand.

The same is true of those glands which are set apart for the elaboration of their particular products from elements contained in the blood. It is quite as impossible for the gastric glands to secrete the proper solvent for the food from blood, the quality of which has been impaired in the manner just indicated, as for the muscular and serous, or other tissues, to repair themselves out of a like material. The mammary glands do not form an exception to this rule. This woman's milk is impoverished and injurious to the child, because in the blood which was brought to them the breasts failed to find the materials out of which they could manufacture a wholesome product. Those elements were drained away in the critical discharge from the glands and follicles of the vagina and of the uterine cervix.

Illness of the infant from leucorrhœa in the mother.

Moreover, in consequence of the mammary glands having become eliminative, as well as secretory, it is not impossible that some of these abnormal elements may also escape with the milk from the breasts. Such a product would be both non-assimilable and noxious. The infant would become impoverished and poisoned from nursing it. It could not thrive upon such aliment. Hence the vomiting, indigestion and diarrhœa which have resulted in the case of this woman's child. The rapid improvement in its health from changing its diet to good cow's milk confirms the view we have taken.

Indirect poisoning of the child.

In rare cases it sometimes happens that the nursing child becomes diseased in consequence of the mother's milk having been poisoned, through the absorption of drugs that have been injected into the vagina for the purpose of arresting a leucorrhœal flow. I am quite confident that I have seen more than one such infant in great suffering, and ill with an obscure disease, which was properly chargeable to the acetate of lead, alum, tannin, etc., that had been used in the manner indicated.

Reserving the differential diagnosis of uterine from vaginal leucorrhœa for another lecture, I will call your attention to the significance of one or two objective symptoms presented in the case now under consideration. If this patient's flow, which is sometimes profuse, and has continued for two years, came from the uterine cervix, in all probability she would have remained sterile; for, as I shall doubtless have occasion to show you, this form of leucorrhœa is a frequent cause of barrenness. And, besides, had it been uterine, and not vaginal, there would surely have been a partial or complete arrest thereof during pregnancy. Sometimes, however, both varieties may exist conjointly, or they may even alternate in the same patient.

Uterine leucorrhœa and sterility.

Treatment.—In all cases of leucorrhœa which are incident to gestation and lactation, you should bear in mind that the blood is being drained of its assimilable material for the growth of the offspring. For this reason it is sometimes quite impossible to cure the affection radically until these functions have ceased by limitation. In either case, indeed, the leucorrhœa may be critical, and it might therefore be injurious either to mother or child to arrest it while these processes are going on. This is a forcible argument against the use of astringents which are designed to seal up this flow, and to close a species of safety-valve to the general economy.

There are two reasons that may justify, and even necessitate, the weaning of the child for the cure of a leucorrhœa which is incident to the nursing period. If the draught upon the mother's resources while nursing, undermines her strength, it furnishes a cause for this disease which is constant in its operation, and which can only be removed by putting the child away from the breast. And weaning is still more strongly indicated if the child was large and plump at its birth, and the leucorrhœa continued during pregnancy also. Besides, the safety and welfare of the infant may require that it shall be brought up artificially, rather than upon the unhealthy milk that is furnished by the mother.

Weaning the child.

Not unfrequently the cure is half performed when you have prevented a waste which only weakens the mother and injures the child. Stop the leak, and her strength may soon return. For it is a condition of healthy glandular activity, that the blood must be nourishing and stimulating to the glands as well as to other bodily organs.

It is no less important to select a suitable diet for this patient, than to decide upon the appropriate remedy for the symptoms presented. Indeed, the rational method of procedure would be, first, to supply the physiological conditions that are requisite to health, in order that our curative agents may afterwards act more promptly and efficiently.

A proper diet.

Granted that, in the case before us, the function of the mesenteric glands is so impaired that they fail to effect the proper changes in the peptones brought to them from the bowel. The indication is to choose such an aliment as by their aid may be assimilated. The whites of eggs, lean meat, sea-food, as oysters or other shell-fish, or good fresh milk, are more easily digested and disposed of, and also more nourishing, than a mixed diet largely composed of fatty substances, soups, and the like. It is quite as necessary to discriminate carefully in this class of diseases, and to allow only such food as will be kindly received and appropriated, as it is in the case of the infant, whose digestion is very weak, and whose alimentary system is easily deranged. Sometimes the vegetable acids are not only grateful, but really beneficial. The patient may eat grapes, oranges, tomatoes, or baked apples, or she may drink a mild wine, or an occasional glass of lemonade. Now and then the most excellent results are obtained from travel, partly because of the change of scene and surroundings, but also, as the phrase is, "from change of pasture." The same food, cooked differently, may be more acceptable to the stomach of an invalid, and less harmful in every way, than if she had remained at home and eaten it from the same dish and table as before.

But let us inquire if there is any means whereby the important function of lymphosis may be stimulated and encouraged. The salts of potassa, soda, lime, alumina, baryta, iron, iodine, ammonia, phosphorus, and other earths and metals, are all more or less intimately related therewith.

Lymphatic stimulants.

As prepared by the pharmaceutist, or in the form of mineral waters in the great laboratory of Nature, they have long been employed for the cure of all the principal disorders of nutrition. And the almost universal record of the good results so frequently obtained from them, leads us to conclude that empirical observation cannot have gone very far astray in this matter. The hint, at least, is significant. Clinical experience confirms their value in the treatment of leucorrhœa. A majority of the reliable remedies for this disease are of mineral origin. And each of them has a specific, pathogenetic, and curative relation to the lymphatic glands. It is for this reason, doubtless, that they are most serviceable in the treatment of scrofulous and catarrhal affections of almost every kind.

Although these clinical generalities are both analytical and suggestive, they should not be allowed to substitute a more careful selection of the appropriate remedy or remedies. We must choose from among all those named, and many more beside, the proper simillimum for the more prominent symptoms complained of. If you will turn to the pathogenesis of calcarea carbonica you will find it. The indications for this most excellent remedy are so positive and almost mathematically exact, that we need look no further. It is called for by the milky leucorrhœa, with aching in the vagina, and itching in the pudenda, with increased flow after exercise, and also in the case of a woman who is subject to a too copious and oft-recurring menstruation.

In prescribing the calcarea carbonica in similar cases, and indeed ordinarily, my own preference is for the third decimal trituration. And, while I do not question the efficacy of the medium and higher preparations thereof, my experience is certainly opposed to the theory which holds that no curative effect can be obtained from this remedy unless it be given in the sixth or a higher potency. Mrs. —— will take one-and-a-half grains of the third trituration of the calcarea morning and evening, and report at the end of a week.

TOO FREQUENT MENSTRUATION IN INCIPIENT PHTHISIS.

Case. — Mrs. S., aged 32, residing in an adjacent state, gives the following history of her case. She has three children, the youngest of which is four years old. She nursed the latter for a period of twenty months, her menses appearing but twice meanwhile. For two years past she has menstruated as often as once in three weeks, and sometimes every two weeks. Originally, menstruation was regular, and normal in all respects. With a single exception, which occurred about four months ago, the menses have not been very profuse. Eight months ago she lost her voice, and in all this interval has not been able to speak aloud. She has no habitual cough or sore throat, but is subject to occasional attacks of diarrhœa, which is very debilitating, and sometimes quite intractable. Has never had the aphonia before, neither was she subject to the croup, or to any anginose affection during infancy and childhood; is losing flesh rapidly; appetite capricious; perspires freely whenever she sleeps; no thirst; pulse one hundred and ten. Tuberculosis is hereditary in the family.

The relation of the menstrual function to the development of hereditary tuberculosis is more significant than you may have supposed. The interval between puberty and the age of thirty or thirty-five represents the period at which females are most liable to be seized with symptoms of that formidable disease. After this period, if the menses are regular, they generally escape until the great climacteric is passed. The first ten years of menstrual life show the largest proportion of cases and the highest rate of mortality from phthisis pulmonalis. It is not uncommon for this disease to appear in young girls at the time the catamenial function is established. Retention of the menses is very often a premonitory symptom. We shall, doubtless, have occasion to confirm its clinical import.

Menstruation and tuberculosis.

But it sometimes happens, that too frequent menstruation may take the place of an arrest or tardy appearance of this flow in incipient phthisis. The case before us is one of this kind. For fifteen years, or from the age of fifteen to thirty, this poor woman menstruated regularly. Lactation was prolonged to twenty months, the menses appearing only twice before her babe was weaned. For the four months following, everything was normal in this respect. The courses then became too frequent, and have so continued until the present time.

Healthy menstruation depends upon ovulation — the ripening and discharge of the ovum, which takes place every lunar month. It is possible that the physiological condition of this peculiar flow may be supplied in exceptional cases of too frequent menstruation. But in young subjects especially, clinical experience leads us to refer this remittent type of menstruation, as it has been styled by Dr. Tilt, to some severe constitutional or local disease or dyscrasia. Sometimes it is caused by uterine ulceration, which may be either benign or malignant. More frequently it is not organic, but origi-

Menorrhagia and tuberculosis.

nates in the depraved and debilitated conditions of the system that are incident to phthisis pulmonalis, and to chronic diseases of various kinds. When it occurs so frequently, it loses the character of the catamenia proper, and becomes a passive hæmorrhage. Under these circumstances the condition of the blood is such that it very readily escapes from the uterine mucous membrane, which is more than ordinarily congested. Whatever impairs the quality of the blood, may thus directly give rise to a too copious, as well as too frequently recurring menstrual flow. Hence it is that instead of amenorrhœa in the early stage of phthisis, we sometimes meet with cases of troublesome and even dangerous menorrhagia. Indeed my own experience leads me to conclude that uterine hæmorrhage, active or passive, is more frequent in women under thirty-five years of age, and who are predisposed to tuberculosis, than our authors and practitioners have generally imagined. As a rule, however, it is more liable to occur in advanced stages of the disease than in its incipiency, and in child-bearing women than in those who are either unmarried or sterile.

In either sex indiscriminately it is not unusual for phthisis to commence with laryngitis, and consequent aphonia. But the marked sympathy existing between the womb, the ovaries, and the larynx, renders this complication more frequent among females than with males. The loss of voice in this case is significant and serious. If it were hysterical, it would not have persisted so many months. In aphonia from spinal irritation, (unless it be traumatic), the attack comes on abruptly, continues for a few days or a week at most, and is very apt to leave as it came. Emotional causes, menstrual or sexual excitement, or bodily fatigue, may induce either of these varieties of aphonia. The loss of voice that sometimes precedes an apopletic fit depends upon congestion of the medulla oblongata about the ganglion of the pneumo-gastric nerve, and is a very different affair. The obstinate aphonia, the habitual diarrhœa, the menstrual irregularity, and the frequent pulse of this patient, are objective signs, which must be interpreted as premonitory of pulmonary tuberculosis.

Significance of the aphonia.

Treatment.—The remedy for this case is calcarea phosphorica; and you will be surprised to observe how promptly and efficiently it sometimes acts under similar conditions to those presented by this patient. It may be given in the third, the sixth, or if you please, a higher potency. My own preference is for the third decimal trituration, of which this woman will take two grains three times daily.

Not unfrequently the bichromate of potassa, phosphorus, sodium, or spongia, will relieve the hoarseness which is incident to these cases of incipient phthisis. For this purpose they may be given incidentally, or if otherwise indicated, in lieu of the calcarea phosphorica.

It is quite as important to prescribe the proper hygienic conditions suited to this infirmity as it is to determine the choice of the remedy. First and foremost this patient should, if possible, remove to a climate which is less humid than this upon the lake shore. This expedient is especially advisable at this season (February). For the weather of the late winter and early spring months in this vicinity is too changeable, and withal too damp, for persons who are predisposed to laryngeal and pulmonary difficulties.

Season and climate.

She should, moreover, have a good diet, and plenty of fresh air, without fatigue. And what is still more important, she should avoid an excess of family care and worry. Any little fret or friction of the domestic machinery has a wonderful influence in keeping this class of patients always on the doctor's hands.

Mental worry.

BURROWING ABSCESS OF THE MAMMARY GLAND WITH A SINUS.

Case.—Mrs. ——, aged 28, has two children, the youngest of which is three months old. She complains of a "gathered breast," which began to trouble her seven weeks ago, or when the babe was five weeks old. She first noticed what appeared to be a small "cat-boil" on the right breast, which was not very painful and did not in the least interfere with nursing. It, however, continued gradually to increase in size, and to become more tender. Three weeks ago her physician advised that it should be poulticed and afterwards freely lanced. The former part of the prescription was tried, but she would not consent to its being opened. As a consequence, the abscess broke at the end of another week, and although it seemed but a small affair, discharged a large quantity of healthy pus. The orifice through which this fluid escaped has continued to enlarge until it is now about the size of the nail of my index finger, and, only yesterday, she was startled by discovering that whenever the child nurses, or she swallows anything, and sometimes when she moves the right arm, the milk escapes quite freely from it. Two days since, another "boil" made its appearance at the lower and outer margin of the same breast, and now, you see the hardened, smooth, glossy and convex outline of the surface at that point, as the redness, and also the pain of which she complains, indicate that the suppurative progress is still going on. She is weak and feeble, with slight hectic, unrest, anorexia, and is withal very much discouraged.

Unless it be located in the loose cellular tissue about the nipple, the mammary abscess which points like a boil is apt to be a serious and deep-seated one. This is especially true if the local and constitutional symptoms indicate that the gland has been inflamed for a considerable time. Under these circumstances, pus may form and collect at the base of the breast, or in the areolar structure that separates the lobules, long before there is any external sign preparatory to its escape. The size of the abscess proper is, therefore, no criterion of its extent or gravity. Boils situated about the margin of the breast, and especially at its lower border, not unfrequently give vent to the contents of a burrowing abscess which may have existed for some weeks, and committed great havoc with the gland itself. There may be only one of these, but usually there are two or more which ripen successively.

We occasionally meet with superficial abscesses that only involve the integument covering the gland, but these are not necessarily, or indeed frequently, seen in nursing women. They occur in young girls, in consequence of tight lacing, the wearing of hard and unyielding pads over the breasts, or of bruising those organs in some accidental way, and scarcely deserve the name of abscess.

The form of milk abscesses of which this is an excellent illustration, is peculiar to depraved conditions of system which constitute a species of cachexia. They are very prone to become sinuous, and the canals which are formed may be either superficial or deep-seated, running through or beneath the gland in every direction. Multiple abscesses may communicate in this manner. Unless relieved by proper means, these sinuses may even become fistulous. It has happened that the entire mammary gland has been destroyed and discharged through these openings.

In the case under review, the extravasation and escape of milk is caused by a rupture of one or more of the proper lactiferous ducts, whieh are compressed during suckling, deglutition, and also when the arm is moved. It is hardly necessary to remind you that these symptoms require immediate relief, else they may persist and increase in severity until they destroy the patient's life.

Treatment.—I have more confidence in phosphorus and silicea than in any other remedies for sinuous and fistulous abscesses of the mammary gland. It is best to give them separately. Perhaps you will succeed more frequently with the former than with the latter. They should be given in the sixth, or a higher potency, and the dose repeated every three to six hours. It has been claimed that the local application of the tincture of phoshorus in tepid or cool water is very serviceable also. The phosphorated oil of the shops will sometimes answer an excellent purpose as an external application.

A domestic expedient.

My practice has been, in most cases of this kind, to resort to the topical use of granulated sugar, which is a simple and unobjectionable domestic remedy. Applied directly to the surface of the ulcer at the mouth of the sinus, whence the pus or milk, or both these escape, it stimulates fresh, healthy granulations, and closes the unnatural outlet. It operates kindly and speedily, is a good antiseptic, and is always available. It may be insinuated into the canal without doing any possible harm, or causing severe pain.

If this simple expedient fails, you may inject a weak solution of tincture of calendula into the sinus by means of a clean urethral syringe. And the same solution may also be applied over the ulcer at the site of the abscess. Calendula is sometimes wonderfully efficacious where there is considerable loss of the integument, and where an extravagant quantity of pus is formed.

The knife.

The old plan of slitting up these sinuses with a knife was cruel, barbarous and unnecessary. It is undoubtedly true that, in a majority of cases, these deep-seated abscesses once formed would seldom become sinuous and fistulous if they were promptly and properly opened, but this fault does not justify the subsequent slashing and hacking of these delicate organs. There is a proper time for all things, including the lancet. And the same is true of the caustic and astringent injections which have been thrown into these passages heretofore.

As in other abscesses that involve a considerable drain upon the patient's strength, we must counteract the loss and fortify against it. This woman should have a good, nourishing diet of eggs and lean meat. Beef is preferable, and may generally be taken in the solid form. Of all vegetable substances which are appropriate to cases of this kind, oatmeal is best. Bread made from unbolted wheat flour, — thus securing the phosphorus which is contained in the hull of the grain, — is also advisable. According to Agassiz's theory concerning the large relative proportion of the same element in fish, we may sometimes select from this class of food. The fish should also be lean. Fresh air and sunlight, with freedom of the mind from all harassing cares, are excellent and available tonics.

A good diet.

Mrs. —— will take of phosphorus 6th, a dose every four hours during the day. The granulated sugar to be applied twice daily. The diet to consist of brown bread and butter, and rare roast beef, with dry, mealy potatoes. She must nurse her babe from the left breast exclusively. The right one should, however, be well drawn by means of a breast-pump each morning and evening, and then kept soft and warm. Let her report at the end of a week.

ABORTION WITH MISPLACED PAINS.

Case.— In consequence of over-exertion, Mrs. G., aged 30, aborted at the end of the third month. She had twice before miscarried at the same period of pregnancy. Immediately after violent exercise at house-cleaning, she began to flow slightly, and to experience an occasional sharp pain in the left hypogastrium. After a restless night she awakened at 6 A. M. with an acute, lancinating headache. This pain in the head was accompanied by an extreme soreness and tenderness in the nape of the neck. The pupils were dilated to nearly the whole extent of the iris. She complained of photophobia, with a shower of sparks before the eyes, and in a species of semi-delirium declared herself in the immediate neighborhood of a fearful conflagration. These latter symptoms would disappear in the intervals between the paroxysms of headache. When the pain in the head returned, she would scream and shriek and beg to be held firmly, in order that no terrible accident might befall her. These paroxysms returned every ten minutes for about two hours, or until I came and relieved her with a few doses of belladonna 3rd.. Upon examination, the os uteri was found but slightly dilated. The pain subsided, and finally ceased.

The same train of symptoms came on the second morning at six o'clock. They were, however, less violent in degree and of shorter duration, lasting in all not more than an hour. The os uteri was a little more patulous. The passive flow continued, but there were no uterine pains whatever.

The third morning she had half a dozen of the same paroxysms of pain in the head. They were repeated once in five or six minutes, and were as severe as those of the first day. In the intervals she was found to be bleeding much more freely.

The stomach had become exceedingly irritable, and she vomited frequently, each effort at emesis serving so perceptibly to increase the hæmorrhage that the patient remarked it herself. The headache passed off, but during the day she had two pretty severe uterine pains of an expulsive character, and became really quite ill. Early next morning regular labor pains commenced and continued, so that in an hour and a half all was over. The head and nervous symptoms vanished as soon as the proper uterine contractions began. The fifth morning the headache did not return. She made a good recovery.

Abortion from over-exertion.

Perhaps a majority of cases of accidental abortion are caused by undue or unusual muscular exertion. Lifting, scrubbing, overreaching — as in hanging a picture, carrying a child a long distance hurriedly — as when in haste to reach home or to take the train, running the sewing machine for consecutive hours and days, horseback riding, or climbing steep and difficult stairs, as, for example, to the cupola of the city hall, have caused the uterus to expel its contents prematurely.

Remarkable tolerance of exercise.

You will not, however, understand me to say that these causes are invariably followed by such unfortunate consequences. Far from it. In many, and probably most pregnant women, there is a remarkable tolerance of fatigue and even considerable muscular effort, if it be moderately and habitually practised. There are those in whom it would be impossible to bring on abortion by any such means. But in the majority of cases such a mishap is more easily induced. This is especially true of women of sedentary habits, who ordinarily take very little exercise, whether indoors or out, but who, under peculiar temptation, or provocation, exceed the bounds of prudence, and overdo and injure themselves. In the matter of taking proper exercise, as in everything they do, these subjects are fitful and capricious. In them a sudden strain, or any unusual effort, conjoined with extraordinary nervous excitement and impulse, may work mischief that might have been averted.

The "habit" of aborting.

Add to this that, if the woman has aborted once or twice already, and is, therefore, predisposed to this accident, these causes are more harmful, and we have the etiology of this class of cases plainly before us. The *habit* of aborting at a particular date of pregnancy also increases the danger from this variety of accidental causes; for there are women who miscarry at a certain time with almost as much regularity as they menstruate when they are well. And, although this result may happen at any period of gestation, it is extremely liable to occur at the end of the third month. This clinical fact is confirmed in the case just now detailed to you. Our patient had already miscarried twice at the twelfth week, and now, with the arrival of the same period, over-exertion in house-cleaning caused a slight uterine flow and pains, which resulted in the loss of the embryo. You should not fail to recognize that this indiscretion and excess on her part were more mischievous at this particular time than they might have been at any other.

Even a slight flow of blood from the gravid uterus, and especially if it be accompanied by pain in either hypogastrium, or about the loins, may betoken a miscarriage. Under these circumstances the symptoms of impending abortion do not differ, in any essential particular, from those which date the appearance of the menstrual discharge. We are naturally suspicious of them, however, and solicitous concerning their interpretation and results; for their continuance signifies an interruption in the process of intra-uterine development, and the possible sacrifice of offspring.

Intermittent abortion.

But the chief peculiarity of this case was the periodical and regularly recurring headache. This was a good example of *intermittent* abortion.* The headache took the place of the uterine pains, came every morning for three successive days, continued for a given time, and then left.

*Vide U. S. Medical and Surgical Journal, vol. iv., p. 75.

The paroxysms, which were distinctly pronounced, came and went with the regularity of labor pains. And they increased in frequency each day. Meanwhile there was no expulsive uterine effort, or at least none of a painful or positive character. By and by the flow increased, and the stomach became implicated. Vomiting ensued. This was a certain sign that the os uteri had begun to dilate more freely and rapidly. The principal obstacle to delivery, and the indirect cause of the headache also, were removed as soon as the cervix was sufficiently relaxed for the escape of the contained embryo. Proper uterine contractions succeeded. The real labor was short and decisive. The headache vanished, hæmorrhage ceased, and our patient made a good recovery.

Treatment. — There are several methods by which this case could have been brought to a successful termination. The question to decide was, which is the more safe and expedient. I might have given this woman a strong dose of ergot, and finished her labor abruptly, by forcing the uterus to expel its contents through the slowly dilating os. Or, perhaps, a powerful cathartic would have produced a similar result. Or an emetic might have unlocked the cervix, with the mysterious key of reflex action. Or sitz-baths, or the colpeurynter, might have brought about the same end. Or an old-fashioned dose of morphine, or perhaps of quinine, might have arrested the headache until such time as the gradual expansion of the lower segment of the womb should permit the proper pains to come on spontaneously, and terminate the delivery.

But the belladonna was a more appropriate, specific, and satisfactory remedy. Not only did it relieve the headache, which, as I have said, was indirectly due to the rigidity of the uterine neck, but it also relaxed the fibres of the unyielding cervix — which is slow to yield before the fourth month — and thus removed the cause of the suffering and the delay. It was appropriate for the pain in the head, because it was specifically adapted to remedy the condition of the cervix, upon which it depended, and of which it was the consequence. It harmonized the nervous sympathies existing between the body of the womb and its inflexible outlet. It charmed away the impending danger to the brain, and permitted nature to complete the delivery with the least possible risk to the health and welfare of the patient.

LECTURE III.

AMENORRHŒA WITH HYSTERICAL SPASMS RESEMBLING CHOREA.

GENTLEMEN:

No class of diseases to which women are subject is more interesting and important than the disorders of menstruation. They are more frequently encountered, are more intricate and enigmatical, and, all in all, more difficult of cure than any others. Here is a case belonging to this class, which is certain to attract your attention because of some unusual incidental symptoms.

Case.—Miss ——, aged 19, of full habit and general good health; is almost never ill. Her mother says that four days ago, on Sunday last, she took cold while in attendance upon the Mission Sabbath School. In consequence of this her menses were arrested, and the same evening she was seized with a severe headache, which has continued with abated violence day and night until the present time. This pain is described as acute at intervals, extending over the whole head, and aggravated by noise and light. The pupils are slightly dilated, and the face occasionally flushed. She sees objects distinctly, and is rational all the while. Since the onset of the attack, however, she has not been able to sleep more than a very few minutes at a time. Two hours ago a new train of symptoms was developed. These symptoms have alarmed the parents and friends exceedingly, and for their explanation and cure we have been consulted. Her relatives are in great dread of paralysis.

The right hand and arm commenced to jerk spasmodically, so much so that at times it became quite unmanageable. Sometimes the arm and forearm were thrown about wildly, and then extended and flexed quickly and violently. Again, the muscles of the shoulder were so severely convulsed as to threaten the dislocation of the head of the humerus from the glenoid cavity of the scapula. Occasionally, during these paroxysms, the shoulder is thrown high up alongside of the head. These movements are involuntary. It is quite impossible for the patient to control or suppress them, and when they have ceased temporarily she complains of great fatigue in the affected arm and shoulder. The paroxysms recur as often as once in five minutes, and, as you will observe, are somewhat grotesque as well as painful to behold. Excepting the left arm, which is but slightly affected, the remaining portions of the body and extremities are not implicated. The pulse is only 80, and normal in every respect. She urinates freely and frequently, but the catamenia have ceased entirely since Sunday. She thinks that when the nervous twitching and spasm commenced in the arms and shoulders the headache became less severe in degree than it was before.

It often happens that the menstrual flow is suddenly checked by "taking cold." Getting the feet wet, exposure from insufficient clothing, or from sitting in a draught of air, may induce a complete arrest of the discharge. In the case before us this result was produced by some such apparently trivial means.

Difference between suppression and retention.

Practically speaking, there is a distinction between suppression and retention of the menses, which you should never forget. *Suppression* of this function implies its complete arrest, or rather, that the ovaries and the uterine mucous membrane have failed to furnish the products which constitute the true menstrual secretion. *Retention* of the menses signifies that, although the catamenial fluid has been secreted into the cavity of the womb, yet, for some especial reason, or reasons, its escape has been prevented. In the one case it is not poured into the uterus; in the other it is not poured out of it through the vagina. This distinction corresponds with that made between urinary suppression and retention. In the former, the urine is not secreted, its elements are not selected by the renal organs from the blood which is brought to them. In the latter, although the kidneys have done their work, the ureters, the bladder, or the urethra, are in a condition which obstructs the flow and prevents the discharge of their proper product.

Remote disease from arrest of menses.

A sudden arrest of the menses, "while the flow is on," is likely to re-act either upon the circulatory or the nervous system, or upon both together. This is a fruitful source of ill health among women. While this function is being performed, it is the easiest thing imaginable, by such means, to convert a physiological injection of the ovaries, and of the uterine mucous membrane, into a pathological state of congestion and inflammation. This is a short step, and it is taken in a twinkling. The most serious and intractable results may follow. Other and remote organs with which the pelvic viscera are in sympathy, may be implicated. Here we have evident determination of the blood to the brain, which is directly attributable to this cause. Sometimes this result is even more pronounced and alarming. There are those in whom the slightest and most temporary arrest of the menstrual flow will induce cerebral lesions that threaten to destroy both reason and life. Our patient has suffered extremely from symptoms of this kind. Fortunately she has escaped the delirium which is usually present in such cases. In its stead, however, there is the insomnia which implies great nervous perturbation and derangement.

Symptomatic nervous phenomena.

The spasmodic phenomena have followed indirectly. They are symptomatic. In their production it is probable that the cerebellum has been especially implicated. For, according to Flourens, Dalton and others, it is the particular function of that part of the brain to preside over and co-ordinate, or harmonize the voluntary muscular movements. In these choreic jerkings we have evidence that this function is disordered. This young lady suffers from what has been improperly styled "insanity of the muscles." The muscles of the right shoulder and arm are in a state of insubordination to the will. She commands, but cannot control them. Their irregular and forcible action is exhaustive, and it is not strange that a temporary arrest of the spasms is accompanied by a sense of weariness of the affected parts. Excepting from extreme exhaustion, there is no danger of her becoming paralyzed.

If, instead of the cerebellum, the cerebral lobes were involved in this case, there would have been marked delirium, and perhaps a mild and self-limited form of mania. Cerebral troubles, dependent on sudden interruption and arrest of the menses, are apt to be characterized by wakefulness, and oftentimes by utter inability to sleep. The hysterical peculiarities which this case presents are also due to the menstrual complication.

Treatment.—The choice of remedies for the symptoms just detailed and analyzed is between belladonna and gelseminum. I prefer the former, because it corresponds more nearly to the patient's habit and temperament; to the probable cause of the menstrual suppression; to the brain symptoms dependent on the same, in all their minuteness; and to the reflex spasms of the voluntary muscles of the shoulder and arm. It is better adapted to the congestive tendency dependent on the arrest of the catamenial flow than any other remedy. If this patient had been seized immediately with the spasms; if the choreic symptoms had developed the moment the menses ceased, we would have ordered the gelseminum. For, in that case, the suppression would have depended on a sudden contraction of the cervix, analogous to that which sometimes takes place in labor. And the gelseminum is even better fitted to overcome that contraction than the belladonna. But here the nervous symptoms were preceded by an evident afflux of blood to the brain. This was the primary lesion, and the order of sequence is a significant factor in the choice of a remedy for any given class of symptoms. Belladonna not only corresponds with the cerebral lesion, but is equally applicable to the relief of the muscular symptoms arising from it.

Should the flow be forced to return?

Precisely what degree of importance should attach to a restoration of the menses in these cases, it is sometimes difficult to determine. The old method was to force their return by the use of emmenagogues, cathartics, hot herb teas, and the warm bath. And this under the impression that the symptoms which had their origin in the arrest of the flow could not be so promptly or effectually relieved as by its re-establishment. In many cases, where they were resorted to at once, and if they were not too powerful, these means were, no doubt, efficacious. Patients were cured in what was called a common-sense sort of way. But where, as in the case before you, a considerable time has intervened between the cessation of the proper menstrual flow and the making of the prescription, it is certainly prejudicial to the health and welfare of the patient, indeed, unphysiological, to attempt to bring it on again. Relieve the indirect symptoms by direct remedies, as speedily as possible, and trust to the natural powers to restore the function at or near the next "period." Where there is evident determination of blood to the head, I can see no valid objection to foot and hip baths as adjuncts to our remedies.

Subsequent trouble from suppression.

This one thing you may bear in mind with respect to this form of amenorrhœa. When some exciting cause has suppressed the discharge suddenly, and when, after a few hours, or days at the farthest, the flow is not resumed, *the chances of trouble at the next* "*period*" *will vary with the degree of congestion and inflammation of the uterus and ovaries consequent upon that suppression.* If the mishap has reacted upon these organs exclusively, the mischief is likely to be perpetuated in the form of dysmenorrhœa, menorrhagia, permanent retention, sterility, etc. But if, on the other hand, the brain is involved, any subsequent irregularity of menstruation will not be so apt to follow. Symptomatic disorders of the nervous system, dependent on this variety of menstrual arrest, are self-limited, and seldom interfere very seriously with the resumption of the flow at the next and subsequent periods. The importance of this rule is shown in the treatment which it is proper to pursue under these varying circumstances. In the former case there is manifest need of treating the patient during the monthly interval, so as, if possible, to avert more serious consequences, and to secure the punctual appearance of the accustomed discharge. In the latter, the present symptoms should be relieved, and the general system regulated by attention to the diet, and by exercise in the open air, after which we may safely leave the rest to nature.

Rest and quiet.

I might spend the whole hour, most profitably, perhaps, in insisting upon the especial need of rest in this class of cases. When you visit such a patient, you will very likely find her in an illy-ventilated apartment, surrounded by a host of anxious relatives, including one or more lovers, and neighborhood gossips enough to discourage her or drive her crazy, and to consume the oxygen to which she alone is entitled. Your first duty, in such an extremity, will be to clear the room of its unwholesome contents. If these "friends" are adhesive and pertinacious, and you cannot devise any better expedient, you may quietly hint that these symptoms are very peculiar, and may possibly develop into some contagious affection, as, for example, the small-pox. This will have the effect to scatter those mischievous comforters, whose sympathy is a curse instead of a blessing, and you can then forbid their return. In similar nervous states the most trivial causes may perpetuate the difficulty. A noisy door-bell, a talkative nurse, too much light, or sound, or stir in the room, or house, the doctor's creaky boots, and many other things may counteract the influence of the most appropriate internal remedies. It is a very important part of your duty to recognize and remove all these obstacles to recovery.

The patient will take a dose of belladonna 3rd, once in three hours during the day, and we shall see how promptly and satisfactorily she will recover.*

ABDOMINAL CRAMPS AND PAINS IN PREGNANCY.

Case.—Mrs. S—— is six and a half months advanced in her second pregnancy. For three weeks past she has complained of occasional pains and cramps in the abdomen. These sufferings are increased by exercise, slight pressure, emotional causes, and especially by the too vigorous movements of the fœtus in utero. Upon examination I found the abdominal parietes somewhat attenuated, and the uterus in the position of right lateral obliquity. Otherwise I discovered nothing abnormal.

Cramps, etc., after the fourth month

Unless the uterus is very decidedly displaced, abdominal and sacral pains, cramps in the limbs, and like symptoms, are not very apt to worry the pregnant woman prior to quickening. After the fourth month, however, and in exceptional cases as early as the third, they may be the cause of much suffering. They depend on the changes which the uterine and abdominal structures necessarily undergo in consequence of the development of the fœtus. As you would naturally suppose, these symptoms are most frequently met with in primiparæ—those who have never borne children before. Occasionally we find a patient who always experiences them during pregnancy.

As the uterus enlarges, there is a gradual distention of the abdominal walls. A very natural consequence of this distention is the production of muscular and neuralgic pains. These pains, which are sometimes general, again local—as in certain forms of hysteria—sometimes shooting and cramp-like, and again more constant, are very likely to be referred to the points of attachment of the various muscles which comprise the parietes of the abdomen. They may be felt in either the right or the left hypochondrium, in the iliac or umbilical region, and finally may settle into the permanent lumbar distress which in many cases precedes abortion. Not unfrequently, on account of its tension and

* At the end of twenty-four hours the headache had ceased; and at the end of the second day (the sixth from their commencement) the spasms left also. Three weeks later, at the usual time, the menses returned spontaneously.

extreme tenderness, when the belly has become hard and full, the skin is the seat of the difficulty. In such a case there is a neuralgic affection of the cutaneous nerves, which is frequently mistaken for inflammation of the womb and its appendages.

In most cases like the one before you, and whatever its seat and character, the suffering is increased by motion. Any exercise which renders it necessary for the patient to breathe more deeply and frequently than natural; coughing or straining at stool; riding or walking, turning in bed, or getting into an upright from a horizontal position; the rolling of flatus in the bowels, or the movements of the fœtus in utero; may produce or aggravate it. It is usually worse when upon the feet than when sitting, and when sitting than when lying. There are, however, many exceptions to this rule. Excepting towards the end of pregnancy, say after the seventh month, it is generally worse in the day and better at night. It may be increased by mental emotions, as fright or anxiety; and is more annoying and obstinate in those who are of sedentary habits than with the active and industrious. Lean women are more liable to it than the more robust. In rheumatic and neuralgic subjects it may depend upon vicissitudes of wind and weather for an exciting cause. Puny, nervous, and delicate children are more active and restless in utero, and therefore occasion more suffering of this kind, than those that are strong and vigorous.

Motion increases the suffering.

Diagnosis. — With respect to the prognosis and treatment, it is very important to be able to differentiate between the several varieties of abdominal pains to which pregnant women are subject. Among the lesions to which they are especially liable, we should separate the peritoneal from the neuralgic, the muscular from the uterine, and the ovarian from the intestinal.

There is a spurious or false peritonitis, which rarely occurs except at the menstrual period, or at the time in the month which corresponds to it during gestation. It usually commences with a chill and local pain of an acute, lancinating character, in the region of one or both ovaries. The corresponding limb is flexed, and cannot be straightened without great increase of suffering. The affected part is exceedingly tender to the touch, and pressure, slight or severe, is insupportable. This pain becomes gradually more diffuse. These

Spurious peritonitis.

symptoms are accompanied by more or less fever and constitutional disturbance.

In the cutaneous neuralgia, although the diagnosis is not difficult, the most unpardonable blunders are frequently made. Tarnier's remarks upon the subject are exceedingly appropriate, and I quote them:* "Having for some time made a special study of these abdominal, inguinal, and lumbar pains, we are convinced that very often they are due to neuralgia of the cutaneous nerves from the collateral branches of the lumbar plexus. To be assured that such is the case, it is only necessary to test carefully the sensibility of the skin in these regions, either by rubbing it rudely with the end of a pencil, or by raising it in the form of a fold which is to be gradually pinched between the fingers. Pressure ought also to be made all along the crest of the ilium, in the direction of the genito-crural nerve. Should we be satisfied with merely questioning the patient, or depressing the walls of the abdomen by the hand, we would incur the risk of obtaining very little information, or of suspecting the existence of deep-seated visceral pain when the skin only is affected. This mistake, which we see committed every day, would be avoided by taking the trouble to make the above-mentioned examination, and we cannot recommend it too highly. The principal parts affected by this neuralgia are the lumbar, iliac, hypogastric, and inguinal points, though the pain may appear in some other portion, of greater or less extent, of the skin of the abdomen. Sometimes confined to a circumscribed point, it occasionally invades an entire half of the abdominal walls. It very rarely affects both sides at the same time with equal intensity."

Diagnosis from cutaneous neuralgia.

If the abdominal muscles are the seat of the suffering, the pains are cramp-like, and accompanied by knotting of the fibres, which is worse upon pressure or motion. The suffering between the severest paroxysms is referred to the points of origin and insertion of separate muscles. This form is most frequent in rheumatic subjects, in whom there may be a sudden metastasis to either of the larger articulations. It sometimes arises from traumatic injuries, as, for example, a blow or fall upon the abdomen.

Characteristic symptoms.

* Cazeau's Midwifery, Revised and Annotated by S. Tarnier. Phila.: 1868. p. 521.

Metritis is a rare concomitant of gestation, but we not unfrequently encounter a species of uterine colic that is apt to be mistaken for one of the former affections. Hysterical women, who are highly emotional, and, I may add, exceedingly impulsive and imprudent also, are liable through some indiscretion, to attacks of this kind, and more especially about the period of quickening. So, also, are those who have been martyrs to dysmenorrhœa. The pain is referred to the uterine region and remains there. It may be intermittent, but it is not erratic like the muscular variety. It is prone to assume some of the characters of labor pains, and if long continued or extreme in degree, may really precipitate a miscarriage.

Uterine colic.

If we except their peritoneal envelope, the ovaries are singularly exempt from disease during pregnancy. From the date of conception their function is physiologically suspended and the condition which threatens their healthy action while menstruation continues is withdrawn. From various causes, however, their investing membrane may become inflamed, in which case the symptoms need not be confounded in your minds. The pain which is referred to the ovarian region, is sharp, and sometimes intense, or pressing, throbbing, burning, and paroxysmal. It may radiate over the abdomen, or extend into the back, or down the limb of the affected side. This limb is generally flexed, or if the patient tries to walk, she is lame with it. In exceptional cases pregnant women are, however, liable to a form of ovarian neuralgia.

Exemption from ovarian disease.

The gastro-intestinal disorders incident to pregnancy are more annoying and frequent before the fourth and after the seventh month than between these two periods. Whenever they occur, however, they are accompanied by such marked digestive derangement that you will have little trouble in their differential diagnosis.

Gastro-intestinal disorders incident to pregnancy.

Prognosis. — I recommend you in no instance to regard a case of this kind as trivial. For there is not one of them which is altogether exempt from the liability to abortion and its fearful consequences. Throughout its whole course, the state of pregnancy is beset with contingencies which it is your duty to avert. And not the least serious among them are such as may develop from symptoms like those of which our patient complains.

Treatment.—This is one of those cases which we often encounter in private practice, and which are distinguished by this peculiarity—*they are better managed by simple domestic expedients than by the most scientific prescriptions.* Yet, as I have said, we must discriminate. For example:

If the pains are muscular, the part may be bathed quite frequently with hamamelis. Perhaps as large a proportion as one-half of all the pregnant women who complain of these symptoms may be relieved by this means alone. It is equally appropriate in ovarian irritation and inflammation. In some cases the rhus toxicodendron answers a good purpose. I generally direct a table-spoonful of the strong tincture to be put into a teacupful of tepid or cool water, and then applied through one or more layers of flannel.

If the suffering has been caused by mechanical means, or is the result of injury, the tincture of arnica may be applied in the same manner.

If it is caused by undue pressure against the attenuated walls of the abdomen, you may counteract this effect by enveloping the abdomen in several layers of an elastic bandage of rubber-cloth in such a manner as to support its parietes. A bandage of linen would be too unyielding, and might indirectly induce abortion.

Toward the latter end of pregnancy the feeling of extreme distention and discomfort in the abdomen, will often yield to the old and simple expedient of anointing it with sweet oil. I have seen the most threatening symptoms of premature labor relieved in this manner. If the pains are cramp-like, the camphorated oil is an excellent application.

If the suffering is neuralgic, you will charm it away by directing that the affected part be covered with simple, dry, uncarded cotton, or cotton batting. In some cases, several layers of flannel will answer equally well. Belladonna, or atropine, internally, may hasten the cure.

In the ovarian neuralgia which sometimes complicates the symptoms, and greatly increases the suffering in these cases, I know of no remedy to compare with the valerianate of zinc. I shall have more to say in future of this contingent of pregnancy.

It is very important always to regulate the exercise of the patient, and as far as possible to prevent too much of mental friction and anxiety on her part; for, although anatomists have failed to demonstrate a nervous connection between the mother and the fœtus in utero, her mental emotions do influence it greatly. It is a bad habit for those who are pregnant to take care of, and to lift and carry around, other children in the family. Although tight-lacing is popularly believed to contribute to an easy and safe labor, it is often prejudicial to the comfort and welfare of the pregnant woman, by inducing abdominal pains and cramps which may result in abortion.

Internally, a variety of remedies may be indicated. Where, as in this case, the suffering is aggravated by motion, however slight, bryonia will sometimes afford almost instant relief. Nux vomica, pulsatilla, belladonna, rhus tox., ignatia, and chamomilla, are also useful under appropriate indications. This patient will take bryonia 3d, three times daily.

EXCESSIVE ABDOMINAL DEVELOPMENT IN PREGNANCY.

It sometimes happens that symptoms which are analogous to those afforded by the patient who has just left the room, depend on other causes than those already named. Only yesterday I was consulted by letter in a case of this kind. My patient writes:

Case.—I had called myself seven months advanced in pregnancy, but many things conspire to make me think it probable that I am at least eight months along. I am *exceedingly* large, and from my extreme size, suffer greatly from faintness. For a fortnight I have endured severe pain in my left side, which nothing will relieve, although sitting up aggravates it. It has become almost unbearable, wearing my life and strength away, and giving me no rest, day or night.

"My little ones have always been large, weighing ten or eleven pounds, and you know I am a wee bit of a woman. But now the doctor thinks it probable that there may be two of them, which are small, but amazingly strong and active, while there is evidently a great quantity of water contained in the womb. The child was in such a position as to cause much suffering and uneasiness, it being apparently *across* the pelvis. The doctor gave me pulsatilla, and whether it produced the effect or not, one week later it was pronounced 'all right.'

"Will you be so kind as to inform me if there is anything that will relieve this pain in my side? If it should continue, would it not be well to hasten delivery, before I am altogether worn out? I frequently have severe and almost unbearable contractions, which cause the abdomen to feel as if turned into stone."

This case presents several points of practical interest. As you will observe, it supplies additional details, and is an excellent appendix to the former one. Gestation is more advanced, and the symptoms are different.

Size of the abdomen as a sign and sequence of pregnancy.

During pregnancy the size of the abdomen is relative. There is no actual scale of measurement or development for all, or even for single patients, who are successively pregnant. Hence the absolute impossibility of judging by this sign whether a woman is in the seventh or eighth month. The abdomen is proportionally larger in short than in tall women, in multiparæ than in primiparæ, in those who are pregnant with twins than in case the womb contains but a single fœtus. Its prominence varies with the laxity of the abdominal walls, the position of the uterus, the size of the fœtus, and possibly its position, and with the quantity of amniotic liquor that surrounds the child or children. It may also become very large from intestinal indigestion and tympanites, abdominal dropsy, uterine or ovarian tumors, and malformation or dropsy of the fœtus.

Whatever their cause, these symptoms give rise to suffering and apprehension. They convert a natural process into a species of martyrdom, which, luckily, is self-limited.

Diagnosis.—You will sometimes find it extremely difficult, and, indeed, quite impossible, to determine the cause or causes of these symptoms and the lesions, functional and organic, of which they are the token. A pendulous belly, with undue size of the abdominal tumor, occurs more frequently in spare, ill-conditioned women than in those who are short, plump, and well nourished. The muscles are thin and flabby, and the patient is more or less anæmic.

If the extraordinary size depends on the position of the uterus, that organ will be found to incline forwards, over the pubes, or to one or the other side of the abdomen—usually to the right side. If upon the size of the child, its outline can be felt through the abdominal walls. Note should also be taken of the size and weight of former children, if the patient has ever been pregnant before. The chances are that, having always had very large children, my correspondent is carrying one now, and that most of her symptoms are referable to this fact. Women who have had children that weighed nine pounds and over, very rarely have twins in a subsequent pregnancy.*

The position of the fœtus in utero would be more apt to modify the shape than the size of the tumor. The position of the child is so frequently changed, even up to the time that labor commences, that a constant and uniform increase in the size of the abdomen could hardly depend on this cause.

The characteristic symptoms by which you would recognize an extraordinary enlargement of the abdomen, dependent on dropsy of the amnion, are the following. It is an acute affection, the tumor is circumscribed, disproportionate, is developed rapidly, and is most likely to occur in those who have previously had, or at the time are having, dropsy elsewhere. It almost never occurs in those who are not of a dropsical diathesis. To the hand, when placed upon the abdomen, the movements of the fœtus seem distant and indistinct. The fœtus is almost always small, feeble, and illy-developed, and generally survives its birth but a short time. The tumor may develop to such an extent as to occasion the most alarming dyspnœa and syncope, by pressing upon the diaphragm and adjacent viscera.

Intestinal disorder may produce an excessive enlargement of the abdomen in pregnant women, either by causing dropsy of the peritoneum, or by the inflation of the bowels with gas. In the former case the hepatic function is almost always implicated. In the latter the intestinal glandular apparatus. The symptoms would vary, and you would not fail to recognize them.

Uterine and ovarian tumors would have a history that commenced before pregnancy. Neither mal-formation, nor hydrocephalus, nor general anasarca of the fœtus, could be diagnosticated with certainty prior to delivery. Twin pregnancy might be detected through the fœtal heart sounds.

Prognosis.—It is an exceptional case for any woman to pass through the state of pregnancy, from beginning to end, without complaining of these or analogous symptoms. And, strange to say, the rule appears to be that, with certain qualifications, those who are most prone to these sufferings are least liable to have

* At birth this patient's child weighed eleven pounds.

difficult labors, or tedious and dangerous convalescence in their lying-in. The chief danger from any of these symptoms, at whatever period of gestation they may occur, is from abortion. If you can avert this calamity, the patient will probably do well. The greater the perturbation of the nervous system, or the more the urinary and hepatic functions are deranged, the more decidedly this unfortunate result is threatened. Dropsy of the amnion is more fatal to the child than to the mother. In all cases you should inspire your patient with courage, and with the hope that all may yet be well. A lugubrious, long-faced doctor would always be an additional affliction to her, but especially under these circumstances.

Treatment.—The general indication is to make the woman as comfortable as possible, to turn aside the contingencies that threaten miscarriage, and to bring her through to term as quietly and safely as we may. To this end the directions which I gave you in my remarks upon the case that preceded this are equally appropriate here.

The remedies indicated will vary with the special pathology of the case, or as the phrase is, with the symptoms presented. If the enlargement is due to abdominal or to amniotic dropsy, those remedies would be called for which are suited to the dropsical diathesis, and you would select from among them that one which is most appropriate to the symptoms of each individual case. I should caution you, however, against prescribing the apis mellifica in a low potency in case of dropsy of the amnion, lest it should precipitate a miscarriage.

Incidental disorders of the intestinal tract suggest their own remedies, among the more prominent of which are arsenicum, chamomilla, nux vomica, mercurius, china, colocynth, belladonna, and veratrum.

The pressure from a misplaced gravid uterus may sometimes be greatly relieved by a change of position on the part of the patient. Or bandages and supports, if properly adjusted, may tend to make life more tolerable, by allowing the patient to move around and to take exercise. They may also be made to add to the strength of the abdominal walls in case the child is preternaturally developed, or where there are twins.

I think that the induction of premature labor would not be justifiable in a case of this kind, unless the patient were in imminent danger from suffocation by dropsy of the amnion. I can imagine, although I have never met with such an example in practice, that this expedient might be necessary as often, perhaps, as once in a thousand cases. Be sure you do not resort to it, gentlemen, on your patient's prescription instead of your own.

The induction of premature labor.

Concerning the alleged power of pulsatilla to correct a malpresentation of the fœtus at any period of gestation, or in labor at term, I am wholly skeptical. Up to this date (Feb., 1869) there is not a single case on record which clearly proves it to be possessed of any such properties. In every published instance the testimony is as invalid and fallacious as in that which we have just had under review. This patient's physician was not certain in his diagnosis. First he said she had twins, then dropsy of the amnion, and finally the (one) child was "apparently across the pelvis." Pulsatilla was given, a spontaneous change followed — as has probably happened with every fœtus from the time of Cain until now — and the result was accredited to the remedy that had been swallowed! Such things may not be impossible, but they are exceedingly improbable.

Pulsatilla in mal-presentations.

SUDDEN SUPPRESSION OF MENORRHAGIA BY ASTRINGENTS THE CAUSE OF SUBSEQUENT ILLNESS.

Case. — Mrs. R—— desires relief from attacks of what has been diagnosticated as bilious colic, from which she has suffered at frequent periods for eight months. The paroxysms almost always come on at night, immediately upon retiring. For a week past they have returned every evening. The pain is referred to the epigastric region, and is described as sharp, cutting and colicky in its nature. It also intermits, and, when most severe, there is a slight inclination to vomit. The paroxysm generally lasts about an hour, during which time she cannot lie down, but must sit upright in the bed. After the fit she sleeps soundly, and, with the exception of a loss of appetite for breakfast, and occasional headache, is quite well next day. It sometimes happens that unusual excitement or fatigue will induce a paroxysm in the daytime. This trouble is greatly aggravated at each menstrual period. At present, the menses recur regularly every four weeks.

Prior to the commencement of these attacks she had, for some months, suffered from too frequent and too profuse menstruation. The flow returned every two or three weeks, and the loss of blood was sometimes extreme. To arrest the hæmorrhage, her physician ordered vaginal injections of strong alum water. This expedient arrested the flow, but induced a severe attack of metritis, from which, in the hands of another physician, she barely recovered. The menstrual interval was subsequently extended to about four weeks, but the flow was still too profuse. All sorts of expedients were tried to arrest it, but without effect, until the patient, becoming wearied with it, took the responsibility of resorting again to the alum injections. As soon as she did so, the excessive flow ceased, but in lieu of it she began to have these attacks of excruciating pain. During the eight months which have intervened she has had three other physicians, none of whom has succeeded in clearing up the diagnosis, or in curing the disease.

Intra-uterine astringents.

The temptation to resort to astringents, topically and internally, in case of hæmorrhage, is a very strong one. This is especially true in those forms of uterine hæmorrhage which are connected with menstruation. The arguments against their indiscriminate employment are few and simple. In the first place, unless connected with abortion or labor at term, the excessive flow is symptomatic. In this case, to check it, and to arrest it by styptics, is not to cure the patient, but to complicate matters and make them worse instead of better. The more rational method would be to address our treatment, external or internal, or both, to the removal of the lesion, or condition upon which this flow depends. Take away the cause and the effect ceases. To strike this single symptom out of existence would be to lose time and work mischief.

Menorrhagia sometimes critical.

Again, a copious menstruation, like a free diuresis or diaphoresis, may be critical, and in a sense salutary. It may represent a species of safety-valve which, for the welfare of the general organism, should not be too abruptly closed. It is quite probable that the menstrual secretion is partly eliminative, and designed to expel certain noxious matters which would prove harmful if retained. To suppress the flow voluntarily might induce the very symptoms which are present in case of retention from diseased states, a consequence which it is our duty to avert.

You will readily perceive that the sudden application of a solution of alum to the vascular mucous membrane of the superior vagina and uterine cervix, for the arrest of the hæmorrhage, would be very apt so to derange its capillary circulation as to cause inflammation. If you desired to produce an attack of metritis, no more certain and expeditious method could be devised. It is no marvel that this poor woman suffered greatly, and almost died in consequence of this unwarrantable expedient. Thousands of lives have been sacrificed in this very manner. These harsh astringents are often thrown into the vagina, and sometimes even into the womb itself, for the same purpose as in this case. With utter disregard of the delicacy of the structures involved, of the danger of inflammation and its sequelæ, of the risk of throwing the fluid through the Fallopian tubes directly into the cavity of the peritoneum, of damming up the blood upon the ovaries, of pelvic hæmatocele, and other consequences a hundred fold more serious than the hæmorrhage itself, this practice is still sanctioned by the profession. I have brought this case before you, in order to impress upon your minds some of the possible consequences that may result from such treatment; also to show you "a more excellent way."

Physiological argument against intra-uterine astringents.

We shall doubtless have frequent occasion to refer to the reflex relations existing between the uterine cervix and the stomach. There is much that is curious and suggestive therein. But there is a clinical hint connected with the history of cases like this, the significance of which you should appreciate. A large proportion of the cases in which astringent injections of various kinds have been thrown into the vagina, and thus brought into contact with the neck of the womb, are characterized by peculiar and inveterate disorders of the stomach and bowels. Some of the worst examples of gastric indigestion that I have ever treated were chargeable to vaginal injections that had been resorted to for the cure of leucorrhœa. In other cases, the ill effects have been observed in the production of intestinal colic, dyspepsia, and constipation.

Digestive disorders from vaginal and uterine injections.

Here the irritant is applied to the superior vagina and about the cervix. Through nervous sympathy the stomach and bowels are implicated. Their functions are deranged, and more or less of actual suffering is induced. Such a train of consequences is all the more certain and characteristic, if the drug with which the injection was medicated had also a specific relation to some portion of the intestinal tract. And, upon reflection, you will find that a majority of the substances used in this manner have such a relation to the alimentary system especially. It is true of tannin, alum, the acetate of lead, the salts of silver, of copper, and of iron, the oil of turpentine, and many other remedies which have been used in this way. This explains the possibility that our patient first experienced her attacks of "bilious colic," falsely so-called, in consequence of the alum injections, which had been taken to suppress the hæmorrhage from the womb.

Menorrhagia from polypi, etc.

But there is another item which we must not pass over in silence. I allude to the fact that menorrhagia sometimes depends upon the presence of uterine polypi, which, being very vascular, occasion the increased and prolonged hæmorrhage at each menstrual period. And not only so, but they sometimes cause a species of menstrual colic, which greatly torments the patient. I have repeatedly had occasion to witness the most extreme suffering, sometimes gastric, again gastro-intestinal, or perhaps uterine chiefly, which was entirely due to the presence and pressure of a polypoid growth within and upon the cervix. Indeed, when I find a patient complaining of these symptoms, and learn that she has not been in the habit of taking vaginal objections, I am suspicious of the existence of some intra-uterine growth, which may be sufficient to account both for the menorrhagia and the spasmodic colic. And I recommend you, gentlemen, to be upon your guard in all cases of this kind. Do not trust too exclusively to objective symptoms, which might mislead you, and bring down reproach upon your school and your skill. Examine the case thoroughly, and do not forget the practical hints of which I have just spoken.

Treatment. — This is a case of neuralgia of the cœliac plexus, induced by the alum injections. How shall we treat it? Is it worth while trying to antidote the poison thus introduced, when so long a time has elapsed since it was taken? Or shall we prescribe for the symptoms as we find them? This is a point upon which doctors would assuredly disagree. My own opinion is that, if the attack were more recent in its origin, and we had a reliable antidote for the toxical effects of alumina, the "chemical treatment," as it is called, might promise good results. But, under the circumstances, we must base our prescription upon present indications.

The character of the pain, the period of its recurrence, the causes that induce it incidentally, and the aggravation at the menstrual period, are the prominent and most significant symptoms. Pulsatilla is the remedy. I recommend that she take a dose of it every three hours during the day. If the paroxysm returns at evening, it may be repeated every twenty or thirty minutes until the attack has passed. When the symptoms are relieved, the medicine may be given at longer intervals. I have sometimes cured this species of neuralgic colic, dependent upon maltreatment of uterine affections, by giving a few doses of atropine 3d, and again with colocynth of the same potency.

Intolerance of vaginal injections.

There are cases of reflex disorders in other organs, as for example the stomach and bowels, the head, the heart, and the general nervous system, but more especially in the ovaries, that will not yield to the best chosen remedies until the habit of taking vaginal injections is proscribed. This remark applies not only to injections that are harsh and decidedly irritant, but also to such as are ordinarily harmless. These cases are exceptional, and should not tempt you into an indiscriminate denial of the efficacy of such means under proper indications. It will be best for this patient not to take any kind of vaginal injection until she has recovered her health, and then only for the purpose of cleanliness.

Should these means fail, it would be proper to proceed upon the hint which I have given you concerning the possibility that there is a foreign body, a polypus, within the womb. The os should be so dilated with a sponge or other tents, that the proper exploration can be made. This should be done slowly and carefully, in the manner which will be detailed when I come to speak of the treatment of uterine polypi.

LECTURE IV.

UTERINE HÆMORRHAGE AFTER TWIN DELIVERY.

GENTLEMEN:

I will embrace this opportunity to speak to you of the following interesting

Case. — Mrs. ——, in her fourth labor, was delivered of twins, the united weight of the children being eighteen pounds. The labor was of only three hours' duration, both children presenting by the head. The placenta, which was a very large single mass with two separate cords, was carefully removed twenty minutes after the birth of the second child. Considering its great size, the womb appeared to contract properly while the placenta was being extracted. But, two minutes after it was taken away, the patient was seized with vomiting, which was immediately followed by a fainting fit. The retching and syncope continued to alternate every few seconds. She became pale and pulseless. I placed my hand over the uterus and found it flaccid and relaxed, instead of firm and contracted as before. It felt as if the finger could be thrust through it with very little effort. Blood was flowing fearfully from the vagina, and my patient was insensible. The pains had entirely ceased.

I removed the pillow from beneath her head and placed it transversely under the hips, after which I at once resorted to friction and kneading of the abdomen with my left hand, while, with the right one, large pieces of ice were passed high up into the vagina, and even through the gaping cervix quite into the womb. In all, a lump of ice as large as the nurse's head — the chignon included — was thus applied. The patient made no resistance and offered no complaint, being meanwhile more like a dead than a live woman. Just in proportion as the womb contracted upon itself, the flow ceased. After more than half an hour of the greatest anxiety to the husband and family, and of extreme danger to my patient, she opened her eyes, in a semi-conscious state, and asked "why everything that flowed from her was so cold?" As soon thereafter as it was safe to move her in the least, the binder was snugly and firmly applied over a dry compress, and, with great subsequent care, she made a good recovery.

In the whole range of medical and surgical practice there is nothing more alarming and serious than a bad case of flooding after delivery. And there is no position in which the doctor can be placed where his coolness and skill, his self-reliance and tact, may be of greater service to his patient. Although they are by no means frequent, still, since it is possible that such a case may be one of the first to which you will be called, it is alike your duty and mine to consider this subject carefully. For the physician must be *au fait*, ready at a moment's notice, to act promptly and efficiently.

Alarming nature of uterine hæmorrhage.

In general, uterine hæmorrhage is more apt to occur after rapid labors. In this respect the same rule holds as in the case of after-pains — the shorter the labor (in multiparæ), the more severe and protracted the subsequent pains, and *vice versa*. The cause is probably the same, both in case of the hæmorrhage and of the after-pains. When the labor is quickly over, and the uterus has been rapidly emptied of its contents, its muscular fibres have contracted less firmly than they would have done in an opposite state of things. Hence the mouths of the vessels, which were ruptured at the site of the placenta, are not closed and sealed as tightly as they should have been. A sudden and fearful hæmorrhage may be due to this cause alone.

Incident to rapid labors especially.

This accident may also be occasioned by adhesion of the placenta throughout nearly its whole extent. If it begins to be detached at the border, and then remains partly adherent, alarming hæmorrhage is very apt to result. If it is first separated from the uterine wall at the middle of the placental mass, a clot may form at that point, and arrest the flow of blood by direct compression. This last is the usual manner of separation of the after-birth. If the placenta is very large, as in this case of twins, and so extensively attached as almost to cover the entire surface of the womb — as in certain of the inferior animals — the liability to hæmorrhage when it is torn off, or comes away, is very much increased. The larger the extent of uterine surface exposed, and especially if the womb has been very much distended, and its walls are flaccid, the greater the danger of and from post-partum hæmorrhage. Hence this mishap is a more serious affair in case of twins than where there is only one

Adherent placenta a cause.

child, and the larger the children the greater the danger therefrom. If only a small portion of the secundines remains, it may be sufficient to cause the most dangerous hæmorrhage.

Hæmorrhage is sometimes due to uterine inertia. Here the entire expulsive power of the organ has been spent in effecting delivery. To fold the womb upon itself, and to constringe and compress the gaping vessels, requires an additional supply of motor force. But it is not forthcoming, and flooding is the indirect consequence of protracted, tedious, and difficult labor. These cases are exceptional, but they do sometimes occur.

Hæmorrhage from uterine inertia.

The presence of clots in the uterus, or of a clot in the os uteri, may give rise to flooding. They operate by interfering with and preventing the complete contraction of the womb. Other causes to which this result may sometimes be referred are a cough, distention of the bladder, partial inversion of the uterus, rupture of the placenta, cancer of the womb, uterine polypi, and albuminuria.

Women of a hæmorrhagic diathesis are predisposed to this complication of labor. Those who have had hæmoptysis, or hæmatemesis, need especial care during and subsequent to delivery, in order to avert it. The same is true of those who flow very freely at each menstrual return, or who have ever had menorrhagia. It is my habit, when the patient is a stranger to me, always to inquire, before the delivery of the placenta, whether she has been subject to either of these forms of hæmorrhage, and also whether she flowed profusely in her previous confinements. For those women who have had one attack of post-partum hæmorrhage, are exceedingly liable to another.

The hæmorrhagic diathesis a predisponent.

Prognosis. — In all those cases in which the loss of blood is not promptly recognized and proper measures taken for its arrest, there is great danger. Other things equal, the more rapid the labor the greater the danger. So, also, of the relative size of the womb. Vomiting is salutary, and not by any means a bad sign, when it *follows* the hæmorrhage, for in this case it may stimulate uterine contractions, and thus help to save the patient. But when it *precedes* the hæmorrhage, it is less favorable. Here it depends on the emptying of the womb and the removal of the accustomed pressure by other organs. Patients sometimes swoon away and die in the first fit of syncope. If, however, they survive one or more of these fits, the case becomes more promising. It is a bad sign if the fainting and flooding continue to alternate.

In all cases the danger is proportionate to the atony of the uterine muscular fibre, the irregularity of its contraction, the pain which the patient experiences (if she is not insensible) the more or less complete delivery of the placenta and the membranes, and the time that has elapsed since the close of labor. The harder, more unyielding and globular the womb feels, through the abdominal parietes, the less the danger. If, however, the fundus is felt near or above the umbilicus, and the womb does not contain another fœtus, there is great risk from internal hæmorrhage, which may be due either to great distention of the bladder, or to a retention of a part of the placenta, or of the membranes. With certain qualifications, the greater the pain, resembling labor pains, the less the danger from hæmorrhage. The danger is also diminished by the length of time that has elapsed since the labor proper was completed. Convulsions, due to a sudden hæmorrhage of this kind, are almost invariably fatal.

Signs of danger.

The risk to the patient is not always removed when the hæmorrhage is under control. It may take months, or even years, for her to recover from the loss of so much blood. There is danger from puerperal phlebitis, cellulitis, pelvic hæmatocele, pyæmia, and also from the formation of abscesses in various parts of the body. Added to this are the mischievous contingencies which beset the suppression of the milk and the lochia, and the fact that the nutritive system of the mother has long been taxed severely for the development of the fœtus in utero.

Sequelæ.

You will not, therefore, be justified in promising to cure every case of this kind, even although you may have been so skillful and successful as entirely to control the hæmorrhage. It is best in every instance to qualify your prognosis, and to allow sufficient time for your patient to recover, providing she really does get well.

A qualified prognosis.

Treatment.—Bear in mind that I am speaking of a very extreme case of post-partum flooding, not of placenta prævia, nor yet of those mild cases of hæmorrhage which are more frequently met with and more easily managed. Teachers and authors almost always confound them, to which fact we may attribute the confused ideas in theory and practice that are generally entertained.

Internal and local treatment.

Authors are not agreed concerning the relative value of internal and external, or constitutional and manual means for the arrest of the flow in a case like this. Some insist that local measures are indispensable and sufficient, and that medicines internally given have little or no effect. Opposed to this class are those who hold the extreme view that this accident should be treated by internal remedies exclusively.* As usual, the proper course appears to lie between them. Both classes of measures may be requisite, and we should not extol the one at the expense of the other. *Passive* hæmorrhage from the womb implies a diseased state, which may have developed into, or from, a dyscrasia, and therefore comes properly within the domain of constitutional treatment. But in a case of sudden flooding, directly connected with delivery and rupture of the vascular attachment between the uterus and the placenta, where the blood flows from the vulva like water from a pump, and where life is jeopardized, and may be lost in a twinkling, other and very different indications are presented. Let us see what those indications are.

Obvious indications.

Whether from a sudden emptying of its contents, or from the exhaustion consequent upon protracted and difficult labor, uterine inertia always implies an imperfect contraction of the womb. Labor proper being passed, the uterine effort is brought to a stand-still. The veins, or sinuses, at the site of the placental attachment have been mechanically ruptured. Unless these torn vessels are compressed, and ligated, as it were, by the uterine contractions, there is nothing to prevent or to obstruct the flow, and death may speedily ensue. Hence the paramount indication is to bring on these contractions as speedily as possible. "A pint of blood saved, and a pint of blood lost to the patient, may make all the difference between a rapid and a tedious convalescence — may make all the difference between a successful and a fatal issue."

* Vide Dr. Guernsey's paper and the discussion thereon, in the Transactions of the American Institute for 1869.

The first thing to be done is to lower the patient's head to a level with, or even lower than her hips. Then grasp the uterus, through the abdominal walls, with one or both hands. Hold it firmly. Make steady and equal pressure, noting carefully if it contracts regularly, is becoming smaller in size, and less flaccid and relaxed. If it is, all is going on well; if it is not, otherwise.

Promote uterine contraction.

If the flow continues, leave one hand (usually the left) on the abdomen, and explore the uterus internally with the other. If the placenta has not been delivered, and is only partially detached, give the patient a plump dose of brandy and water, and then pass the hand into the womb and remove the after-birth. Peel it off by insinuating the fingers between it and the internal uterine surface. And don't bring away the hand until you bring the whole placenta along with it. Be careful, however, not to invert the womb. In these cases the placenta is frequently retained in consequence of the paralysis of the uterine muscular fibre, and not always because it is morbidly adherent. Remove the clots from the os and uterine cavity also.

Remove the placenta.

The proper course is not to put on the binder while the hæmorrhage continues so profuse. The hand, when applied over the abdomen, may first have been dipped in cold water. Or cold cloths may be applied to the vulva. Pieces of ice, when they can be had, may be introduced into the vagina, and, in exceptional cases, even carried up to the fundus of the womb. Or ice-water may be injected into the uterine cavity, the vagina, or the rectum. Pouring cold water from a height upon the abdomen, although efficient, may do mischief indirectly, by wetting the clothing and causing the patient to take cold. Colpeurysis, which consists in introducing the colpeurynter per vaginam, and filling it with ice-water, is also an available and excellent expedient. It not only supplies the shock from the cold, which is so useful, but also serves to stimulate the reflex contractions of the uterus, much as the child's head would do, if it were still in the vagina, and thus to put a stop to the flow.

Available expedients.

There is a great aversion on the part of many physicians to the introduction of the hand into the uterus. The danger therefrom is more imaginary than real. It is true that the cases of uterine hæmorrhage in which this expedient is requisite are not very numerous, but they do certainly occur. Earle, who is very emphatic on this point, says:* "I have noticed, and it is what we should expect, that the men who deprecate the procedure are generally those who possess big hands." When the hand is placed within the womb, it stimulates immediate contraction. The organ closes around the hand just as it did around the fœtus, and this involution, closure or contraction, is *the* great hæmostatic.

The hand in utero.

Now, since the os sometimes closes very soon after the delivery of the secundines, and since the longer you delay the greater will be the difficulty in inserting the hand at all, and the greater the danger from internal hæmorrhage also, if the symptoms do not yield readily and promptly to other measures, the sooner you resort to this expedient the better. If any portion of the placenta remains, remove it; if the womb contains one or more clots, remove them. If you can find the spot from which the flow comes, and can compress it between the hand within the womb and that upon the abdomen and over it, do so. Firm pressure over the fundus and towards the pubes will help to empty the womb of the clots which it may contain.

Gooch, who is excellent authority, gives the following testimony concerning the efficacy of pressure by the hand directly upon the denuded portion of the uterus: †

"My belief now is, that when hæmorrhage occurs after the removal of the placenta, the quickest way to stop it is to introduce the left hand closed within the uterus, apply the right hand open to the outside of the abdomen, and then between the two to compress the part where the placenta was attached, and from which chiefly the blood is flowing. When the hand is introduced merely as a stimulant, there is an interval of time between its arrival within the uterus and the secure contraction of this organ, during which much blood is often lost. By directing the hand to the very vessels from which it issues, and compressing them as I have described, this quantity is saved. If I may judge by my

* On Flooding after Delivery, etc. By Lumley Earle, M.D., etc. London. 1865; p. 77.

† An Account of some of the most important Diseases peculiar to Women. By Robert Gooch, M.D. Philadelphia. 1848. Second Edition; p. 300.

feeling, the blood stops, in a great degree, even before the uterus contracts; the hand acts first as a tourniquet, then as a stimulant. It is true we can not tell with certainty where the placenta was attached, and consequently where the pressure should be applied, but as it is generally attached to or near the fundus, if the pressure be directed there, it will generally be right. Besides, after the child is born, it is often several minutes before the placenta separates and descends; if, during this interval, we pass the finger along the cord and observe, at its entrance into the uterus, whether it turn towards the front, the back, the right or left side, or straight up to the fundus, we shall form a tolerably exact idea of the spot to which the placenta has been attached in this individual case."

Where the uterine atony is very marked, and there is reason to fear that the hæmorrhage may return, the ergot is an excellent remedy. You may give it in a low potency, or, if you please, in substance. The fluid extract, the tincture, and the wine of ergot are not reliable. If you prescribe the drug with a view to its prompt, tonic effect, and with the intention of causing the womb to contract firmly and securely, give ten to twenty grains, freshly powdered, in a little warm water. It may happen that you will not have occasion oftener than once in ten or twenty years to resort to this expedient, but I charge you not to forget it.

In these extreme cases of post-partum hæmorrhage, stimulants should be given very freely and frequently. This is especially requisite where the flow occurs in those who have been under the influence of chloroform or ether. Brandy is best of all, after which come whisky, ammonia, and camphor. There is no danger from the reaction which may soon after follow. Fresh air is equally necessary.

Stimulants.

Do not, for any possible reason, allow the patient to sit up in the bed, or she may fall at once into a mortal syncope. Keep her as quiet as possible. If she faints, lower the head still more. If she vomits, turn it gently, but do not raise her shoulders. Examine from time to time, and learn *for yourself* if the flow is ceasing.

Keep the head low.

If she has not urinated for some time, or there is reason to believe that the bladder contains a considerable quantity of urine, draw it off by means of the catheter. And do not forget that this condition is apt to be pres-

Emptying the bladder.

ent whenever the uterus, instead of contracting in a globular form just above the pubis, is high up towards the umbilicus, and pointed in its outline.

The value of the binder.

Although for more than thirty years an effort has been made on the part of some prominent members of the profession to do away with the use of the obstetric binder, the general sentiment and practice is still in favor of its employment. When carefully and properly applied, there is really no valid objection to it. The arguments against its use are founded upon its abuse in the hands of those who have been careless and are unskillful. In cases like the one we have just studied, it affords an additional safeguard, and a means of comfort, which, while it does not in any manner interfere with the internal treatment, could not be substituted by anything else. As I have already hinted, in general the bandage should not be applied until the globular form of the uterus has been recognized through the abdominal parietes, and the hæmorrhage has measurably ceased. Until this period, in a bad case of flooding, the hand should not be removed from the hypogastrium.

The compress.

The objections that have been urged against the binder apply more properly to the compress which is beneath it. If not carefully adjusted, this may do real mischief by interfering with the proper circulation of blood in the pelvic and abdominal organs, and by displacing them. You should never make use of it without being careful to recognize any change in the position of the uterus, especially in the direction of latero-version, in which case it will be necessary to replace the bandage directly over the front face of that organ, wherever that may be. Of course it need not be of so firm and unyielding a texture as to injure the soft parts. In most cases it may consist of an ordinary dressing towel, folded several times. In ordinary labors, without subsequent hæmorrhage, I dispense with the compress and make use only of the binder. Yet in, or rather after flooding, I have great confidence in the additional application of the compress with the binder.

A rare expedient.

In illustration of the value of these adjuvants, the following case occurs to my mind. One of my medical friends, while riding past a farm-house on the prairie, was hastily summoned to the bedside of a lying-in woman, who had just been delivered of a bouncing baby. She was almost dead from the loss of blood, which had run through the bedding, and stood in pools upon the floor. She was bloodless, pale, cold, and gasping for breath. Equal to the emergency, my friend seized the family bible and bound it very tightly over the womb with a coarse towel. This severe compression stopped the hæmorrhage almost instantly, and saved the woman's life. I do not recommend you, gentlemen, to employ books as uterine hæmostatics in ordinary cases of flooding, but to carry about with you, and to cultivate, that species of inspiration which seizes upon every variety of remedial resource, and puts it to the best possible use.

PSEUDO-PROLAPSE OF THE UTERUS.

Case.— At five P.M., of June 4, 1866, I was summoned in haste to visit Mrs. ——, who, the husband wrote me, was "almost dead with prolapse of the womb." In his note he requested me to bring the necessary instruments for replacing that organ. The patient, aged 52, had been ill one week, under the care of two physicians who had diagnosticated the case as one of prolapsus uteri, and who, I was told, had several times restored the womb to its normal position. These operations had caused her great pain, and she had a mortal dread lest I should think it necessary to repeat them. The day previous, the doctor had succeeded in introducing a Hodge's lever pessary, which, after a little, dropped out of itself. Although she had taken opiates freely and frequently, she had not slept for two days and nights. There was retching and bilious vomiting, and, although she had taken cathartics, the bowels had not been opened for four days. There was much ineffectual tenesmus, and with each effort at stool she complained of feeling as if the uterus and neighboring organs would be expelled from the body. She was exceedingly nervous, and at intervals of five to fifteen minutes suffered acute pains across the inferior portion of the abdomen. These pains were aggravated by motion and by any considerable degree of mental excitement. She described them as short, sharp, spasmodic, cutting and colicky in nature. She was greatly depressed in spirits—"must have relief or she should die."

I enjoined rest, as first and most important. Belladonna 3d, and nux vomica 3d, were to be taken in hourly alternation until the symptoms improved, after which they were to be repeated every two hours. If she slept, she was not to be awakened or disturbed. If the bowels did not move before daylight, they might give her an enema of tepid water. I made no examination per vaginam.

June 5, 5:30 P.M.—Patient better. After taking the first dose of the belladonna she slept for some minutes, and had but one more spasm of the pain. The remedies were repeated only at long intervals, for she slept quietly during the greater part of the night. At daylight, not having had a stool, the enema was administered with good effect, although the passage was very painful, and she was much exhausted in consequence. The tenesmus and vomiting were relieved, and she declared herself well. Continued the same remedies once in four hours. The "touch" revealed the uterus *in situ*. The husband and family were delighted with the promptness of the relief afforded.

Two days later this patient was able to attend to her household duties.

Frequency of uterine prolapse.

Nothing is more common than a temporary prolapse of the womb. Some women have it at each menstrual period; others after any extraordinary fatigue, as in walking or riding, some from a fit of mental anxiety or of coughing: others after a stool; and others again after coitus. When induced by these causes it is a self-limited affection, and may pass away with rest in the recumbent position. This is a very different thing from a chronic and inveterate prolapse, and requires very different treatment. If my predecessors had recognized this fact, this patient would have improved before I came; for in that case they would have forborne to do anything mischievous. A correct knowledge of special pathology on the part of the physician is sometimes an excellent safeguard for the patient.

Consequences of incorrect diagnosis.

One of two ill results may follow a wrong diagnosis in cases of this kind. Either the slight and temporary displacement may be converted into a permanent one, with all its consequent suffering and disorder, by reason of a harsh and inappropriate treatment; or it may happen that harmless and inefficient means may get the credit of holding some specific curative relation to uterine deviations of whatever kind.

Unnecessary manipulation.

Nothing could be more cruel, harmful and unnecessary, than to resort to manual treatment in such a case as this, in the stage in which I found it. Why explore and worry such a sensitive womb with the sound? Probing will not relieve these acute symptoms, and a pessary would be about as useful as a fracture box in inflammatory rheumatism.

Opiates might deaden the sensibilities, but they are possessed of no curative relation to the symptoms detailed, and would indirectly unhinge the nervous sympathies more and more. If the cathartics operated at all, the effect would be, by increasing the peristaltic action of the intestines, to increase the uterine displacement and to render it more permanent. There is no question, in my own mind at least, that very many examples of confirmed prolapsus have been entailed upon our patients by such inappropriate and inexcusable treatment at the hands of those who have preceded us.

Harmful medication.

On the other hand, the fact that such cases may get well of themselves, providing we do nothing to interfere therewith, is too frequently lost sight of by our physicians. Every kind of remedy has thus been given and extolled as a specific for uterine deviations. You will find the most incredible stories of cures with this or that dilution detailed in our books and journals. Perhaps a single dose has worked the most marvelous results, the womb being replaced, according to the report, almost as soon as the medicine was swallowed, no allowance being made for the tendency to a spontaneous reduction of the dislocation, the self-limited nature of the attack, or the good effect of rest in the proper position.

Spontaneous cures and quackish claims.

When carefully chosen, it is reasonable to suppose that our remedies are capable, in many instances, of curing what might otherwise develop into a troublesome case of uterine prolapse. We may sometimes avert such a consequence of neglect, or of ill treatment, in much the same manner as we prevent a case of pulmonary congestion from resulting in pneumonia. It is possible, by this means, to spare our patients much suffering, and frequently to turn aside what would otherwise be a real calamity. I cannot claim that belladonna is a specific for any form of uterine luxation, but I may insist that it was adapted to the relief of the peculiar incidental symptoms of which this patient complained. Nux vomica will not go to work like an intelligent agent to restore the fallen womb to its proper position, but it holds a specific, pathogenetic relation to the incidental symptoms in many cases of the

What remedies may do in prolapsus.

kind. And so of podophyllin, sepia, calcarea carb., and many other remedies. We must select the remedy according to the symptoms that are present, just as in case of incipient pneumonia, or pleurisy. In this stage, the proper treatment is medical, and not surgical.

Alternation of remedies.

Whether you should alternate remedies, as it seemed best for me to do in this case, your own observation must help you to decide. It would be very wrong to claim that cures have not been effected in this manner, and equally at variance with truth to assert that careful study and close observation do not lead a majority of practitioners more and more to prefer the single remedy.

HYSTERIA IN A WOMAN AGED SIXTY.

Case.—I was called, during the night of August 20, 1857, to visit Mrs. ——, aged 60. She was in a semi-conscious state. At intervals of from two to five minutes she had spasms which affected chiefly the neck and superior extremities. During these spasms both the fingers and the wrists were very much flexed. The arms and hands trembled constantly. The pulse continued quite regular and uniform, both during the paroxysm and in the interval. The eye was slightly suffused, but otherwise natural; the pupil being neither dilated nor contracted. When the paroxysm subsided, she became very restless, and moaned and wept immoderately. I observed that by directing the conversation to other matters, leaving her condition and surroundings for foreign topics, the duration of the interval between the fits could be considerably prolonged. She had been very much exercised and excited over the proposed marriage of a daughter, to which she was opposed, and for three days had neither slept nor eaten.

I ordered a cup of strong coffee—for I knew that she could not drink this beverage in health without becoming exceedingly nervous and wakeful. Of this she took two teaspoonfuls once in ten minutes. She had only a slight spasm after the first dose, and in half an hour had fallen quietly asleep.

The next morning she felt greatly refreshed by her night's rest, but was still somewhat weak and exhausted. She had an indistinct recollection of my having been in her chamber the night previous, but knew nothing of having taken the coffee. I ordered tea instead of coffee, a generous diet, and for the future less excitement and fatigue. She recovered promptly without medicine.

As a rule hysteria occurs only in those women who have not

ceased to menstruate. Occasionally, however, we meet with well-marked examples thereof before puberty, and after the climacteric. It is rare to find an example of this strange affection in one who is more than fifty years of age. I will not detail the clinical history of this disease at the present time, but direct your attention to one or two points of practical interest in the case before you.

Hysteria incident to menstrual life.

We make a distinction between spasms and convulsions, which it will be well for you to bear in mind. Spasms are not necessarily, or even generally, accompanied by an entire loss of consciousness. Their manifestation is local and temporary. They leave the patient quite decidedly, and she becomes almost, if not altogether, rational in the interval. Convulsions, on the contrary, are soon, if not from the outset, characterized by a complete obliteration or suspension of the perceptive faculties. The patient knows nothing of what is going on around her. She may remain as oblivious during the interval as in the paroxysm. Convulsions are accompanied by a more general derangement of muscular action. The spasmodic movements are less apt to be local, and more frequently implicate the different sets of voluntary muscles in succession, beginning with those of the head, neck, and superior extremities.

Spasms *or* convulsions?

If you examine the eye of an hysterical subject, you may find that it is not changed in its appearance. The pupil is neither dilated nor contracted. Sometimes the eye is suffused, and the ball may be rolled upwards. Now and then there will be a marked difference in the size of the pupils, but this may or may not be pathognomonic. I am not aware that any author has observed this as a symptom of hysteria, but I am inclined to think that it is possessed of some significance as a diagnostic sign.

The pupil in hysteria.

Add to this that you may sometimes detect the patient looking at you askant, or slyly listening to what you say, breathing more regularly and freely, or having her spasms at longer intervals, when she discovers that you are quietly busying yourself with other topics of conversation. A little tact will sometimes enable you to cut the Gordian knot of diagnosis in the most complicated cases of this kind.

The patient's manner.

If the pulse is not perturbed, but keeps the even tenor of its way, during both the paroxysm and the interval, it is an almost positive sign of hysteria. If the attack is referable to emotional causes, acting upon a too susceptible organism, the nervous symptoms that follow will almost certainly be tinted with some peculiarities. Loss of sleep is a powerful predisponent of this disease.

The pulse

Treatment.—Tact is no less important in the treatment than in the differential diagnosis of hysteria. In no other disease is it of more practical moment to be personally acquainted with your patient. If you know her peculiarities beforehand, the case may be said to be half cured at the outset. There are a thousand little items which the physician who is observant gathers up and stores away against a time of need. And it often happens that what would appear trivial, turns out in the end to be most significant and useful. For, in this manner, he may not only interpret the meaning of certain extraordinary and alarming symptoms, when they are present, but may be led at once to the selection of the remedy proper to the case.

Value of tact.

However much we may pride ourselves upon our scientific attainments, I assure you that our patients are prone to estimate our professional capacity and skill, by our ability to turn all sorts of expedients to the best account, at the shortest possible notice. They will think more of you, if you can effect a cure with some simple and harmless domestic remedy which they have overlooked, like the coffee in this case, than if you go through the labor and take the time and pains to select the appropriate simillimum. Keep your quiver full of arrows, and be ready for any emergency.

Value of impromtu resources.

I know of no remedy so well adapted to the relief of nervous symptoms, caused by mental fret and friction, and accompanied by insomnia, or wakefulness, as coffee. A characteristic indication for it is found when the patient "cannot sleep for thinking." The mind will not rest. The mental faculties are more than usually and incessantly active. The fact that coffee disagrees with a person when she is well, may afford you a clinical hint which will be available in prescribing for her when ill. The coffee may be administered in the crude form, in the lower, medium, or even the higher potencies, with equally good results, as in the case I have cited. In some forms of hys-

Coffea.

terical neuralgia, you may effect a prompt cure with caffeine in the third decimal trituration. In one form or another, coffea has appeared to me to be very well adapted to many of the nervous affections of old people, and of old ladies especially.

PROCIDENTIA UTERI FROM PERTUSSIS.

Case.—At the eighth month of pregnancy, Mrs. ——, aged 32, was seized with a violent attack of whooping cough. The paroxysms of coughing were so frequent and severe as to threaten premature labor; but by careful management she was finally brought to term without any serious mishap. After delivery she got up well, the violence of the cough gradually abating until, at the end of two months, it had almost entirely ceased. With the exception of a slight cough, and an habitual constipation (which she always has while nursing), she felt herself well. At the end of the third month, and while taking her usual afternoon drive, she took cold, and the consequence was, a recurrence of the whooping cough. The fits returned with their former severity, and she "felt as if she should cough herself to pieces." The second evening after the return of these trying symptoms, while at stool, and during a paroxysm of the cough, she suddenly felt something escape the vulva. I was summoned, and arrived shortly. The womb had been forced entirely out of the pelvis, and was lying between the thighs. It was easily reduced by appropriate taxis and the proper treatment was instituted. She made a good recovery.

Antagonism of the diaphragm and perineum.

Pertussis is a rare contingent of pregnancy. This case is, therefore, somewhat extraordinary. I have cited it in order to make a few clinical points particularly clear to your minds. It illustrates the antagonism of the diaphragm and the perineum, the former of which, you remember, is the muscular floor of the thorax, and the latter of the abdomen, or, more properly, of the pelvis. In consequence of gestation, and after delivery, the lateral and inferior supports of the womb are not always sufficient to retain it *in situ*. The ligaments have been stretched and off duty for so long a time that they are lacking in tone and strength. The vaginal and muscular column resting on the perineum has been so relaxed and distended as to yield it but little support from below.

This state of things predisposes to downward displacements of the womb after delivery. If the patient is upon her feet too early and too frequently, if the womb folds upon itself very slowly, and its involution is imperfectly accomplished, such mishaps are more likely to follow. Constipation in some lying-in women, and diarrhœa in others, are predisponents of prolapsus and procidentia uteri.

Among the exciting causes of these particular displacements in lying-in women, and in those who have recently been delivered, a violent cough is, perhaps, the most serious. Hence, we may have prolapsus in a slight or extreme degree as a concomitant of pneumonia, pleurisy, bronchitis, or whooping cough. The pectoral lesion proper has nothing to do with causing the displacement. The cough alone is responsible for it. It acts through the spasmodic and forcible contractions of the diaphragm, which it necessarily induces. And the more violent the coughing fit, the greater the danger of this unfortunate result.

Cough a cause of uterine displacement.

During the fit of whooping cough the convulsive action of the diaphragm is sometimes prolonged and painful. In children it is very apt to be followed by retching and vomiting, and sometimes by severe and intractable tenesmus of the bowel. In the case of my patient, who had just been straining at stool, its effect was to overcome the slight resistance offered by the sphincter vaginæ and the perineal muscles, and to empty the pelvis of the womb itself. Of course, this accident would be much more likely to happen at the second or third month after confinement than after the vagina and perineum, as well as the uterine ligaments, had recovered their tonicity, and were better able to sustain the womb, and to retain it in its proper place.

Labor a predisponent.

Treatment. — The treatment proper for a case of this kind is preventive, postural, and remedial.

The occurrence of a severe cough during gestation, and especially towards its close, should cause you to take especial pains to prevent such a sequel to the labor as happened in this case. After delivery the patient should be kept in the horizontal position for a longer period than usual. The binder should be snugly and firmly applied, and she should not be allowed to stand upon her feet until three or four weeks have elapsed. She should be cautioned against straining at stool,

Rest.

or in urinating, and counseled to suppress the desire to cough, as much as possible.

Where the womb has really been expelled, the first thing to be done is, of course, to replace it. This may be easily accomplished in recent cases. Place the patient on her back, raise the hips and lower the head. Then, having anointed the hand, grasp the tumor firmly, and insinuate it gently within the vulva, passing it first in the direction of the vaginal axis, and afterwards in that of the pelvic axis proper. When *in situ*, apply a perineal bandage and pad, which should be worn for some weeks, even after the patient has left her bed. There is no more natural and effectual support, in a case of procidentia, than this. You can extemporize such a support out of the simplest materials.

Taxis and reduction.

The most appropriate and efficient remedies should be given for the cough, and every precaution taken to prevent a relapse. This is especially important in case of whooping cough, the effects of the paroxysm being so disastrous and prejudicial to permanent recovery. Cure the cough, and its indirect consequences will cease. Stop the convulsive action of the diaphragm, and the uterine displacement may not return.

LECTURE V.

CHLOROSIS.

GENTLEMEN:

I will open my lecture with some remarks upon the following

Case. — Miss ——, aged eighteen, complains of a complete loss of appetite, and of headache. She is listless, and suffers greatly from palpitation of the heart, especially after exercise. At times, she has a dull, dragging pain in the cardiac region. The anæmic murmur (*bruit de diable*) is easily recognized. Until about a year ago she felt very well, but since that time these symptoms have been steadily increasing in severity. The skin is pale, of a greenish-yellow tint, and almost transparent. Her lips, tongue, and alæ nasi are almost colorless. The eyelids and features are slightly œdematous, particularly after sleeping. The teeth are decayed, the finger nails brittle. She has never menstruated, and says that her mother and her elder sister were more than nineteen years old when their menstrual function was first established.

In rare instances chlorosis is a congenital affection. A large proportion of cases occur in the young and unmarried. Absence or suppression of the menses is so frequent and almost invariable an accompaniment of chlorosis, that some authorities have regarded it as identical in nature with amenorrhœa. Others are not decided as to which is cause and which effect — whether the chlorosis is the cause or the consequence of the menstrual derangement.

Chlorosis and amenorrhœa.

We remark in chlorosis a decided impairment of the vegetative functions. There is always more or less of headache, anorexia, gastric derangement, dyspnœa, fluttering, palpitation, timidity, general malaise, constipation, and hypochondria. In some cases these symptoms persist for years without proper recognition and relief. They are exceedingly common among young, delicate girls, especially among those who work in shops and factories, and who follow sedentary pursuits, as

Digestive symptoms.

seamstresses and school-teachers. Their persistence and the accompanying ill health frequently lead physicians to decide that such patients are suffering from inflammation of the brain or its membranes, ulceration of the stomach, phthisis pulmonalis, organic disease of the heart, of the liver, or of some other organ.

The headache is very prone to take on the form of hemicrania, and is not unfrequently mistaken for neuralgia. Sometimes it is regularly periodical. It is always paroxysmal, and is greatly aggravated by emotional causes, over-anxiety, and too much of mental labor or worry. In rare cases it is so severe in degree as to produce delirium, spasms, and even mania. And thus it happens that the patient may suffer a temporary loss of memory, or she may decline into a state of mental torpor, and general insensibility. Chorea, hysteria, partial paralysis, and epilepsy, are among the possible concomitants and sequelæ of this headache in chlorotic subjects.

Cerebral symptoms.

While they are really the least serious, the heart symptoms are the most alarming to the patient and her friends. Chlorotic palpitation, as it is termed, is due to a functional change in the rhythm of the heart's action; this change is of nervous origin, and has no necessary connection with organic disease of the heart. It may continue for years without inducing any structural changes, or the prolonged functional disorder may insidiously injure the heart's texture.

Cardiac symptoms.

There is a strange relation or sympathy between the generative system of the female and the heart. One woman has menstrual retention from dysmenorrhœa, and all her sufferings are referred to the cardiac region. Another has menorrhagia, and she complains only of similar symptoms. A third, who has chronic ulceration of the os uteri, tells the same story. In a fourth, the sole pathological result of an excess of sexual indulgence is disclosed in the same identical symptoms. The same may be true of amenorrhœa, prolapsus, ovaritis, and chlorosis. By physical exploration we can detect no difference in the incidental conditions of the heart. The whole præcordial trouble is symptomatic, nor will the objective cardiac symptoms enable us to differentiate between them.

Sympathy between generative organs and the heart.

In chlorosis the pulse is usually, but not in every case, slower and weaker than natural. It may not exceed fifty or fifty-five beats in the minute, and is sometimes as low as forty-five or forty-eight. Now and then, however, you will encounter a case in which it is considerably quickened. As a rule, the more marked the anæmia the more frequent the pulse, providing, of course, that the impoverished condition of the blood is not the result of sudden and excessive hæmorrhage. In chlorosis, as in hysteria, the pulse has this characteristic, that whatever its usual rate of frequency, no matter what the condition of the patient, or the circumstances in which she may be placed, that rate is but little, if at all, changed thereby.

The pulse.

The anæmic murmur, (*bruit de diable*,) which, in most cases of chlorosis, may be heard over the præcordial region, but more distinctly along the course of the great vessels, as the carotid and femoral arteries, is a curious and suggestive symptom. Some authorities believe it to be caused by an impoverished condition of the blood, in which there is a deficiency in the proportion of red corpuscles. Others ascribe it to a diminution in the volume of the blood contained in the vessels. It occurs in anæmia as well as in chlorosis.

The anæmic murmur.

There is not unfrequently a total loss of appetite. The patient may subsist for months upon an incredibly small quantity of food. In other cases the most unheard-of caprices are likely to be indulged. She craves such *outré* articles as chalk, plaster, bits of clay, of coal, or of slate-pencil, cinders, sand, magnesia, grains of coffee, and vinegar. A frequent peculiarity of the appetite is a total disrelish for, and dislike of, every variety of animal food. One of my chlorotic patients had not tasted a mouthful of any kind of meat for more than ten years. In some the appetite is fitful. They will fast for a long time, and then eat excessively. Generally, they do not anticipate or enjoy their meals, but "go through the motion" of eating at stated periods, simply because it is expected of them in the family and in society.

The appetite.

In consequence of this impairment of the digestive functions, a train of symptoms is sure to follow. The bowels become inveterately constipated, or there may be alternations of constipation and diarrhœa. The breath is sometimes disagreeable, or even fœtid. In a few cases observed

Incidental symptoms.

by Marshal Hall, it had the odor of new milk. In very rare and extreme cases hæmatemesis or malæna may ensue. Sometimes there is obstinate and persistent ulceration of the stomach, with intractable vomiting of ingesta. The cellular and muscular tissues become flabby. There is general and progressive emaciation. She becomes bed-ridden, and is believed to have passed into a hopeless decline. A species of dropsy, either general or local, may supervene. Some patients with chlorosis suffer great torture from gastralgia. In others there may be successive attacks of gastro-enteritis. Organic lesions of the liver and spleen are frequent concomitants of chlorosis, especially in the west and southwest, and in all malarial regions.

Menstrual irregularities in chlorosis.

It is unusual for this disease to exist without more or less menstrual derangement. The most ordinary complication of this kind is with amenorrhœa. The chlorosis may set in before the menses have appeared, at puberty, and they may fail altogether. Or there may be an incidental and prolonged arrest of the flow in those who have menstruated before. In either case, the menses do not appear for months, and perhaps for years. The suppression may date from the commencement of the chlorosis, but most frequently it follows in the train of other symptoms. The chlorosis is very apt to come on stealthily and insidiously, so much so that neither the patient nor her family remark anything wrong with her health until the disease is pretty well developed. She may have complained for a considerable period of symptoms of which I have spoken, and in addition have noticed that her catamenial discharges were less free than natural, but it is not, perhaps, until the flow has ceased altogether that any alarm is excited, or counsel desired in her case. It has frequently happened that the co-existence of amenorrhœa and gastric derangement has given rise to suspicions of pregnancy; while in other cases, the arrest of the menses with troublesome chest symptoms has aroused suspicions of incipient tuberculosis.

Hereditary amenorrhœa.

Although she is eighteen years of age, this woman has never menstruated. But in her case there is a family or hereditary idiosyncrasy which may explain this fact. Her mother and sister were nineteen years old before the menses appeared. We cannot, therefore, charge the non-appearance of the flow to the chlorosis, or *vice versa*. From which you will infer that although they may and do frequently co-exist, these disorders have no necessary relation with each other.

Chlorosis and dysmenorrhœa.

You will sometimes meet with chlorosis in a patient who is subject to dysmenorrhœa. In such cases, the incidental hysterical symptoms are more pronounced and persistent. They are very troublesome and difficult of cure. The menstrual flow often becomes so scanty as to increase the difficulty by its retention, and we may thus have a case of painful menstruation resolving itself more and more into one of entire suppression. Or the dysmenorrhœa may develop into menorrhagia, which will further complicate the chlorosis.

Chlorosis in pregnancy, etc.

Chlorosis is also incident to those states in which menstruation is physiologically suspended. It may occur during pregnancy, in child-bed, during lactation, or after the grand climacteric.

Discoloration of the skin.

The peculiar discoloration of the skin, which is very marked in this case, is pathognomonic. In mild and recent attacks it is of a pale greenish tint. Hence the popular name, "green sickness." The lips, alæ nasi, the gums, and the tongue, lose their vermillion hue. The skin is sometimes of a yellowish cast. (Sauvage called chlorosis "white jaundice.") In later stages of the disease, and in very bad cases, the discoloration is more marked. The skin becomes of a waxy, dull leaden, slate-color, sallow, or dirty-white hue, and there are dark lines beneath the eyes, and at the angles of the mouth. The white of the eye has a peculiar pearly, translucent appearance. The face becomes tumid, and the eyelids, especially the upper one, puffy and œdematous. The general surface of the body appears dry, bloodless and opaque. The hands are shriveled, the nails split, brittle and broken.

The mental state.

Patients with this disease are averse to exercise, and to society. They become listless, and sometimes pass into a state of pseudo-narcotism; or they are low-spirited, and look upon life and the future with the most gloomy forebodings. They are disposed to melancholy. They lose interest in their studies, permit their accomplishments to grow rusty from disuse, and, in brief, are really wretched.

Etiology. —The causes of chlorosis are predisposing and exciting. Among the former, the most prominent is the lymphatic temperament. It is extremely rare to meet with it in any other class of subjects. This predisposition is strengthened by a tendency to scrofula. In these persons the blood-making function is liable to such disorder as results in a deterioration of the quality of that fluid. Hence the relative diminution of the red corpuscles, and the proportionate increase in the watery part of the blood, which are almost always present in chlorosis. This predisposition is fostered by whatever hygienic influences may tend to lower the standard of health, and to vitiate the process of sanguification. These causes are usually classed as exciting ; but they are only remotely so. They include an exclusive diet of indigestible, inappropriate or unwholesome food, confinement in damp, shady, illy-ventilated apartments, deficient exercise and clothing, unrequited affection, nostalgia, ennui, chagrin, jealousy, fright, sexual excitement, and uterine and ovarian disorders.

Chlorosis and scrofulosis.

Most authors will tell you that chlorosis arises from "a disease of the blood," a phrase which is utterly destitute of meaning. It is true that in many cases the proportion of the red globules is deficient: but unless it be traceable to a loss of blood by hæmorrhage, that is a symptom merely. In anæmia from hæmorrhage of any kind, the poverty of the blood is accidental, and due to an actual loss or withdrawal of the colored corpuscles. In chlorosis, the change in the composition of the blood has been gradual, is the work of disease that has implicated and impaired the process by which the blood itself is made. In the one case it is a chance effect; in the other a natural and necessary consequence of diseased action.

Blood-changes in chlorosis.

I have already explained the physiology of hæmatogenesis.* You are familiar with the function of the lymphatic glands and their duties in this relation. Without their aid, the blood could not be manufactured. It is a peculiar predisposition to disease in them which constitutes the chlorotic diathesis. But these glands cannot operate independently of the nervous system, any more than the liver or the pancreas. And so we must go back of them for the prime cause of the disorder.

Hæmatogenesis.

* See Lecture II, pp. 41-2, of this volume.

It is "begging the question" to refer the essential pathology of chlorosis to an impoverished condition of the blood. That fluid may contain seven-tenths, or even nine-tenths serum, as found in Jolly's analysis of the blood of chlorotic subjects, but it will not suffice to declare that all the symptoms in this disease are due to, and depend upon, this condition alone. Nor does the relative loss of the red globules represent the disease. The special pathology and etiology of chlorosis are not to be found in the hydræmia, spanæmia, or the chloro-anæmia, which in most cases are attendant upon it. For occasional well-marked cases of this disease are certainly met with, in which there is no manifest change in the composition of the blood.

The spanæmia in chlorosis incidental.

Numerous reasons have been adduced for a belief in the nervous origin of chlorosis. Thus Eisenmann* assigns the following: "(*a*) In certain cases Becquerel and Rodier failed to detect any changes in the blood. (*b*) Chlorosis is much more frequent in females than in males, and it is a well-known fact that the nervous system predominates in the former. (*c*) The incipient symptoms of chlorosis, those which anticipate any change in the blood are nervous, and those nervous symptoms continue through the whole course of the disease. (*d*) Chlorosis yields to those remedies which are known to act favorably in affections of the spinal cord, as morphia, strychnia," etc.

The nervous theory.

To these we may add that many attacks occur in those who are predisposed to chlorosis, in consequence of fright, the exercise of strong mental and moral emotions, sexual excitement, masturbation, and the nervous tension incident to city life and society among the better classes. Dr. Clotar Müller bases his assumption of the nervous origin of chlorosis on (*a*) "the great influence which mental emotions and certain depressions of the nervous system exert upon the origin and development of chlorosis; and (*b*) the powerful curative influence of remedies acting directly upon the nervous system, and manifesting an influence corresponding homœopathically to the depression and general prostration of vital power peculiar to this disease."†

The same author says: "If I may venture to draw a conclusion from my own observations, I should assume as most probable that

* *Bulletin de Thérapeutic*, Sept. 30, 1859.
† Vide North Am. Hom. Quarterly, Vol. VII, p. 158.

chlorosis is originally an affection of the spinal and ganglionic systems of nerves, having a character of weakness and exhaustion combined with erethism and excessive excitability." Becquerel and Rodier confirm this view: "For us, as for some other authors, chlorosis is a disease which has its beginning and its seat, its point of departure primarily, in the nervous system, giving rise consecutively to disorders of digestion, of menstruation, and of the circulation. If this definition is correct, the change in the blood in chlorosis is not a constant and capital fact, but a secondary, incidental phenomenon, which is not absolutely indispensable to the disease."*

Gabalda says emphatically, "We regard this disease as a perfectly distinct neurosis." M. Jolly and Dr. Tilt insist that chlorosis is a neuralgic affection of the ganglionic system. Dr. H. Jones, that "in many cases, occurring among the poorer classes in London, the action of malarious influences upon the ganglionic system is the first link in the chain of causation."

Upon this theory, which is so well supported by facts and by medical authority, we are able to explain the insidious and peculiar character of this complaint Its seat is in the nervous system. Back of all the symptoms disclosed by the solids and fluids, the cause is at work to undermine the general health. And thus it happens that in confirmed chlorosis "there appears to be not a system, an organ, a texture, or even a fluid, in the animal economy, which does not suffer."

I have already said that the menstrual disorders incident to chlorosis are generally considered as the cause, and not the consequence thereof. The argument against this hypothesis is short and simple. In a majority of cases the manifest signs of chlorosis appear before there is any derangement of the monthly periods. In some instances the menstrual function escapes all implication, and the patient has chlorosis without any catamenial irregularity whatever.

Chlorosis precedes amenorrhœa, etc.

Now, if the non-appearance of the flow, or its suppression, or even its excess, were the cause of this disease, one or the other should always precede the pallor of the skin, and the nervous, circulatory, and digestive symptoms of chlorosis; this affection could never

Menstrual complications symptomatic.

* Traité de Chemie Pathologique appliquée a la Medicine Pratique. 1864; p. 155.

exist in one who menstruates regularly; nor could it ever occur, as it really does, in the male subject. We therefore conclude that the menstrual complications incident to chlorosis are symptomatic, and not idiopathic. The real disease is the chlorosis, and not the amenorrhœa, the dysmenorrhœa, or the menorrhagia. It is said that in the West Indies many male negroes formerly sickened and died of a disease which, in all of its principle features, was identical with chlorosis.

With characteristic originality, Prof. Meigs styled chlorosis an "endangial disorder." He referred all the symptoms, but more especially the changes in the composition of the blood, to a pathological state of the endangium, or lining membrane of the circulatory vessels.

Dr. Von Maack* holds that, in chlorosis, it is impossible for the iron of the food to be changed into hæmatin and fixed. And this because the saccharine function of the liver is either disordered or arrested. But this must suffice for the etiology of chlorosis.

Chlorosis and jaundice.

Diagnosis.—You will not be very likely to confound chlorosis with jaundice. The pearly look of the white of the eye in the former disease, and its yellow cast in the latter, will enable you to differentiate between them.

I have drawn the following table, which may help you to diagnosticate chlorosis from anæmia:

CHLOROSIS.	ANÆMIA.
1. Is an idiopathic affection.	1. Is an accident, or sequel of other diseases.
2. Is not caused by the loss of blood, or other debilitating discharges.	2. Is frequently caused by hæmorrhage, suppuration, leucorrhœa, diarrhœa, colliquative sweats, etc.
3. May result suddenly from mental causes alone.	3. Never does.
4. The mental and nervous symptoms are especially prominent.	4. Not so in anæmia.
5. The nervous symptoms initiate the attack.	5. The opposite occurs in anæmia.
6. Fugitive neuralgic pains in the head, the spine, the stomach, the chest, and especially in the side, are almost invariably present.	6. These pains are lacking.
7. May be accompanied or followed by hysterical spasms, chorea, paralysis, or epilepsy.	7. These complications and sequelæ are not incident to this affection.

* L'Union Medicale, February, 1859.

CHLOROSIS.	ANÆMIA.
8. The skin is of a greenish, or greenish-yellow tint.	8. The skin is blanched, palid, puffy, and doughy.
9. Hæmorrhages are not very frequent.	9. Hæmorrhages are very frequent.
10. Is very rare in male subjects.	10. Affects the sexes indiscriminately.
11. Rarely happens in those who are under twelve or over thirty years old.	11. May occur at any age.
12. Is limited to women of lymphatic temperament.	12. May happen to women or men of any temperament.
13. Is very liable to be accompanied by suppression or retention of the menses.	13. Is more likely to be accompanied by too frequent and copious menstruation.
14. May exist and run its course without any perceptible change in the composition of the blood.	14. Is always characterized by an impoverishment of the blood.
15. The degree of change in the blood bears no necessary relation to the severity of the disease.	15. The impoverishment of the blood is in direct ratio with the degree of functional disorder.
16. Is most common among the better classes of society.	16. Is most common among the poorer classes.

Although these symptoms are sufficiently distinctive, it sometimes happens that a diagnosis between these affections is extremely difficult, if not altogether impossible. There are, doubtless, exceptional cases, in which they co-exist in the same patient.

Prognosis.—In the milder forms, and under proper management, chlorosis is curable. The chief danger is from incidental organic diseases, the most serious of which are cardiac and pulmonary affections, myelitis, tuberculosis, dropsy, paralysis, epilepsy, and repeated hæmorrhages. The disease is of a lingering, tedious nature, and patients get well or worse very slowly, But now and then one who has been ill with this disease for a long time dies suddenly without any premonition. For this reason, your prognosis should be guarded.

Danger from incidental disease

It is a favorable sign if, under treatment, the appetite and spirits improve, and also if the menstrual irregularity is corrected without forcible measures. Relapses are frequent.

Treatment.—After this analysis of the disease in question, you are prepared to appreciate the difficulties in the way of its most appropriate and successful treatment. Its Protean phases and multiform complications sometimes embarrass the practitioner exceedingly. The rule, however, holds, that the more carefully the remedy is chosen, providing other very necessary conditions are complied with, the more certain and satisfactory is the result.

Remedies for general states.

In general, you should give especial prominence to remedies which are suited to derangements of the nervous functions, or of the circulation, or of digestion, or of menstruation. These are cardinal points in the special therapeutics of chlorosis. In most cases, the characteristic indications are discoverable in them. In one person the nervous symptoms may predominate; in another, the digestive; in a third, the sexual, and so on. Or, if they are mingled, try to learn the order of their sequence, their cause or causes, and what constitutional or accidental agency serves to perpetuate the mischief.

Treatment for emotional cause.

You may often find the proper remedy by selecting one that is appropriate to the mental or emotional condition which induced the attack. Our works on materia medica teach you what these remedies are. Most prominent among them is ignatia. After this, there are belladonna, hyoscyamus, coffea, opium, aconite, and some others. In selecting from this, and a much larger catalogue, the indications are very similar to those which call for certain remedies in hysteria.

Remedies for the chlorotic cachexia.

Calcarea carbonica, sepia, sulphur, natrum muriaticum, graphites, ferrum, phosphorus, plumbum, and similar remedies, are often appropriate for the chlorotic cachexia, and in chronic cases may sometimes be given temporarily with good effect, in lieu of other medicines. The first two are especially useful in the menstrual irregularities incident to chlorosis. The same is true of cyclamen and pulsatilla. Other remedies sometimes employed are kali carb., arsenicum, lycopodium, conium, nux vomica, china, chamomilla, helonine, and senecin. Indeed, as in hysteria, almost any remedy in the whole range of the materia medica may be called for. It would be a work of supererogation, as inappropriate as a paternoster, for me to detail all the symptoms which might indicate them in this connection.*

Upon the theory that chlorosis and anæmia are identical, and

* For particulars see N. American Hom. Quarterly, Vol. VII, p. 152, *et seq.*

that both affections are due to a deficiency of iron in the blood, iron is regarded by many physicians as a specific in chlorosis. It is almost as universally given in this disease as quinine in intermittent fever, or mercury in syphilis. But, for the best of reasons, it frequently fails to cure. In order to be useful, it should be prescribed upon pathogenetic indications, and in such form and quantity as to be available. When there are only about thirty grains of iron in the whole mass of blood contained in the body, it surely is irrational to attempt to supply any deficiency thereof by thrusting large quantities of the crude metal, or any of its salts, into the stomach. Iron is not appropriate to those cases of chlorosis which are of nervous origin, or in which, from the onset of the disease, the nervous symptoms have been especially prominent. In anæmia proper it is more generally useful.

Iron in chlorosis.

In many cases of chlorosis there is, however a preparation of iron in which I have great confidence. This is the citrate of iron and strychnia, a salt which came into use some years ago. I give it empirically in the third decimal trituration. In my experience nothing is so well adapted to control the whole train of symptoms in most cases, although it is by no means an invariable specific. It seems to combine the good qualities of iron with those which belong to the strychnia group. It will accomplish more than ferrum metallicum, ignatia, nux, or strychnia, when given separately. I could detail several cases of this disease cured with this remedy alone. In this compound form it certainly merits a proving.

Citrate of iron and strychnia.

For an interesting paper on chlorosis arising from mental shock, I refer you to Dr. Hammond's recent report of several cases of this kind cured with arsenic and strychnia.*

Much harm is sometimes done by attempting to force the menstrual flow. You should be careful to avoid this, remembering that the menses will appear as soon as the general health warrants and favors it. Relieve other and more urgent symptoms, restore the physiological equilibrium, and this function will probably resume its accustomed order. There is good reason for believing that the non-appearance of the menses in many cases of chlorosis is a conservative

Wrong to force the menses.

* Quarterly Journal of Psychological Medicine, etc., Vol. III., p. 417.

precaution, designed by nature to economize the patient's strength.

An exception to the rule just specified is found in those cases of spasmodic dysmenorrhœa, which are incident to chlorosis.

Spasmodic dysmenorrhœa.

Here the most sensible and successful plan of treatment is to address our remedial measures to the cure of the stricture of the uterine cervix, upon which the nervous symptoms depend for a local cause. We may give belladonna, gelsemiuum, caulophyllin, or some analogous remedy. The warm sitz-bath, or vaginal injections of warm water, may facilitate the flow, and relieve the suffering and the remote nervous symptoms at the same time. But if the spasm of the cervix is particularly obstinate, I know of nothing to compare with the careful and appropriate use of the sponge-tent.

Much relief may sometimes be afforded by domestic adjuvants. In case of spinal irritation and tenderness, the back may be sponged

Adjuvants.

once daily with salt and water. Friction along the spine is sometimes very useful. For the relief of local neuralgic pain, in the side and chest especially, the part may be covered with a layer of cotton batting, oiled silk or flannel. If the pain is very acute, dry heat will suffice. If it is rheumatic, the local use of hamamelis may be prescribed.

The diet should be selected with great care. It should consist of digestible and nutritious articles, both animal and vegetable.

The diet.

If the patient has a distaste for meat, she may cultivate an appetite for it, by beginning with salt meat of some kind, as, for example, cod-fish, mackerel or herring, dried beef, lean ham, and the like. Or sea-food, as oysters or other shell-fish, may be taken. Eggs or milk prepared in various ways, may tempt the appetite. Bread from unbolted flour, animal broths, chocolate or malt liquors, may be chosen. She should not be ordered to ride or to exercise upon an empty stomach.

Moderate exercise in the open air is indispensable. Riding, on horseback or otherwise, is preferable to walking or performing

Exercise and travel.

manual labor. And when your chlorotic patients go for an airing in their carriage, be sure they have the light as freely as they have the air. These hothouse productions need it as much as the pale plants that have grown in the cellar. Boating, billiards, croquet and calisthenics may be very useful. But best of all is a change of scene and surroundings. If to these can be added the health-giving influences of cheerful society, so much the better. These hygienic means will frequently accomplish more than our best chosen remedies. Sea-bathing has its advocates, and mineral waters, especially those which are chalybeate, are strongly recommended.

Whatever the cause may have been, it should be removed, and the utmost pains taken to keep the patient from under the dominion of all perturbing influences. Marriage is sometimes salutary, but is of questionable utility, excepting where the attack has resulted from disappointed love.

Miss —— will take a small powder of the citrate of iron and strychnia, 3rd dec. trituration, twice daily, with out-door exercise and a generous diet.*

AMENORRHŒA WITH SUPRA-ORBITAL NEURALGIA.

Case.—Mrs. R——, aged 36, with light hair, blue eyes, and mild disposition, complains of a peculiar form of neuralgia associated with the return of menstruation. The menses are tardy; sometimes delayed one, two, or even three days. Their appearance is invariably preceded by a violent neuralgic pain, which is located over the left eye, along the superciliary ridge. This suffering usually begins when the flow should commence, and continues with increasing severity until menstruation sets in, after which it gradually subsides. In the interval her health is excellent. She has never had any other form of neuralgia, but has been subject to this for ten years past. It has never been located over the right eye, or in any other than its present seat. She "expects to be sick" three or four days hence.

Varieties of menstrual neuralgia.

This case is an anomalous one. It is by no means rare to hear women complain of neuralgia which is most troublesome "at the month." Sometimes it affects the head, the face, the teeth, or the ears. There are those who have occasional attacks of angina pectoris at this period. Ovarian and mammary neuralgia are frequent

* At the end of one month, the menses made their first appearance. She had much pain, with scanty flow. The second period was regular, the flow free enough, with little relative suffering. The headache and cardiac symptoms had entirely disappeared; the skin became natural; the lips and cheeks had resumed their proper color. She took no other remedy.

accompaniments of menstruation. Incidental, shifting local pains often torment women whose courses are due but are somewhat delayed. But a circumscribed neuralgia of this sort, in this particular locality, recurring with the regularity of an ague paroxysm, in immediate relation with the menses, and subsiding as soon as they have commenced, is by no means common.

Local peculiarity.

A strange peculiarity contingent on all these cases of menstrual neuralgia, is that the pain is more likely to be seated in the left than in the right side of the body.

Local treatment.

Treatment. — These pains are reflex. The cause that produces them is a temporary retention of the menses. Remove this cause, and the suffering is at an end. This indication may be met, temporarily at least, by a variety of domestic expedients. A drink of gin, a warm sitz-bath, the application of a bag of hot salt to the hypogastrium, the operation of a carthartic or an enema, chloroform, or opium, may promote the menstrual flow and arrest the pain. But these expedients are only palliative and transient in their effect. They will exert no influence over the function at the next period. In anticipation of the menses the neuralgia will return again.

Specific treatment.

In order to effect a radical cure thereof, we must look to the seat and character of the pain, its particular relation to the menstrual nisus, whether it comes on, or is worse before, during, or after the flow, and to like symptoms, for especial indication for our remedies. I have never seen but one well-marked case of this kind before. It was the exact counterpart of this. I gave that woman pulsatilla 3rd. The flow commenced almost immediately; the neuralgia vanished; and although five years have elapsed, it has never returned. Mrs. R. will take the same remedy three times daily, until the menses appear, and I prophesy that she will be free from this unwelcome neuralgia in the future.

HYSTERIA AT THE CLIMACTERIC.

Case. — Mrs. S——, a strong, healthy-looking woman of 50, relates the following history: She was taken ill while pregnant with her sixth and last child fourteen years ago. This illness she attributes to neglect and unkind treatment on the part of her husband. Despite much trouble, suffering and anxiety, she went to term, and her child is still living. Her chief symptoms were a feeling as if she were dying, with great prostration, sinking, choking at the throat, and partial unconsciousness. She would weep and sob for hours together, and her gloomy feelings could not be dissipated. These attacks came irregularly, but increased in severity toward the close of gestation.

Two years later an eruption resembling "salt rheum" made its appearance on the right arm, above the elbow, and on the same side of the neck. The cropping out of this eruption, which is worse in cold weather, was followed by manifest relief of the nervous symptoms. She soon remarked that when it was out most freely, she felt best in other respects, and *vice versa*. This alternation has continued for twelve years. Whenever the eruption disappears, the nervous symptoms are very distressing.

Menstruation continued regularly until four years ago, the patient being at that time forty-six years old. It then began to be irregular, sometimes being absent for two, three, or even four months, and when it returned, it was liable to be profuse and long-continued. Twice she went only two weeks between her periods. Once, as they did not return from October to the following July, she supposed that they had entirely ceased.

Skin disease and hysteria.

I have brought this patient before you to illustrate the possible relation between a cutaneous eruption and the existence of hysterical symptoms. For twelve years this eruption has alternated with intractable nervous symptoms, more alarming than serious. She has been questioned very thoroughly, but we cannot learn that she ever had any eruption which had been repelled prior to the date of her present illness. Nevertheless, the evident relation between the disease of the skin and the other symptoms complained of will not be doubted.

Repelled eruptions are, in general, more likely to produce some structural disorder of the mucous membranes than to give rise to functional or organic lesions of the nervous system. But instances are not wanting in which serious neuroses, as, for example, insanity, epilepsy, paralysis, neuralgia, have been due to this cause. And so, also, with hysteria. I have seen the most obstinate cases refuse to yield to the best affiliated remedies, because they originated in the repercussion of some apparently trifling eruption. If you will take this clinical hint at its proper value, it may be of great service to you by and by. These cases are exceptional, it is true, but such a one may be the very first on the list of your private patients.

The menstrual irregularity in this case is referable to the critical period through which the patient has been passing during the last four years.

Treatment. — We should, so far as is possible, ascertain the especial nature of the eruption which has caused, or is so nearly related to, the disorder for which we are to prescribe. Is it vesicular, papular, pustular, or squamous? Has it always preserved the same character? Does it itch, or burn, or what are its peculiar sensations? What accidental circumstance is likely to bring it out, or aggravate it? These and similar inquiries may influence the choice of a remedy, especially in chronic cases. The key to the cure may be found through them.

Character of the eruption may indicate the remedy.

In this case the eruption was originally vesicular. Each time it reappears a crop of vesicles forms. They soon break and discharge, and the serum dries and forms a yellowish crust. This is followed by slight itching, especially when the part is exposed to the air.

These symptoms indicate rhus tox., and it alone may be sufficient for the cure, not only of the eruption, but of the incidental affection also. I prefer the thirtieth attenuation of this remedy for chronic cases. In exceptional cases, it answers very well to alternate two potencies of this remedy, as, for example, the third and the thirtieth. If the rhus fails, we may give sulphur in a similar manner.

Mrs. S. will take a dose of the rhus tox. 30th, every morning and night, and report in two weeks. She must be careful to avoid pastry, spices, fats and indigestible food of all kinds. And also to forbear applying any wash or ointment that might repel this eruption and increase the difficulty.

LECTURE VI.

OVARITIS.

GENTLEMEN:

Inflammation of the ovaries has been designated in medicine as ovaritis, oöphoritis, oaritis, ovarite, and ovarian folliculitis. There are two excellent reasons why you should study the medical history of this affection most carefully. In the first place, the disease occurs more frequently than is generally supposed; and in the second, our literature is lamentably deficient in respect to its pathology and treatment.

Ovaritis may be acute or sub-acute. Some authors speak of a chronic variety, but this is included in the sub-acute, which is the more common form of the complaint. Indeed since they differ only in severity and duration, one description must answer for all. Most authorities are agreed that the left ovary is more frequently inflamed than the right one. Out of forty cases collected by M. Chereau, the affection was double in four cases, seated in the right ovary in eleven, and in twenty-five cases in the left one. Tilt found the right ovary inflamed in but five out of seventeen cases. M. Tanchou suggests that the nearness of the left ovary to the rectum, and the mechanical pressure of fæcal matters upon it, may account for its greater liability to inflammation.

The sub-acute form most frequent.

Causes. — Ovaritis is rarely an idiopathic affection. It is liable to occur immediately before, during, or immediately subsequent to the appearance of the catamenia. In many cases, every return of the menstrual period is characterized by marked symptoms of ovarian irritation and inflammation. The ovaries bear much the same relation to the uterus, that the Malpighian tufts do to the tubes of Ferrein and Bellini in the kidneys. Bearing in mind this intimate functional relation, you will readily perceive that amenorrhœa, or retention

Generally symptomatic.

of the menses, from occlusion of the vagina, by an imperforate hymen or os, or atresia of the vagina, or of the uterine cervix, would be likely to induce congestion of the ovaries, as well as of the uterus and Fallopian tubes. The repletion occasioned by the non-exit of the menses might be harmful in various ways, but the most painful symptoms incident thereto would be those of ovarian inflammation.

Ovaritis from dysmenorrhœa.

A sudden suppression of the menstrual flow, as from cold, or coitus, has sometimes caused a severe attack of ovaritis. It may be due to spasmodic, obstructive or mechanical dysmenorrhœa, arising from partial obliteration of the uterine cervix. It is a frequent consequence and complication of membraneous dysmenorrhœa; and Drs. Rigby, Simpson, and others treat of a variety of painful menstruation under the title of Ovarian Dysmenorrhœa. If the monthly return is characterized by very considerable suffering, neuralgic headache, fugitive and erratic pains, and hysterical symptoms, one may suspect that the focal point of the disorder is in the ovary.

There are perhaps few examples of menorrhagia of long standing that are not dependent upon or associated with ovaritis.

From medical and mechanical causes.

A frequent cause of the disease under consideration is the improper and harmful use of emmenagogues, which are given with a view to relieve menstrual suppression, or to induce abortion. The resort to mechanical expedients for the same purpose may produce a like result. These villainous appliances all act as irritants to the delicate structure of the ovary, tending to derange its innervation, circulation and nutrition, and thus, directly or indirectly, to induce the inflammatory process. Inordinate sexual indulgence, especially after prolonged or unusual abstinence, may cause ovaritis. I have met with several examples of this kind in women whose husbands had but just returned home after a long absence. Ungratified sexual desire, in those who are of amorous disposition, may likewise cause ovaritis. Some most painful attacks, due to this cause, are met with in young widows. The same result has been witnessed in prostitutes when placed in confinement. The employment of unnatural means for the gratification of the sexual passions; nymphomania;

gonorrhœa; or blenorrhagia in the female; a too forcible coitus, as in rape; falls or blows upon the iliac region; the use of astringent vaginal injections, causing the sudden suppression of leucorrhœal, or a hæmorrhagic discharge; the employment of escharotics in ulceration of the os uteri; the extension of endometritis through the oviduct to the ovary; retroversion of the womb, and constipation, especially at the menstrual period; sudden exposure to cold, and check to perspiration; emotional causes, as the reading of novels by those who are young and of sedentary habits; unrequited affection; the abuse of aphrodisiacs and alcoholic liquors, are among the more frequent and ordinary causes of ovaritis. Scanzoni reports having observed many cases in which this disease was developed in consequence of an inflammation of a portion of the intestinal canal, and especially of the rectum. I have known it result from a sudden and intentional suppression of milk in a mother who had been sucking her child.

Epidemic ovaritis.

The intimate relation existing between the functions of the mammary glands and the ovaries is significant of ovarian lesions incident to the puerperal state. If the lacteal secretion does not appear at the proper time, the ovary is very liable to become irritated, and even inflamed. This inflammation extends by continuity of surface, to the peritoneum. Hence arises a common sporadic and insidious form of puerperal peritonitis. In 1746 an epidemic of this form of puerperal fever prevailed at the Hotel Dieu, in Paris, and another in Vienna in 1819. Of fifty-six females who had died of puerperal fever, Dr. Robert Lee found that in thirty-two cases the ovaries were red, swollen and softened; and in two hundred and twenty-two cases of the same fever M. Tonellé found evidences of ovaritis in fifty-eight. Kiwisch remarked that, as contingent upon lying-in, ovaritis occurs generally in groups of cases, an observation that corresponds with the idea advanced by certain authorities, that it is sometimes epidemic. Kiwisch has often "made from ten to twenty consecutive autopsies without meeting with any considerable inflammation of the ovaries, after which the disease was observed, in more or less considerable development, in from six to ten individuals consecutively."

Traumatic causes, incident to labor, sometimes give rise to

ovaritis. Metritis may supervene upon delivery, and the inflammation extend through the generative intestine to the ovary, in some such manner as inflammation of the duodenum may indirectly extend to the liver.

Traumatic ovaritis.

It is possible that, by reason of being compressed against the bony pelvis, the ovaries are sometimes injured during labor, but, as the gravid uterus occupies the superior strait, this result could happen only in exceptional cases. In the puerperal state, the absorption of post-organic matters from the cavity of the womb sometimes gives origin to a painful and dangerous form of this disease. Pus and other deleterious products may be conveyed by the oviduct from this cavity direct to the ovary, or lodged in the peritoneum, and thus serve to light up the inflammatory process.

In rare cases, the rheumatic diathesis acts as a predisponent of ovaritis. This is an inveterate form of the complaint. In an example of the kind that I now have under treatment, the patient has, for six years, suffered almost martyrdom from rheumatism. For six months past she has had amenorrhœa, with prolapse of the left ovary, and ovaritis. A peculiarity worth mentioning is that an elder sister of hers died of rheumatism with menstrual suppression that had persisted for more than a twelvemonth.

The "hysteric constitution," as it is styled by Robertson, is a marked predisponent of ovaritis. The class of patients most liable to this inflammation are recognized as the nervous, irritable, and hysterical, those whose temperaments are mercurial and volatile.

Symptoms.—In acute, post-partum ovaritis, the constitutional symptoms are marked and decided. As in inflammation of the serous tissues generally, the attack commences with a chill, followed by fever, acceleration of the pulse, and local pain. This pain is sometimes described as sharp and intense; again it is forcing, throbbing, or dull, sickening and paroxysmal. It may be seated in the upper and posterior portion of the vagina, in one or both of the iliac fossæ, the groins, the lumbar region, the sacrum, the hips, or in the thighs, and occasionally reaches to the end of the toes. Sometimes, in lieu of a positive pain, there is a disagreeable feeling of weight and smarting in the region of the ovary, and patients not unfrequently com-

Peculiar pain.

plain of a burning sensation in the same locality. On applying the hand to the hypogastric region, you may discover that there is really an increase of heat in the part affected.

When decidedly paroxysmal, the sufferings may either remit or intermit. The iliac and hypogastric regions become exceedingly sensitive to the touch, so that pressure, palpation and percussion are insupportable. The least motion, more especially the attempt to sit upright in bed, increases the suffering, and syncope may result. In milder cases, riding and walking have a similar effect. One of my patients complains most of riding in a railway car. The thigh that corresponds with the affected side is sometimes flexed, cannot be extended without causing much suffering, and on this account is rendered almost useless. She cannot sit, or stand erect, without extreme pain. When in the horizontal position, she prefers to keep the thigh flexed on the abdomen, and the leg on the thigh, in order to procure ease by relaxing the intra-pelvic and abdominal muscles, and thus relieving pressure upon the tender and inflamed ovary.

Exercise — position.

If the lesion involves any considerable portion of peritoneum, you may expect general abdominal tenderness, with tympanites, and other symptoms of true peritoneal inflammation. In post-partum ovaritis, whether it be a sequel to labor at full term or to abortion, the disease has its origin in this membrane (which is reflected over the ovary), whence it spreads rapidly.

Peritoneal ovaritis.

In consequence of its increased weight, produced by a species of strangulation and inflammation, the ovary is liable to a hernia or descent, posteriorly into the recto-vaginal space or cul-de-sac, laterally along the sides of the vagina, anteriorly between the uterus and the bladder, and even occasionally into the labia majora. In rare cases, this hernia of the ovary is congenital.

The following interesting case of this kind is cited by Billard, (Traité des Maladies des Enfants nouveau-nés. Paris, 1833, p. 474).

"Josephine Romer, seventeen days old, was brought to the Infirmary, September 12th. She was strong, and seemed possessed of a good constitution; the abdomen was somewhat tense; and at the left inguinal region there was a round tumor of the size of a filbert, somewhat hard to the feel, which could not be returned to the abdomen, neither reduced in size by pressure, nor was its volume increased by the crying of the child. Its direction was obliquely towards the labium of the corresponding side, which it did not quite reach. On considering the location of the tumor, and although the sex of the child forbade the supposition, one could hardly resist the conviction that it was a congenital inguinal hernia. Our judgment was accordingly suspended until, at the end of twenty-six days, the death of the child from pneumonia allowed us, by dissection, to ascertain the nature of the tumor. * * * * The hernial tumor was formed by the left ovary, that had descended through the inguinal canal and ring, which were much larger than one usually finds them in girls. The uterus, drawn by the round ligament, and by the ovary that formed the hernia, had left its natural position, and was inclined to the left side of the bladder. The left kidney, instead of being on a level with the other, was drawn downward by an enveloping cellular tissue, and also by a fold of peritoneum, intimately connected with the orifice of the sac; the renal artery and vein had also yielded to this traction, and both were elongated and narrowed; and finally, the ovary and the fimbriated extremity of the Fallopian tube, somewhat reddened and swollen, were lodged at the base of the sac formed by the prolongation of peritoneum, with which cavity it communicated. There were no adhesions between the intestinal convolutions and the surrounding parts, and the opposite ovary was in its usual situation.

"A careful examination of the round ligament on the side where the hernia was, satisfied me that it was much shorter than that of the opposite side, and that, in place of losing itself in loose filaments, it terminated in the labium by an aponeurotic expansion; from which it would seem that the ligament, shorter, and more firmly fixed to the labium, had, in the first place, caused the uterine displacement, and subsequently drawn the ovary through the inguinal ring. It followed, from this abnormal adhesion, that all the movable, connected and contiguous parts on the left side of the abdomen were drawn to the side of the hernia, for they were not separated from each other, nor did they follow the abdomen in the intra-uterine development and enlargement of the fœtus."

The benign tumor formed by the displacement in ovaritis,

may vary in size from that of a large almond, to that of a hen's egg, or even larger. It is more swollen and sensitive at each menstrual period. This drawing, on the blackboard, will give you a pretty correct idea of the posterior and more frequent dislocation of the ovary, which you will remark has dropped into the recto-vaginal pouch, so that it is situated between the anterior wall of the rectum and the posterior wall of the vagina.

The swollen ovary feels like an enlarged gland, is convex, and sometimes throbs and pulsates beneath the finger. The anal and vesical symptoms correspond with the variety and extent of the ovarian displacement. As a rule, the lower the organ, the greater the suffering. The tumor may press upon the broad ligaments and cause uterine deviations, or upon the veins and nerves within the pelvis, and occasion great suffering, paralysis, and, according to Carus, convulsions of the inferior extremities.

But since, as Becquerel insists, these symptcms are common to inflammation of all the organs contained within the lower pelvis, how are we to decide, in a given case, if they depend upon ovarian inflammation and consequent displacement? In the more acute attacks of ovaritis, and particularly in lean persons, it is sometimes possible to detect the tumefied organ by examination through the abdominal parietes. In this case the swelling is circumscribed and extremely painful to the touch. This is the most severe, or peritoneal form of the disease, which Scanzoni teaches "is the only form accessible to palpation."

In diagnosticating the sub-acute and chronic varieties, it is necessary to resort to the "touch." Upon making an examination per vaginam, we find the "tender spot" complained of to correspond with the position of the prolapsed ovary. We may discover the tumor at the right or left sacro-iliac symphysis, or in one of the sacro-sciatic notches. If the displacement is a lateral one, we may confirm our suspicions by an examination of the corresponding groin, or iliac region, through the abdominal walls with one hand, while with the other we explore the vagina.

The vaginal "touch."

It frequently happens that the patient winces or complains when the finger touches the uterine os or cervix—a circumstance that, unless one is very careful, may mislead in the diagnosis. Pressing the vaginal portion of the

Characteristic pains.

cervix, backwards and laterally, occasions acute pain in the affected ovary. She declares that "she cannot bear to be touched just there," and may proceed to tell you that the same suffering is sometimes caused by contact of the male organ with that spot during coitus. One of my patients made a similar complaint in consequence of having touched the posterior vaginal wall at its superior portion, with the pipe of her syringe, which she had been told must be introduced high up into the vagina.

The rectal "touch."

The displaced and inflamed ovary is most easily felt upon examination by the vagina when that canal is short, and the uterus and its appendages are not far removed from the vulva. But when the vagina is long, and the womb high up in the excavation, it is necessary also to resort to the expedient of exploration by the rectum. Placing the patient in the obstetric position, with the thighs well flexed, the finger introduced into the rectum may be made to reach further, and acquaint us more fully with the degree of ovarian swelling and displacement, than any other means at command. This end is facilitated by the thinness and elasticity of the coats of the rectum, and the possibility of exploring the posterior surface of the womb, and even of the ovaries, in their normal state. And this mode of examination may be rendered still more valuable in certain cases, by the employment of the free hand in abdominal manipulation — it being sometimes possible thus to press the tumor upon both its anterior and posterior surfaces at the same moment.

The "double touch."

In the worst examples of prolapse of the ovary into the recto-vaginal space, the same end is gained by a resort to what has been styled the "double touch" of Recamier, which consists in the introduction of the index finger into the rectum, and of the thumb of the same hand into the vagina. By forcing the perineum upward, this expedient permits us to compress the morbid growth between the thumb and finger. The character of the resulting pain, and the shape, position and mobility of the tumor, are believed to be pathognomonic of the disease in question.

One of the most painful and persistent symptoms consequent upon a posterior prolapse of the inflamed ovary is an intolerable sense of strangulation and obstruction of the bowel, following the effort at stool. Rigby compares the character and quality of this suffering to that proper to orchitis, which, as you know, is almost insupportable. It is undoubtedly due to the pressure of fæcal matter, and to the peristaltic movements of the rectum upon the dislocated, swollen and excessively tender ovary. It may continue for hours after defecation has been accomplished. The symptoms induced thereby are sometimes mistaken for those of retroversion of the womb, and of stricture of the rectum. Constipation is an almost necessary consequence; and it is possible, as has been claimed, that, in some cases, it may even tend to produce the displacement of the ovary. The whole alimentary system is liable to be deranged. The tongue becomes coated, the patient complains of thirst, anorexia, and, in rare cases, of obstinate heartburn, and even vomiting, as in the early months of pregnancy. The febrile symptoms correspond with the suddenness and severity of the attack.

Feeling of strangulation.

The vesical symptoms are sometimes so pronounced as to lead to suspicion of idiopathic disease of the bladder, and possibly of the kidneys also. When there is strangury, dysuria, heat and pressure in the bladder, and these symptoms are greatly aggravated, or recur, only at the menstrual period, they signify that a sub-acute inflammation of one or both ovaries may be the cause of the suffering. You are not to conclude that they are necessarily the result of anteversion of the uterus, which affection, I repeat, exists more frequently in imagination than in fact.

Vesical symptoms.

The menstrual irregularities incident to ovaritis will not fail to attract your attention. The physiological theory that menstruation consists essentially in the ripening and discharge of the unfecundated egg, or the "parturition of the ovum," as Tyler Smith most appropriately terms it, is now the generally received explanation of this process.

The ovary is *par excellence* the organ of menstruation; the maturation and extrusion of the ovum, the first direct step in the process. This little organ, at once the most diminutive and important of all the pelvic viscera, is a species of alarm clock, that introduces the element of time into the generative system, and presides over this function with respect to its occurrence and regularity. Its organic symptoms are wonderful, and almost unlimited in their range and significance. Physicians are accustomed to speak of the " uterus and its appendages;" a more correct phraseology would be, " the ovaries and their appendages."

Retention of the menses is one of the most common and serious symptoms of sub-acute and chronic ovaritis. Young women are especially liable to that form of amenorrhœa, described by the older writers as emansio mensium, a condition in which the menstrual flow has never been established. When a simple suppression of this discharge — suppressio mensium — occurs during the course of other diseases; as, for example, in phthisis pulmonalis, and the protracted fevers, or from incidental causes, it may signify that one or both ovaries are inflamed. The cause has operated indirectly. The lesion is secondary or symptomatic. The effect is none the less palpable, and equally prejudicial to a complete recovery.

Menstrual disorders incident to ovaritis.

It is impossible to treat properly such cases of menstrual irregularity without a knowledge of their special pathology. Some slight obstruction prevents the escape of the menses from the uterine cavity or the vagina. The new and abnormal pulse is reflected upon the ovary. Inflammation is the result, and the regularity and completeness of the function is disturbed for months, and possibly for years. Not to speak of the harmful consequences supposed to result from the non-elimination of certain matters contained in the menstrual blood, the suspicious character of the vicarious hœmorrhages sometimes induced, or the liability in many cases to the development of pectoral disorder from this cause, there is no question but that, in the great majority of instances, amenorrhœa is intimately connected with, and dependent upon, ovaritis.

The varieties of dysmenorrhœa known as spasmodic, mechanical, and obstructive, implicate the ovaries in a similar manner, and are, therefore, to be regarded as incident to, and not dependent upon, the disease under consideration. The ovarian form of dysmenorrhœa is always accompanied by ovaritis. The physiological injection of the organ, so necessary to its functional activity, becomes excessive and exaggerated. The first stage of the inflammatory process is present, and the congested viscus is tender and painful.

Dysmenorrhœa and ovaritis

All the suffering, which is paroxysmal, tormenting, and neuralgic in character, may be referred to the ovary. The lower part of the abdomen becomes extremely sensitive, and the patient undergoes a monthly martyrdom, accompanied by a distressing headache, neuralgia, and hysterical symptoms of every shade and variety.

Menorrhagia and ovaritis.

In my lecture on menorrhagia, you will recollect that I called your attention to the clinical fact that the most inveterate examples of that affection had their origin in sub-acute and chronic ovaritis. To members of our school of medical faith, this fact is especially significant. The recognized superiority of our remedies for the arrest of profuse flooding can only be explained by their power to regulate, harmonize and restore the delicate vascular sympathies that exist between the ovaries and the uterine mucous membrane. In illustration, I will read you the notes of a case upon which my advice was desired by Dr. B., a member of the class from Wisconsin.

Case. — Mrs. ——, aged 18, married one year, came under my professional charge about three years ago. She is troubled with menorrhagia. The attacks have recurred at intervals for a period of two years, for the relief of which she has taken domestic and allopathic medicines in large quantities. She was formerly strong and robust, but, on taking a sudden cold during the catamenial period, the menses were suppressed for nearly a year immediately preceding her last illness. The attacks of flowing last for a period of one or two weeks, and weaken her so much that she can scarcely raise her hand. The interval varies from three to four weeks, but is sometimes extended to eight or ten weeks. The flow is always long-continued, and profuse in amount. She had lost all reckoning as to the time for the recurrence of the regular flow.

The discharge is sometimes dark and clotted, but more frequently of a thin, fluid character. Sometimes — and especially when the clots are passed — it is attended by much suffering, but, excepting in the region of the ovaries, there is in general no pain. Both ovaries are tender and exceedingly painful, but only *during the flow.*

She had been taking internally, and also by injections into the womb, most of the astringents laid down in the Materia Medica. In three months, by the use of pulsatilla, sulphur, nux vomica and sabina, giving the first two night and morning for a fortnight, and the last two for a like interval, and then repeating, I succeeded in establishing the regular "periods." Menstruation would then seem to be natural, the proper flow to continue for three or four days, after which, instead of decreasing, it would increase, and consist of clots with arterial blood. The discharge would then continue for ten days or a fortnight, despite my best efforts to suppress it. For a time, drop doses of hamamelis seemed to check it, but after a little it lost its effect.

This patient has never had any children, or, to her own knowledge, ever been pregnant. At times she has leucorrhœa, which is readily relieved by appropriate remedies. When I first saw her, the appetite was morbid, and she had lived upon rich and highly-seasoned food. She craved pickles especially.

In this case, the nature of the exciting cause, the amenorrhœa, and the ovarian tenderness, assure us that the hæmorrhage could not have been due either to prolapsus uteri, hydatids, or a cancerous affection of the womb. The doctor's success in establishing a periodical return of the menstrual flow is confirmatory of the view that its essential pathology was to be sought for in the ovaries. The throwing of astringent injections into the uterine cavity, by his predecessor, was a species of malpraxis which, besides being a positive injury, demonstrated the ignorance of the practitioner.

Gonorrhœal ovaritis.

Gonorrhœal ovaritis is, I am persuaded, more frequent than is generally supposed. According to M. de Meric ("London Lancet" for September, 1862), it is most liable to occur during the acute stage of gonorrhœa in the female. In this it differs from the onset of orchitis in the male, which occurs towards the decline of the gonorrhœal discharge. This rule has many exceptions. The same author states that such an effusion and induration as takes place in the epididymis, when the testicle is inflamed, does not occur in the ovary in consequence of gonorrhœal ovaritis. Nevertheless, the character of the suffering induced is very similar. However much the patient may complain of the vaginitis and urethral symptoms in case of gonorrhœa, the acuteness and severity of the pain in one or both ovaries, when they are the seat of this specific inflammation, is still more marked and decided. It closely resembles that of orchitis.

As a concomitant of gonorrhœa in the female, ovaritis may undoubtedly result, as Dr. Tilt suggests, from "the immediate application to the ovaries of the blenorrhagic pus which has been conveyed by the same capillary attraction by which the seminal fluid is conducted;" from extension of the disease from the vagina; or possibly from inoculation of the whole glandular system, including the ovaries themselves, with the specific poison.

The excessive tenderness of the vagina in cases of this kind, interposes a barrier to the employment of the "touch" in making a careful diagnosis, and hence this affection has been overlooked by a majority of writers and practitioners. I can not give you a better idea of this form of the disease than by quoting a case from M. de Meric's excellent paper.

"On October 27, 1858, I was asked to see the wife of a wealthy tradesman in one of the metropolitan suburbs. She was said to be very ill, and I found her in bed. The patient was then about thirty-two years of age. She stated that, for three weeks at least, she had noticed an abundant discharge, which had considerably stained her linen with large yellow spots. The discharge had of late increased, and she had been obliged, on the day of my visit, to take to her bed, owing to a severe pain in the left iliac region. There had been a certain amount of uneasiness in micturition, but that had passed off. The last menstruation had occurred about three weeks before.

"On examination, I found the patient suffering from feverishness; the linen shown to me was marked with large yellowish spots, and pain on pressure over the left ovary was very acute. The diagnosis of a case of this nature was seemingly easy enough. I suspected sub-acute metritis, the inflammation having suddenly extended along the Fallopian tube, and reached the ovary. This latter circumstance was explained by an imprudent exposure to cold, viz., driving home from the theatre in an open carriage. The pain was so acute that I did not propose a vaginal examination, but at once ordered fomentations to the left iliac region, a gentle purgative, an antimonial mixture, low diet, and rest.

"It should be noticed that the lady was suckling a child about seven months old.

"On leaving the house, the husband accompanied me, and inquired about the state of his wife, hoping it was nothing serious. As he had been under my care, some years before, for gonorrhœa, I thought it my duty to ask him whether anything of the kind had happened again; and I learned that he had been suffering from a slight discharge, which was going off.

"The case now took a different aspect; and, after weighing all the circumstances, I came to the conclusion that my patient had been infected, and was laboring under gonorrhœa, the inflammation having traveled to the ovary by way of the uterine cavity.

"On the 29th, two days after my first visit, I saw the lady again, and found the discharge had diminished; the pain over the left ovary was still severe, though the pulse had somewhat come down. I proposed leeches, but so much repugnance was expressed that I advised counter irritation by mustard poultices, and the use of the same lowering means. The case progressed very favorably; a few astringent injections were made as soon as the acute inflammation had gone by; and in about three weeks the patient had so far recovered as to resume her household duties. I did not think it necessary to advise the weaning of the child. The father also regained his health in a short time."

Some most painful attacks of gonorrhœal ovaritis arise from the use of strong astringent injections designed to stop the vaginal flow. I have recently treated a case of this kind, in which the husband ventured to prescribe the same injection for his wife that had been ordered for himself by a quack doctor. After a few hours she did penance for his infidelity and presumption, in a most severe attack of inflammation seated in both ovaries. Women sometimes resort to such harmful expedients at their own suggestion, and in a fit of desperation. I am greatly mistaken if in the future your professional experience does not prove that ovaritis is a frequent and most painful contingent of gonorrhœa in the female, Dr. Simpson and others to the contrary notwithstanding.

At my next lecture I shall speak of the pathological anatomy, the differential diagnosis, prognosis, sequelæ, and treatment, of ovaritis.

LECTURE VII.

OVARITIS — (CONTINUED).

GENTLEMEN:

In my last lecture your attention was directed to the nature, causes and symptoms of ovaritis. As related to the history and treatment of this disease, other points remain to be noticed. And, first, of its

Pathological Anatomy. — You will not be surprised to learn that, until quite recently, the physiological anatomy of the ovaries was so little understood that distinguished physicians have been known to mistake healthy for morbid appearances, in these organs, at *post mortem.* It is related of the eminent anatomist Vesalius, that he referred the origin of symptoms of uterine strangulation, amenorrhœa, and chlorosis, to the presence of yellow spots, the modern corpora lutea, in the ovaries of four unmarried women, upon whose bodies he conducted an autopsy.

The lesions vary.

The structural changes incident to ovaritis vary with the acuteness of the attack, the brevity of its course, the seat of the lesion in one or another of the ovarian textures, its relation to the last menstrual period, to labor, whether premature or at full term, and to the grand climacteric. As with inflammation seated in other organs, so in ovaritis, the more rapid the course of the disease, and suddenly fatal the attack, the more marked are the evidences at *post mortem* of congestion, and its immediate consequences.

The line of demarcation that separates the physiological changes proper to the maturation of the ovum and the dehiscence of the follicle at each menstrual period — *id est*, the escape of a small amount of blood into the cavity of the Graäfian vesicle, the retraction of its walls, the formation of a clot, the fading hue of the coagulum, and the final cicatrix — from the more marked engorgement and effusion proper to acute attacks of ovaritis, is very indistinct and illy defined. In this connection, the following differential diagnosis between healthy and morbid ovisacs, as detailed by Dr. Farr, and re-arranged by Dr. Clay, in his notes to Kiwisch,* is of practical interest :

NATURAL FOLLICLE.	MORBID FOLLICLE.
1. Always near the surface when preparing for dehiscence, and often projects considerably above the level of the ovary.	1. Often not peripheral, but more or less central in its position in the ovary. It may attain to the size of one-third or half of the ovary, without necessarily causing any distinct prominence above the surface, especially when occurring singly.
2. Coats unequally thick ; thinnest at the most prominent part of the follicle.	2. Walls are equally thick, and exhibit at no part any evidence of attenuation or absorption.
3. Considerable vascularity above the elevated part, plainly visible externally.	3. No preparation for rupture is indicated externally, by any peculiar arrangement of vessels, or by any marked increase of vascularity.
4. Walls of follicle at this stage, of a bright yellow color.	4. The walls do not exhibit the remarkable yellow color, or the cerebral foldings, characteristic of the advancing normal ovisac, the tissues being composed of the undeveloped Graäfian follicle.
5. The liquor folliculi is either clear and limpid, or intermixed with blood, or the center of the sac is filled with a coagulum, which is at first bright red, and afterwards becomes pale, and at length nearly white. The coagulum may adhere to the walls, and undergo fibrillation and subsequent conversion into a solid body, or into a dense white membrane ; or it may be rapidly absorbed.	5. Contents of the sac are neither the clear liquor folliculi, nor the bright clot, nor the developed fibrin, but generally a collection of dark coffee-ground matter, resulting from the admixture of a quantity of decomposing blood corpuscles, and fragments of membrana granulosa, intermixed with a dirty fluid.

The discoloration and the clot.

Any considerable engorgement of the ovary with blood, occasions an increase in the size and weight of the organ. The tumefaction is accompanied by softening of tissue, increased vascularity, and a change of color to a rusty dark red or blue, or even a mahogany hue. In idiopathic cases, which are rarely the subject of post mortem examination, an apoplectic effusion of blood into the follicles, and the subsequent formation of a coagulum therein, sometimes results. As in cerebral apoplexy, the size, complexion, and character of this coagulum varies in different cases and in different stages of the disease. The masses are irregular or rounded,

* Kiwisch on the Diseases of the Ovaries, by Clay, London, 1860, p. 63.

and sometimes as large as a cherry. The softer the clot, and the lighter its color, the more chronic or protracted has been the inflammatory process. Recent effusions may supervene upon those of earlier date, in which case different follicles will be occupied with coagula of varying hues and consistency. Sometimes the wall of the follicle is hypertrophied, and rendered more firm than natural. In rare cases it is friable, and this species of hæmatic cyst may be ruptured, and its contents extravasated within the stroma, and the enveloping membrane (tunica albuginea) of the ovary, or into the peritoneal sac. Scanzoni details the case of "a young girl of eighteen years, who died suddenly during menstruation, with all the signs of an internal hæmorrhage. The autopsy demonstrated in the right ovary, which was slightly amplified, a pocket of the size of a pullet's egg, filled with coagulated blood, in the posterior wall of which was found an opening of nearly nine-tenths of an inch long, through which nearly seven pounds of blood had penetrated into the abdominal cavity." In septic states of the blood, as in the ovaritis of lying-in women, caused by the absorption of post-organic matters from the cavity of the uterus, the ovary may be engorged with effused blood from passive hæmorrhage. These, and similar disclosures by the knife of the anatomist, have sometimes caused the ovarian lesion to be entirely overlooked, and an off-hand, uninstructive diagnosis of pelvic hæmatocele to be made by the physician.

Hæmorrhage into the ovary.

Any of the various "terminations" of inflammation may sometimes be recognized in the ovary. A very considerable effusion of serum into the peritoneal investment of the organ, or the collection of the same fluid in the distended vesicles, discloses a dropsical condition that may have escaped notice during the life of the patient. In the former case the tumor is unilocular, in the latter multilocular. It is more than probable that, as in pleurisy and pericarditis, this serum is at first exuded as a critical means of relief to the inflamed structure, and that subsequently the absorbents are not capable of removing it.

Dropsy as a sequel.

When resolution has taken place, the structure of the ovary is changed. The retracted cicatrices make it more solid in consistence, with an irregular, bosselated surface. The glandular structure disappears, and may be substituted by various forms of heteroplastic growth; as, for example, the cartilaginous, calcareous, cancerous, and possibly the tuberculous. Nearness to the grand climacteric increases the liability to atrophy of the whole organ.

Liability to suppuration.

Puerperal ovaritis, whether peritoneal, parenchymatous, or follicular, and whether it occurs as a contingent of labor at full term, or in abortus, is most liable to terminate in suppuration. Abscesses of the ovaries are by no means uncommon. Their history is of the greatest clinical interest and importance. After death from puerperal fever, the puriform exudation may sometimes be found deposited in the follicle, which is thus enlarged to the size, perhaps, of a hazel nut. A description of these abscesses is thus given by Kiwisch (*op. cit.* p. 90):

"Follicular abscesses, after a long continuance, may attain a very considerable size; indeed, according to our own observations, they have contained about sixteen pounds of pure pus. The cyst wall may resist perforation for some time, and, in isolated cases, for a long period of years. The parenchymatous abscesses are generally not so large, though we have seen them reach the size of a child's head; and we have also to observe that they commonly increase much quicker than those previously mentioned. These abscesses often proceed from several small foci, which coalesce in the course of time, and the greater part of the stroma of the ovary is destroyed, or a sinuous cavity is inclosed in its rudiments. After a protracted duration of the disease, these collections of pus are surrounded by a membrane; but it is difficult to separate from adherent parts, and it cannot be anatomically demonstrated to any extent. The disposition to perforation is a characteristic feature of these abscesses; in the acute form of the disease, it may take place in the course of a few days or weeks. The cystless abscesses in the neighborhood of the ovaries, are also disposed to perforation. Consecutive collections of pus, in previously degenerated follicles, seldom burst, with the exception of those cases in which the contents have an ichorous property."

Character of the pus.

The pus contained in the ovarian abscess, in most cases, is laudable; but, occasionally, ichorous and corrosive. The danger of rupture and extravasation of the contents of these abscesses, is proportionate to the bad quality of this purulent matter, complicated perforations being more frequent where the pus is of an ichorous and disorganizing character.

The abscess may discharge its contents directly into the abdomen, with fatal consequences. A case of this kind is cited by Dr. Seymour, from Guy's Hospital Reports.*

"The patient was a young woman, of the lowest and most unfortunate class of females. She was greatly emaciated, had a very quick and feeble pulse, a shining red tongue, and constant watchfulness. She suffered from constant and irrepressible diarrhœa, and for many successive days vomited both food and medicine; the catamenia were absent. * * * * After having been in the hospital about two months, she suddenly complained of the most acute pain over the abdomen, and, in a few hours, expired.

"On opening the abdomen, death appeared to have been produced by the effusion of a large quantity of pus into the peritoneal cavity, which escaped from an abscess in the right ovarium, which abscess appeared to arise from suppuration in the substance of the viscus, similar in every respect to phlegmonous abscess in any part of the body, and not connected with any cyst, or change, or addition of structure, the product of morbid growth."

Extemporized outlets for pus.

Collections of benign pus in the ovaries may find an outlet through the bowels, the bladder, the uterus, the vagina, or the abdominal parietes. They seldom perforate the small intestine, but more frequently communicate with the rectum, on the left side, and the colon on the right. Serious consequences, from the escape of the purulent collection, are prevented, by the formation of adhesions between the neighboring structures. Many obscure cases of renal, uterine, and rectal disease originate and culminate in this effort of nature to extemporize an outlet for the contents of an ovarian abscess. Fistulous abscesses of this sort are sometimes salutary, and again intractable, chronic, and necessarily fatal. In rare cases they may discharge, repeatedly, through the unnatural outlet. It should not be forgotten that, although it may take place in the unimpregnated female, ovarian suppuration occurs most frequently, in consequence of post-partum injury or inflammation.

* Seymour on Diseases of the Ovaria; p. 38.

The quantity of pus contained in the ovarian abscess may vary greatly. In most cases it is not very large. Examples are, however, recorded, in which an incredible amount has been observed. Dr. Taylor, of Philadelphia, reports a case of chronic ovaritis affecting the right ovary, in which the sac weighed seventeen pounds, and yielded sixteen quarts of pus. It sometimes happens that the purulent matter, with which the stroma of the ovary and the tissues of adjacent organs are infiltrated, is itself decomposed. In this case the evidences of fatal peritonitis are superadded to lesions already noted. Kiwisch says (*op. cit.* p. 92):

Enormous quantity of pus formed.

"The more acute the progress of an ovarian abscess, the slighter is the thickening of its walls, and the more benign its pus; but much more frequently it happens that, after its contents have been evacuated externally, complete contraction and obliteration of the pus cavity takes place. This is observed particularly after parenchymatous inflammations, and the intraperitoneal suppurations surrounding the ovaries. Those abscesses, however, whose walls are highly organized, which are not excavated for months or years, particularly when the point of rupture has no favorable direction, generally cause exhaustion, in consequence of the frequent renewal of the decomposing pus, or become fatal by the supervention of pyæmia."

The post mortem disclosures in ovaritis, chiefly affecting the peritoneal investment of the ovary, are of the kind proper to serous tissues generally. Sometimes the most extensive adhesions are formed. "Thus the ovary may become agglutinated to the broad ligaments, to the pelvic parietes, the uterus, the bladder, or the rectum and the sigmoid flexure, to the cæcum, the vermiform process, and the small intestine; and it is generally attached to several of those viscera at the same time." The fibrous bands that connect these various organs and surfaces, belong to the variety of pseudo-membrane, classed by Laboulbéne as "permanent," which are themselves subject to diseased conditions. In some cases a considerable increase in the size and weight of the ovary may be due to an excessive development of the fibrinous exudation.

The various lesions we have detailed are seldom found uncomplicated with those of inflammation of adjacent organs and structures. This is especially true of puerperal ovaritis, which, as we have said, is apt to run its course with metritis, endometritis, or peritonitis.

Variolous ovaritis.

Beraud, Trousseau and others, treat of a form of ovaritis which is contingent upon variola, (l'ovarite varioleuse). It may attack either the parenchymatous structure or the peritoneal envelop of these organs.

Characteristic symptoms.

Diagnosis — The diagnosis of ovarian affections is, sometimes, very difficult. This is especially true of the sub-acute and chronic varieties, unconnected with the puerperal state. When the patient is extremely sensitive, and especially where it becomes necessary to explore the rectum, we may resort to the employment of anæsthetics with advantage. I have already given you a full description of the symptoms of ovaritis. The character of the suffering, its periodical aggravation with each return of the catamenia, the menstrual derangements incident thereto, the symptoms of strangulation and inflammation from a hernial descent, or other displacement of the floating organ, the circumscribed swelling, the constitutional effects, and the sequelæ, are sufficient to enable you to distinguish this from other diseases of the female generative system.

The principle of "exclusion."

In making out the differential diagnosis of ovaritis, in its various forms, it is well to proceed upon the clinical principle of exclusion. Having examined if there be any disease of either of the neighboring organs, and not finding it present in a given case, we are confirmed in our diagnosis that the affection is ovarian. As explained in my last lecture, the "touch" is an invaluable aid in all doubtful cases.

Prognosis. — In the milder forms of ovaritis uncomplicated with organic disease of other portions of the generative apparatus, the prognosis is favorable. Very considerable structural changes may be resolved away, and the general health and vigor reinstated. The most obstinate examples of this disease are complicated with menstrual disorders, more particularly with menorrhagia. In the gonorrhœal type, when it does not result in suppuration, the symptoms are likely to become intractable and obscure, although most cases recover sooner or later. When there is ulceration of the womb, and the patient has been under treatment therefor, especially if the os and cervix have been frequently and severely cauterized, the prognosis should be guarded.

The danger from ovaritis after abortion.

When acute ovaritis supervenes upon abortion, the danger is in ratio with the advanced state of pregnancy at which the miscarriage has taken place. The more advanced the period of gestation, the greater the danger. Much depends also upon the cause or causes that have produced the abortion. As the normal stimulus for uterine muscular contraction is derived from the ovaries, so it is reasonable to suppose that any agency that produces a like result, whether medicinal or mechanical, vital or villainous, must operate through the same medium, and thus implicate these organs more or less seriously. The prognosis will vary accordingly.

As a contingent of lying-in.

As a contingent of child-bed, the danger varies with the history of the previous labor, the patient's vigor of constitution, the circumstances by which she is surrounded, the care she receives, and the epidemic prevalence of puerperal peritonitis. The occurrence of rigors that alternate with fever of an irregular type, local ovarian pain and anguish, a frequent pulse, colliquative sweats or diarrhœa, suppression of the milk or lochia, with tympanites, dyspnœa, great prostration, and copious deposits in the urine, are untoward symptoms. Rupture of the hæmatic cysts, and of the ovarian abscesses, and the extravasation of their contents, may prove suddenly fatal. Under these circumstances, the patient sometimes dies as abruptly and unexpectedly as if from perforation of the intestine in typhoid fever, or from the bursting of an aneurismal sac.

Danger from suppuration.

Ovarian suppuration is not necessarily fatal. We should, however, qualify our prognosis most carefully. Where the accumulation of pus takes place rapidly, especially during lying-in, and symptoms of adynamia, and decomposition of that fluid, are present, there is danger from purulent infection and infiltration. Other things equal, the more depraved the state of the blood, the greater the danger from ovarian abscess. If the formation of the "pus cavity" is slower, and its secretion more benign in character, and more especially if adhesive inflammation has served to protect the adjacent viscera from implication, and to afford a means of final discharge, the case may terminate favorably. Sometimes a period of months, or even years, is consumed in this critical process. If the case becomes thus chronic, there is danger from exhaustion, caused by the drainage of the patient's nervous energies and nutritive resources. This is especially true of scrofulous subjects, who present a cachectic appearance, and finally succumb to vital losses of this character. Becquerel* reports the case of a young woman of twenty-three years, in which death followed the discharge of an ovarian abscess into the rectum. Kiwisch says, (*op. cit.* p. 86) :

" The course of these pelvic tumors is various. In favorable cases, the tumor, and with it all uncomfortable symptoms, completely disappears, after a duration of some weeks or months. We have observed tumors the size of an adult head, exceedingly hard, and apparently in direct contact with the external abdominal integument, terminate in that manner. In other cases, suppuration extends, and perforation takes place in various parts of the surrounding structures, finally terminating favorably. On the contrary, when the course is unfavorable, the continued or relapsing acute attacks, or the profuse suppuration, or the dissolution of these tumors, causes the exhaustion of the patient. A rare, fatal termination happened to us in one case, from strangulation of the adherent small intestine, two convolutions of which, strongly distended by gas, burst spontaneously, during violent contraction."

Resolution of ovarian tumors.

A spontaneous removal of ovarian tumors of various kinds, incident to the inflammatory process, sometimes occurs. This may take place even when the tumors has become so large as to be pushed out of the lower pelvis, in order that it may have sufficient room for development, as happens with the uterus, or at about the fourth month. Dr. Meigs† relates several cases in illustration of this fact, from which we select the following :

" May 23, 1852. I this day examined the hypogastric region of Miss M. This lady, who has a very great spinal curvature, was examined by me about nineteen or twenty months since. I then found a very solid, incompressible, and immovable tumor, large as a child's head at term, which occupied the hypogastric region, and which *was not a womb*. It appeared to come up out of the

* Traité Clinique des Maladies de l'Uterus et de Ses Annexes, Paris, 1859. Tom. II ; p. 476.

† Woman, her Diseases and Remedies. Phila., 1859 ; p. 357.

pelvis. I considered it to be an ovarian tumor — and, of course, my opinion was, that it was incurable, and must, in the course of time, destroy her life. To-day, no trace of it is discoverable — nor is there any reason to suppose it exists. I take comfort from this example — one of the most extraordinary I have met with — for all future cases of a similar character. I am wholly at a loss to account for its disappearance, since I am sure it *was not a hypertrophied* womb that I detected nineteen months ago — and that it was not any glandular or hygromatous tumor. She is well in February, 1859."

Drain from excessive discharge.

Apart from the danger from rupture and discharge of its contents into the abdominal cavity, from the pressure and weight of the tumor when very large, and the drain upon the patient's strength to nourish and sustain the mass, some allowance should be made for the liability to recurrent attacks of peritonitis, which always imperil the life of the patient. The same may be said of co-existing lesions of adjacent organs.

Consequences of structural change.

Adhesions, resulting from the formation of adventitious membranes are not more dangerous than those which are incident to other serous tissues when inflamed — as, for example, the tunica vaginalis testis, or the pleura. They may take place in consequence of a slight attack of ovaritis, usually styled "menstrual colic," in the newly-married female, or from metastasis of mumps to the ovaries, as happens to the testicle in the male subject, without any untoward results. This remark applies also to simple hypertrophy, atrophy, and induration of the ovaries.

Cancerous, calcareous, cartilaginous, and tuberculous degeneration of the ovary necessitates an unfavorable prognosis — unless, indeed, the surgical expedient of excision may promise somewhat of good.

Sequelæ. — Besides the lesions already spoken of as incident to ovaritis, there are others that should not be overlooked.

Menstrual sequelæ.

These are chiefly related to the functions of menstruation and generation. Menstrual derangements are very liable to follow ovaritis, whether it involves the follicular or the peripheral structure of the ovary. Many examples of amenorrhœa, dysmenorrhœa, and menorrhagia, are to be regarded as sequelæ to attacks of ovaritis, the more evident symptoms of which may long since have passed away. The textural changes detailed when treating of the pathological anatomy of this disease, are sufficient to explain the menstrual sequelæ which are so often entailed upon the patient. It would not be reasonable to expect that the delicate process of evolution could proceed in an uninterrupted, physiological manner, after the Graäfian vesicles had once been transformed into hæmatic, serous or purulent cysts, and their walls hypertrophied, ruptured, or cicatrized. If blood or pus have infiltrated the stroma, or pseudomembranous adhesions attached the organ to neighboring viscera; if the fimbriated extremity of the Fallopian tube is bound down to the ovary, and that portion of the generative intestine occluded, the menses will either be entirely suppressed, or their escape and discharge become painful, scanty, insufficient, irregular, or too frequent and profuse.

Implication of the uterine mucous membrane.

Nor are the evil results of these ovarian lesions limited to the ovaries. The intimate sympathy existing between these organs and the uterine mucous membrane is certain to implicate the latter in whatever pathological process affects the former. With each return of the catamenial period — no matter whether all its phenomena are present or not — this mucous membrane becomes highly injected and very vascular. If the proper flow is established, at the proper time, and in proper quantity, this physiological afflux of blood is quietly remedied and removed, as in the case of other mucous membranes after their secretions have been poured out. On the contrary, if the natural stimulus, originating in the ovary, is withheld, or perverted in its action or qualities, uterine derangements are a necessary consequence. Hence the intractable nature of many examples of sub-acute and chronic metritis. Moreover, a long chapter of reflex disorders may be indirectly due to the same cause.

Sterility from ovaritis.

I am inclined to the opinion that, as a sequel to ovarian inflammation, sterility is more frequently met with than is generally supposed. The history of menstrual disorders and irregularities, just alluded to, confirms this idea. Indeed, whatever imperils the integrity of the catamenial function may also implicate fecundity. When lesions of the ovaries are sufficient to prevent the completion of the process of ovulation, they also prevent conception. If inflammation of both ovaries were as common as that of a single one, sterility would be as familiar a complaint as almost any other. As it is, while one of them escapes, other things equal, the power to procreate is continued, by a species of compensatory relation, as in the case of the male, when one of the testicles is diseased or has been removed. Induration of both ovaries, when it occurs in consequence of disease, is as inevitable a cause as atrophy from old age. The ovaries may be so displaced as to remove them from the reach and grasp of the fimbriæ of the Fallopian tubes. In this case they would have no communication with the uterine cavity; and if the ovum were furnished by the follicle, it could not be conveyed to the womb. Sometimes, as a result of ovarian disorganization, diseased and imperfect ova are formed and furnished by the female. These may be impregnated, but subsequently are imperfectly developed, and abortion is a natural and necessary consequence. Hyperplastic formations and adhesions about the ovary may interfere mechanically to prevent conception, in some such manner as an excessive deposit of fat in the omentum sometimes prevents women, who are remarkable for their pinguidity, from having children.

Sterility is not an uncommon sequel to gonorrhœal ovaritis. A moment's reflection will convince you that this variety of the disease under consideration is more likely to affect both ovaries at the same time than any other, not even excepting the puerperal form. The lesion resulting therefrom may involve the most serious consequences to the generative function. Hence sterility not unfrequently follows an attack of gonorrhœa; and those who have had gonorrhœa repeatedly, are not apt to become pregnant. Without doubt, this result is sometimes chargeable to the blighting effects of the specific virus upon the ova, which it destroys in some such manner as it does the vivifying influence of the spermatozoa in the semen masculinum. But I apprehend that, in the majority of cases, actual lesions of the ovary are produced by the modified inflammatory process, which lesions are sufficient to account for the sterility that follows.

Barrenness from gonorrhœal ovaritis.

Bernutz styles ovaritis "female orchitis." In the male subject inflammation of the testicle, accompanying or following a severe attack of gonorrhœa, may, and I believe frequently does, prove itself a cause of sterility. The same remark applies to those women who, having suffered from this form of ovaritis, find themselves barren in consequence.

My professional experience confirms this view. Physicians are often consulted for the cure of sterility in the persons of women whose husbands have been wild and profligate in youth, and whose bad habits may have perpetuated themselves. Careful inquiry into the history of such a case, may disclose that the patient has had one or more attacks of gonorrhœal ovaritis, from which, indeed, she may be suffering at the moment of consultation. It is more than probable that such examples of ovaritis are modified by the specific gonorrhœal taint, however faint the impression and remote its cause. This clinical fact affords a plausible explanation of the source of difficulties among the higher families and orders of society, on account of their lack of progeny, with which history and human experience abound.

Nymphomania from ovaritis.

Although it may doubtless be true that, in exceptional cases, nymphomania results from ovaritis, yet experience has demonstrated that the most common effect of the disease is to diminish rather than increase the sexual feeling. Dr. Ashwell* says: "In two instances, I am perfectly convinced that the result of the malady was entire aversion to intercourse, and it is now allowed that nymphomania more generally depends upon the external organs, so far as physical causes are concerned."

General treatment.

Treatment. — This is divided into general and local. Owing to the present imperfect state of the materia medica, the pathogenetic indications for remedies in the treatment of ovaritis are neither very explicit nor very numerous. Its special therapeutics must, therefore, be founded upon our knowledge of its pathology, the proper use of such provings as we have at command, the similarity of textures implicated in this and other well-known diseases, and the results of clinical experience.

In the puerperal form, when the attack comes on a few days

* A Practical Treatise on the Diseases peculiar to Women. Phila., 1855; p. 445.

after delivery, and the symptoms are those of surgical fever, with pain in one or both ovaries, and violent constitutional disturbance, aconite and arnica may be given for some hours, in rapid alternation. If not of traumatic origin, belladonna may be substituted for the arnica.

Treatment of puerperal ovaritis.

The symptoms and conditions which indicate belladonna, deserve especial mention. It is particularly adapted to the early stage of peritoneal inflammation, where the pains are circumscribed and stabbing in character, or darting, lancinating, and such as mark the acute stage of inflammation in other serous tissues — as, for example, in the arachnoid membrane. The diffuse peritonitis that sometimes supervenes, may also require the same remedy. If the attack occurs in consequence of taking cold, or is erysipelatous in character, belladonna is strongly indicated. The same is true of great cerebral disturbance, delirium, insomnia, dilated pupils, also of hysterical complications, neuralgia, and spasms.

Belladonna.

If the attack is ushered in by marked symptoms of local congestion, this remedy is particularly appropriate. This is true of the idiopathic, as well as of the post-partum varieties. In many sub-acute cases, aggravated at each menstrual period, the belladonna may be given for a few hours with manifest advantage. If the pain is somewhat neuralgic in character, it may be equally useful.

Next to belladonna, in the treatment of peritoneal ovaritis, colocynth, I am persuaded, is more useful than any other remedy. This is most marked in ovaritis supervening upon abortion. I am anxious that you should not forget this fact. In this connection it is too frequently overlooked. You will find the symptoms that indicate colocynth detailed in the materia medica. It is especially appropriate to those cases in which the bowels, and indeed the whole abdominal contents, are implicated, with stitches in the ovaries, diarrhœa, colic, pressure in the abdomen, suppression of the lochia, and tenesmus. Also in puerperal fever after vexation. Colocynth is recommended by some authorities for chronic ovaritis.

Colocynth.

The good repute of veratrum viride in puerperal metritis, its apparent capability of restoring the lacteal secretion and the lochia, when they have been suppressed by the inflammatory process, renders it probable that this agent is possessed of some specific relation to the ovaries. As a remedy in ovaritis, it should be given in an early stage of the disease, when the organism is most perturbed by reason of vascular and nervous derangement.

Veratrum viride.

Mercurius vivus is useful at a more advanced period, more especially, it is said, when there is reason to apprehend that suppuration may occur. Many practitioners rely chiefly upon this remedy in alternation with belladonna. The symptoms, mostly abdominal and symptomatic, which indicate mercurius vivus need not be detailed in this connection.

Mercurius vivus.

During the summer term of lectures in this college for the year 1864,* I called attention to the efficacy of the hamamelis virginica in ovaritis. The remarkable effects of this remedy, locally and internally, in orchitis, led me to infer that it would also be useful in some forms of ovaritis. I have prescribed it in numerous cases with remarkable results. It seems appropriate to the sub-acute attacks of this disease, which are incident to pregnancy and menstruation. In the former case, I have no question of its power, in some instances, to prevent abortion, where such a mishap threatens in consequence of ovarian irritation and inflammation. In the latter, it allays the pain and averts the menstrual derangement which is so liable to follow. It is also useful in gonorrhœal ovaritis, in which variety the suffering is sometimes extreme. This affection bears a close analogy to the gonorrhœal orchitis of the male, in which hamamelis is almost specific. For internal use, I prefer the second or third attenuation.

Hamamelis virginica.

The lauded virtues of gelseminum in gonorrhœa and spermatorrhœa of male subjects, suggest that it might also be useful in ovaritis. The same is true of its power to excite uterine muscular contractility, and to allay hysterical spasms.

Gelseminum.

Lachesis is indicated in ovaritis accompanying scanty, tardy, irregular menstruation, vicarious leucorrhœa, and menstrual derangement incident to the critical period. When conjoined with metritis, in sub-acute and chronic cases, this remedy is sometimes very useful. It is recommended

Lachesis.

* See Medical Investigator, Vol. III, p. 62.

by Hering in chronic enlargement with induration or abscess of the ovaries. The following cases were kindly furnished by my friend, Dr. A. H. Botsford, of Grand Rapids, Michigan:

"Miss M—— had suffered many months from dysmenorrhœa, with scanty menstruation. She complained of great tenderness in the iliac region, sometimes on both sides, and at others only on one, and I remarked a fullness in the region of the ovaria, when felt through the abdominal walls. She was so lame and sore that she could not walk. The attacks would culminate in a diarrhœa, the discharges having all the appearance of pus. Under the use of lachesis she gradually improved. Indeed it never failed to relieve her most signally, and the early employment of it invariably prevented the recurrence of the acute symptoms and of the purulent discharge by the rectum. This patient ceased to menstruate at twenty-seven or twenty-eight years of age, and had no further trouble of the kind. She died at thirty-five, of pulmonary congestion.

"Mrs. B——, aged about 35, came under my care five years since. Ten years ago she was ill during the whole summer, with pain, soreness and swelling in the region of the ovaries. Is of opinion that she recovered in spite of medicine. She had chronic diarrhœa, with stools like 'matter, as if from a boil.' She had also an abscess communicating with one of the intercostal cartilages on the left side of the thorax. I gave her lachesis and hamamelis. She was very soon relieved, and now keeps the medicine within reach. She has no family. Menstruation is regular, but she is liable to acute attacks of ovaritis with each monthly return, especially if she overworks or is much fatigued."

In frail, scrofulous subjects, predisposed to excessive purulent discharges, these ovarian abscesses sometimes secrete an enormous amount, and for a long time. This drain produces a species of cachexia in which other remedies may also be of service. The hepar sulphuris, calcarea carbonica, china, and phosphoric acid have been recommended to meet this indication.

Bryonia alba.

Bryonia does not appear to be so well adapted to inflammation of the peritoneum as to that of some other serous tissues — as, for example, the pleura and synovial membranes. So far as we are aware, it has no specific relation to the ovary. In the puerperal form of ovaritis, where the attack sets in with chilliness and rigors, and especially in case of threatened mammary abscess, the breast being large, hard, tense and painful, it may, however, be very useful as an intercurrent remedy. We have sometimes employed it with advantage in rheumatic ovaritis. The same remarks apply to the rhus toxicodendron and the cimicifuga or macrotys.

The menstrual disorder aids in choice of the remedy.

The ovular theory of menstruation is confirmed by clinical experience. Excepting those already named, and a few others which are given for specific reasons, all the remedies of considerable repute, in the treatment of sub-acute and chronic ovaritis, have been prescribed for the relief of menstrual irregularities. Moreover, it is especially significant that each of these remedies is said to have caused abortion, a fact which confirms the idea advanced by Tyler Smith, that the specific stimulus of uterine contraction resides in, or must operate through, the ovaries. From these observations, certain therapeutical deductions are obvious. There is no question but that many examples of ovaritis, complicated with catamenial derangement, have been unwittingly cured by secale cornutum, sabina, apis mellifica, pulsatilla, sepia, platina, cantharis, and caulophyllin. The best criteria for the use of these remedies in ovaritis, will be found in their adaptation to menstrual disorders, as amenorrhœa, dysmenorrhœa, menorrhagia, and also, in many cases, to leucorrhœa.

Ovaritis, complicated with ulceration of the os uteri, requires to be treated most carefully. A resort to astringent injections, or cauterization, is too frequently had, by those who covet notoriety, and are reckless of consequences. The proper constitutional and local treatment for uterine ulceration will be detailed in a subsequent lecture.

Treatment of ovarian atrophy and induration.

For atrophy and induration of the ovaries, with which sterility is almost always associated, jodium, conium, plumbum and baryta muriatica, are in good repute. Change of air, and diet, travel and diversity of scenery, are sometimes of lasting benefit. I have succeeded in curing one case of barrenness, in which there was chronic induration and insensibility of both ovaries, with an almost total atresia of the canal of the uterine cervix. This canal was dilated artificially, while, at the same time, remedies were given to restore the menstrual process. Conception followed, and the ovarian lesion disappeared.

Treatment for gonorrhœal ovaritis.

When there is reason to suspect that either the gonorrhœal or syphilitic taint is present, the mercurius solubilis, mercurius jodatus, nitric acid, thuja, kali jodatum, or aurum metallicum, may be indicated.

Calendula.

The curative virtue of calendula would be available in case of fistulous opening and discharge of the ovarian abscess through the abdominal walls, or into the bowel, bladder, uterus, or vagina.

Local treatment.

In puerperal ovaritis, when the inflammation and tenderness become diffuse and very acute, I know of no local expedient so grateful and beneficial, in a majority of cases, as the application of dry, hot bran to the abdomen. It should be sewed up in bags, heated as hot as can be borne, applied, and then renewed frequently. This application possesses the merit of availability and lightness; it is inodorous, and medically unobjectionable.

After the acute symptoms have yielded somewhat, and the patient is able to lie upon her side, dry heat may still be used, by means of a heated dinner plate, which is wrapt in flannel and kept in constant contact with the abdominal parietes. Cloths dipped in hot water soon become cold, and the patient may be chilled thereby. Hops are sometimes prescribed in extreme cases, in which it is impossible for the patient to sleep, and where nervous symptoms predominate. Emollient cataplasms of various kinds have been resorted to, and sometimes with good results.

Hamamelis virginica.

In acute ovaritis, where the pain is more circumscribed and very severe, arising, propably, as M. Velpeau suggests is the case in orchitis, from strangulation of the organ by its envelop, great relief may be afforded by the external use of the hamamelis virginica. I prefer Halsey's fluid extract of this drug, which may be mixed with hot water, in the proportion of one part to three, and applied locally, by means of cloths or flannels that have been dipped therein. In case the swollen and sensitive organ is prolapsed along the wall of the vagina, a weaker solution of the hamamelis, containing glycerine, may be used as a vaginal injection, or applied by means of cotton wool or charpie saturated with the same, and introduced into the vagina. This application is sometimes remarkably efficacious. It may also be injected into the rectum. If the inflammation is of traumatic origin, arnica may be used in the same manner as recommended for the hamamelis. The local and general employment of aconite is recommended in case of a rheumatic complication, which sometimes involves the most extreme suffering.

Arnica — Aconite.

Vicissitudes of weather and temperature sometimes affect this class of cases so unfavorably, that it is well to protect and insulate the ovaries from their harmful influence. For this purpose a layer of cotton batting, flannel, or silk, should be worn next the abdomen. In very susceptible subjects, where, from taking cold, mild attacks of ovaritis frequently accompany menstruation, this expedient is also serviceable.

Protect from cold and dampness.

Warm baths are better than cold, and the hip bath is preferable to any other. The cold hip bath is sometimes useful, but should be taken quickly, in order to insure reaction. They should not be used indiscriminately. For the relief of pelvic pains incident to severe attacks of ovaritis and ovarian neuralgia, Dr. Aran recommends the expedient of packing the speculum, in vagina, with coarsely powdered ice. Such extreme measures are rarely, if ever, justifiable.

Baths, etc.

Little attention need be paid to restoring the displaced ovary. Remove the inflammation, and the structural changes consequent upon it, and the dislocated ovary will take care of itself. Any attempt to reduce the luxation, farther than by placing the patient in a favorable position, would probably result in more of harm than of good.

As one of the most trying obstacles in the way of a cure is found in the recurrent menstrual congestion; so it is quite impossible, in many cases of ovaritis, to effect a cure while the patient yields to sexual indulgence. She must live *absque marito*. I have found that those patients with ovaritis who come to this city for treatment, and who are thus removed for a time from the stimulus of sexual excitement, recover more rapidly and permanently than others of my patients, who, while being treated, are obliged to remain at home. There are, however, a few exceptions to this rule.

Proscribe sexual intercourse.

LECTURE VIII.

BILIOUS COLIC DURING PREGNANCY.

GENTLEMEN:

We will devote the first part of this hour to the study of a case of bilious colic in a woman who is pregnant.

Case. — Mrs. D——, aged 30, a healthy looking woman of bilious temperament, with black hair and eyes, is six months advanced in her third pregnancy. She complains of repeated attacks of bilious colic, which are accompanied by the usual symptoms of that disorder. Sometimes the paroxysm is very acute, and of brief duration, coming on abruptly and going off in the same manner. Again, the pain is more dull, steady, and persistent, lasting perhaps for twelve hours or more. These paroxysms are not referable to errors in diet, or to excess of exposure, labor or worry, as in ordinary bilious colic, but recur without any obvious cause, sometimes waking her out of a sound sleep. She had them throughout both of her former pregnancies, but never at any other time. She carried both of her children to term. Unless they have continued for six hours or more, the attacks of pain are not followed by jaundice. Her father and two of her uncles were subject to severe fits of bilious colic.

This case illustrates the peculiar relation existing between the uterus and the liver,— a subject of study which is really more important than you may have supposed. For, not only are these viscera organically related through the sympathetic and spinal nervous systems, but their vascular connections also are peculiar and significant.

The vascular relation between the uterus and the liver.

The portal vein receives blood from each and all of the chylopoietic organs. Without this supply of blood from the stomach, the intestines, the spleen, the pancreas, and the mesentery, the curious and complex function of the liver could not be properly performed. But this is not all. The vaginal, hæmorrhoidal, uterine, and ovarian plexuses of veins also communicate, by anastomoses, with the portal system, as well as with the inferior vena cava. A portion of the return current of blood is therefore conveyed directly from the pelvic organs to the liver, *en route* for the general circulation.

Whether this vascular arrangement really implies such a compensatory relation between the hepatic and uterine functions as was insisted upon by Stahl and others, it is foreign to our present purpose to inquire. Its very existence suggests the possibility of diseased conditions which shall depend upon some derangement of the circulation in these inter-communicating vessels.

One of the most marked of the anatomical changes consequent upon conception is found in the uterine veins. They become enlarged into canals and sinuses, with an increase of capacity which is in ratio with the nutritive demands of the contained embryo or fœtus. Being destitute of valves, the only safeguard against a regurgitation and stasis of blood in them is their tortuosity, and perhaps, also, as Köllicker has shown, the temporary supply of muscular fibres to their middle coats.

Vascular changes in the gravid uterus.

A woman becomes pregnant. Prior to this she may have been very healthy. She may or may not be of a bilious temperament. But within the month, and sometimes almost immediately, the hepatic and intestinal functions are deranged. She has nausea and vomiting, which, as in bilious affections uncomplicated with gestation, are worse in the morning. The tongue is furred, the breath foul. She has no appetite for breakfast, there is disgust of water, almost invariably constipation, with bilious headache, highly-colored urine, and hypochondriasis. The matter vomited consists chiefly of mucus, but the paroxysm does not terminate until more or less of bile, it may be only a few drops, is ejected.

Bilious symptoms in early pregnancy.

These symptoms are commonly known as "bilious." That they are contingent upon pregnancy is a matter of every-day observation. But that the extraordinary development of the vascular system of the uterus consequent upon conception is their indirect cause, is not so generally recognized. This functional derangement of the liver may arise from sluggishness of the venous circulation in the pelvic organs. The uterus becomes a diverticulum which receives

The uterus a diverticulum.

and retains an unusual quantity of venous blood. Its weight is increased, it suffers a temporary prolapse, pressure therefrom increases the obstruction in the local circulation, and the parts which are even remotely related through a common vascular apparatus are almost necessarily implicated.

Venous engorgement in uterine affections.

A similar result may happen in the case of uterine deviations of whatever kind, but more especially in prolapsus, procidentia, and retroversion, in uterine scirrhus, fibroids, or polypi; in chronic metritis, dysmenorrhœa, amenorrhœa, and uterine ulceration. As hæmorrhoids and dysentery, and similar diseases in the ano-pelvic region, are very liable to be complicated with some hepatic disturbance, so it is with these different lesions of the womb. And since a proper supply of bile is indispensable to intestinal digestion, we see at a glance what a blow is aimed at nutrition when the function of the liver is thus deranged. In this list of diseases there is not one which is not usually accompanied by more or less of indigestion and inanition.

Cholestræmia contingent upon pregnancy and uterine disease.

Now the chief office of the liver, as an *excretory* organ, is to eliminate the cholesterin, which results from the destructive changes going on in the nervous substance or neurine. This post-organic product would be poisonous if retained in the blood, and it is therefore expelled by way of the hepatic and intestinal outlet, just as urea escapes through the urinary apparatus. And, as we observe that the muscular tissue, of which it was so recently an integral part, is peculiarly susceptible to the toxical effects of an excess of urea in the blood, so the nerve-centers, the brain especially, are extremely sensitive to the action of cholesterin. Hence the hypochondriasis of pregnancy, and of most chronic uterine affections, which owes its origin to torpidity of the liver, and to the imperfect performance of its excretory function. And hence, also, the possibility of such suffering as that of which our patient complains. For biliary calculi consist chiefly of cholesterin, and their existence in a given case is proof positive of hepatic derangement.

Bilious colic is therefore a contingent of pregnancy. There are those who, like Mrs. D., never have it except when they are pregnant. Some, however, are liable to it whenever they menstruate;

others in consequence of excessive sexual intercourse or excitement; and I have known it to be caused by wearing an ill-adjusted or a misplaced pessary.

Treatment. — We have proof that a knowledge of the organic relations between the uterus and the liver is practically important, not only in the clinical history of similar cases, but also in the known common influence of different remedies over these organs. Take, for example, nux vomica, aloes, podophyllin, and chamomilla, as they are most frequently prescribed in uterine and intra-pelvic affections generally. The symptoms which guide to the selection of any of these remedies usually pertain to the liver, or to some portion of the intestinal tract, rather than to the uterus and its appendages.

Common influence of remedies on the uterus and liver

There are, it is true, many exceptions to this rule, but the clinical fact is suggestive. In uterine lesions especially, the dial-plate upon which their characteristic symptoms may be read, and which must be consulted before we can treat them understandingly and successfully, is often located where you would least suspect it, — sometimes in the liver, or in some portion of the gastro-intestinal tract; again in the heart, the brain, or the general nervous system, and even in the eye. Hence a great variety of remedies may be requisite in uterine therapeutics, and the necessity of careful study in their employment must be apparent to you all.

The symptoms of uterine disorder may be remotely located.

Before the termination of pregnancy, and while the cause is still in operation, we should be chary of promising a radical cure in a case of this kind. The disease being self-limited, its symptoms may not wholly disappear until term. In exceptional cases, however, there may be but one or two attacks of the colic. During the paroxysm the indication is to afford prompt relief from the suffering. Among the remedies most frequently employed for this purpose are nux vomica, podophyllin, chamomilla, atropine, and chelidonium. With some practitioners the dioscorea is in excellent repute. Inhalations of ether or of chloroform may be justifiable in extreme cases. In hysterical subjects, with threatening spasms, ignatia, belladonna, or hyoscyamus may be called

This form of bilious derangement self-limited.

Remedies during the fit.

Local palliatives.

for. Dry heat, in the form of hot plates wrapped in flannel, or bottles of hot water, or cloths wrung out in hot water and applied over the seat of the pain, are sometimes most grateful and beneficial. The warm bath is contra-indicated in case of bilious colic occurring in a pregnant woman.

Prophylaxis.

China is perhaps the best prophylactic against bilious colic. It seems to hold some specific relation to the formation and excretion of cholesterin. We do not know precisely what that relation is. Whether it stops the destructive metamorphosis of neurine, and thus limits the production of cholesterin, or helps the liver to eliminate it more readily, is an unsettled question. At all events, we may avail ourselves of the clinical fact that it serves to palliate and to prevent painful attacks of this disorder. When prescribed with this intent it should be given once or twice daily. In a case like the one before us, china will not interfere with gestation. Mrs. D. will take this remedy morning and evening.

Diet: mental and physical exercise.

Her diet should consist of albuminous substances, and fruits. Fats, and all kinds of pastry, would be poisonous. The same is true of coffee and malt liquors. She should have daily exercise in the open air, and be especially careful to avoid all sources of mental anxiety.

PROLAPSUS UTERI, WITH SUPERFICIAL ULCERATION OF CERVIX.

Case.—Mrs. ——, aged 24, began to menstruate at twelve, from which period she dates her illness. The catamenia are irregular, sometimes appearing once in three weeks, again in four, and, occasionally, with an interval of five weeks. The only particular suffering experienced at the period is a dull, aching pain about and in front of the left hip, and a dragging pain across the loins. The flow usually continues three days, and is normal in quantity and quality.

During the inter-menstrual period she complains of a bearing-down sensation within the pelvis. There is great weakness of the back in the lumbar and sacral regions. Standing for any length of time, or walking a short distance, fatigues her exceedingly. When weary, she is subject to a peculiar sensation in the lumbar region, "as if a considerable portion of the back-bone, perhaps six inches long, had been removed." This is soon followed by a faint feeling, and sometimes by actual syncope. At other times, and especially if she is in a room in which there are many other persons, as in a church, or in a concert hall, there is a sense of impending suffocation. Sometimes the unnatural feeling along the spine recurs without any apparent cause or premonition. Then follows an irresistible propensity "to drop down upon the knees." At such times the lower limbs feel numb, insensible, and semi-paralyzed, but the knees are especially weak and powerless.

Another symptom which she has remarked is a sense of coldness on the top of the head, which, whenever she swallows either warm or cold drinks, is curiously changed into a sensation as of "crawling" under the scalp. So marked is this symptom that she has insensibly acquired the habit of placing her hand on that part of the head for its relief, whenever she puts a cup or a glass to her lips.

For some years past (she does not know how long) she has had leucorrhœa. The discharge is habitually more profuse immediately before, but ceases during menstruation. In character she describes it as "catarrhal," creamy, bland, and unirritating.

The touch reveals the uterus prolapsed, the neck of the womb tender and tumefied. When she stands the anterior lip of the cervix rests upon the posterior vaginal wall, directly over the perineum. Upon examination with the speculum, a large, irregular, suppurating ulcer was found to extend within the external os uteri, and over a considerable portion of the anterior lip of the cervix.

Uterine luxations may begin at puberty.

Uterine deviations not unfrequently date from puberty. They are the more likely to follow if menstruation begins at a very early or a very late age. With this patient the flow first appeared when she was but twelve years old. Under these circumstances it must have required more than ordinary effort on the part of the ovaries and the generative intestine to establish this very important function. The ripening, transit, and parturition of the ovum in such subjects resembles labor, and so far as disorders of place are concerned, the consequences to the uterus are of a similar character to those which are contingent upon that process in older women. In the case before you, the afflux of blood to the internal generative organs, the increased weight of the womb, the requisite dilatation and relaxation of the uterine cervix and of the vagina, the contractile effort of the womb to expel its contents, supplied the identical conditions which predispose to uterine displacements following abortion or labor at term.

Irregular menstruation may be a cause or a consequence of uterine deviations. In one form or another they are very apt to co-exist. It is unusual to meet with a chronic case of prolapsus, or of retroversion, in which the menses are not more or less irregular as to the time and method of their recurrence. This state of things is undoubtedly due to a derangement in the local, intra-pelvic circulation. The uterus has become the seat of venous engorgement. Its increased weight has borne it down upon the structures that were designed to sustain it, until they have given way, and it has become displaced. For the uterine ligaments are not fortified against this increase of weight in the womb. An undue or unusual determination of blood to this organ, or sluggishness in its circulation, weakens these supports, and renders them more liable to yield.

Irregular menstruation a cause of prolapsus.

Hence, also, the frequent complications of uterine displacements with chronic disorders of digestion. The connection between the venous systems of the uterus and the liver, explained in my remarks upon the preceding case is significant. There are few examples of prolapsus which are not accompanied by hæmorrhoids, prolapse of the rectum, or by a more or less obstinate constipation.

Uterine luxations and digestive disorders.

Lumbar and sacral pains are incident to most cases of prolapsus, and of uterine ulceration also. But the kind and degree of these pains are modified according to circumstances. As a rule, they are more acute and tormenting in nervous, hysterical and delicate women than in those who are of a different temperament and organization. Among the more robust and energetic there is sometimes a remarkable tolerance of uterine displacements, which may exist for years with little complaint of pain in the loins, or of especial suffering of any kind. But these cases are exceptional.

Lumbar and sacral pains.

In prolapsus, the pains in the lumbar and sacral regions are brought on or increased by standing, riding, or walking, and sometimes by bending forwards and then rising suddenly to an upright position. The back feels very weak, and perhaps as though it were actually broken in two. The more chronic the case the greater the suffering, more especially if at the same time the patient has leucorrhœa, irregular menstruation, or ulceration of the uterine cervix. For, independently of the falling of the womb, these several diseases are almost always accompanied by similar symptoms. This poor woman has them all, and it is by no means strange that such an array of symptoms should present themselves.

Prolapsus and paralysis.

The dropping down of the uterus, and its direct pressure upon the anterior sacral nerves, and also upon the utero-cervical ganglia of the sympathetic, is sufficient to account for the sudden, partial, and temporary paraplegia, or powerlessness in the lower limbs. She falls upon the knees irresistibly. There is numbness and semi-paralysis, which are self-limited. The nervous currents between the spinal center and these parts are interrupted, and the consequence is manifest. Rest, with change from the upright to the horizontal position, causes the womb to lift itself, as the French would say, and the normal nervous circulation returns.

Hysterical complications.

The same physiological reasons explain the peculiar sensation "as if a portion of the spine had been removed," the faintness, the syncope, and the eccentric symptoms which are referred to the top of the head. Through the frequent recurrence of this displacement, the nervous system has acquired a predisposition to hysterical complications. On this theory, the increase of suffering from swallowing cold or warm drinks, which act produces a "crawling" sensation beneath the scalp, as well as the sense of suffocation when in a room full of people, are by no means inexplicable. The relief afforded by pressure upon the top of the head, proves that the peculiar sensation felt in that region is purely nervous.

The reality of "nervous" symptoms.

Let me remind you, however, that these symptoms are none the less real because we style them "nervous," and because it is only through our knowledge of the reflex nervous system that we are competent to explain their existence. In truth, this woman has suffered more from these peculiar sensations in the head than from the pains in the loins, or in the left iliac region, the temporary paralysis, or from any and all of her other symptoms. For, although the element of exaggeration enters largely into the hysterical constitution, we cannot doubt that persons with this temperament are possessed of an increased susceptibility to pain and disease, and that they do really suffer more than others under similar external circumstances.

Symptoms *versus* disease.

But this case has other complications. Some authors will tell you that prolapsus, leucorrhœa, and uterine ulceration, like a cough or a diarrhœa, are not to be considered as so many separate disorders, but as *symptoms* merely. And in the main their view is correct: but symptoms, like quarrels, do not come without cause. When it is possible, we must find out their source, in order to be able to explain their significance and to cure them. There may have been an order of sequence in the coming on of these symptoms, which it is most desirable and necessary for the physician to know.

Leucorrhœa and ulceration from prolapsus.

Our patient has a chronic prolapse of the womb, which in all probability owes its origin to causes already named. Following this displacement, and consequent upon it, she also has leucorrhœa and uterine ulceration. Which of these two contingent affections came first, we do not know. Nothing is more common than a leucorrhœal flow of a catarrhal nature accompanying the slighter and more temporary degrees of uterine prolapse. Here the discharge depends on glandular derangement without structural lesion. There need be, and generally is, in these cases, no ulceration whatever.

Ulceration from abrasion.

But if the uterine deviation is persistent, and especially if the uterus lies low upon the perineum, its friction against the posterior vaginal wall is pretty certain, sooner or later, to cause an abrasion of its investing epithelium. This mechanical cause may induce and perpetuate a superficial ulceration of the neck of the womb, or of the vagina, or of both of these parts together. As the deeper seated textures become involved in the lesion, a more or less copious discharge is poured out, and in future the leucorrhœa will either depend entirely on, or be greatly modified by, the existing ulceration.

Ulceration *sans* inflammation.

The belief is very general that, directly or indirectly, all cases of uterine ulceration originate in the inflammatory process. But I apprehend this view is not correct. Inflammation always imperils the proper nutrition of the organ or tissue in which it is seated. Its chief danger lies in this very fact. But there are many disorders of nutrition, and some of them of a most serious character, which certainly are not in any manner dependent upon the inflammatory process.

It is probable that a large proportion of cases of uterine ulceration commence with simple abrasion of the mucous surface.

Causes of uterine abrasion.

The wearing of an ill-adjusted pessary, or of one which is made of improper material, the careless employment of the female syringe; the abuse of sexual intercourse; horseback riding; mechanical injury of the os uteri during delivery; the use of harmful injections thrown into the vagina, especially after coitus or during menstruation; the contact of corrosive discharges from the uterine cervix, and of vitiated semen, as well as friction from the various uterine displacements, may be sufficient to produce it.

Nature of ulceration from abrasion.

Superficial ulceration of the os following abrasion of its epithelium differs from other varieties of uterine ulceration. It consists essentially in defective reparation of its investing membrane, and not in a destructive metamorphosis of the underlying textures.

Treatment. — The medical management of such cases as this is especially vexatious. We must begin rightly or we shall fail.

Therapeutical reflections.

Any attempt to cure the leucorrhœa without recognizing or relieving the ulceration of the os uteri, or to remedy this lesion without doing anything for the displacement of the womb, would reflect upon our skill and experience. And so also if we were to elevate some of the incidental, irrelevant, hysterical symptoms of which our patient complains to the dignity of characteristic symptoms, when they do not deserve such distinction, and afterwards busy ourselves with curing them.

Rule deducible from order of symptoms.

It is a rule in therapeutics that the symptoms of a complicated, chronic case of disease should be made to disappear in an order which is the reverse of that in which they came — the last first, and so back to the starting point. But when applied to the treatment of uterine affections, this rule has many exceptions. The most stupid blunders have sometimes been perpetrated through ignorance of this fact.

The first indication is to keep this woman as quiet as possible.

She need not lie in bed all the time, but she should assume the recumbent position either upon the side or the back. And, if necessary, she should persevere in this for some weeks, or even for months. For you will not cure these cases so promptly as some enthusiasts would lead you to believe possible. Walking, standing and sitting aggravate her sufferings. She must, therefore, keep quiet.

Postural treatment.

Her shopping and her church-going must be done by proxy. She is no more able to run a sewing machine than she is to run with a fire engine. And, if she were my private patient, I should forbid her dressing her own hair — which is really one of the most tiresome and injurious kinds of exercise for a woman who is suffering from uterine disease. Her clothing should be worn loosely about the waist.

Dressing the hair, etc.

No matter what the kind and degree of the uterine displacement, if the os uteri is abraded or ulcerated, it is wrong to apply any pessary whatever; for, by direct pressure upon, and contact with, the denuded surface, these instruments may work serious mischief. Under such circumstances, they have been known to increase the suffering, to extend the lesion of the cervix, to multiply the reflex symptoms, and to augment the leucorrhœal flow. Keeping the patient in the proper position is a harmless and efficient substitute for these appliances in all cases of this particular kind. (*Exit the patient.*)

Contra-indications for the pessary.

Another requisite for this woman's recovery, of which I have forborne to speak in her presence, is the prohibition of sexual congress. Otherwise it is next to impossible to cure some of these cases. Her separation from her husband will insure against the undue determination of blood to the internal generative organs, which is consequent upon the sexual act, and will thereby remove one of the principal causes that serve to perpetuate the abnormal condition and position of the womb. If we overlook or ignore this item, a cause which may counterbalance all our efforts at cure, will be constantly at work, and we may fail in consequence.

Prohibition of sexual congress.

I do not doubt that much of the boasted efficacy of escharotics in uterine ulceration should really be attributed to the interruption of sexual intercourse, which they necessitate. I can conceive that frequently the caustic might be less harmful than coitus.

Modus operandi of caustics, etc., in certain cases.

And so, also, of similar cures which are ascribed to the use of cold water in the various hydropathic establishments. Without saying a word against this system of treatment, it is quite probable that the benefit derived in many of these cases is due as much to the enforced absence of the patient from the bed and board of her husband as to the baths and remedies that are prescribed.

Calendula topically.

For the cure of a simple, suppurating ulcer of the os uteri, I know of nothing so beneficial locally as the calendula. To a drachm of the strong tincture of calendula add two ounces each of glycerine and distilled water. Of this mixture a tablespoonful may be put into a teacupful of tepid water for an injection per vaginam. This injection, which should be retained as long as possible, may be repeated once or twice daily. The calendula not only heals the abraded surface most kindly, but it also relieves the swelling and tenderness of the cervix, which are so marked in the case under review. In not a few instances it may suffice to arrest the leucorrhœal flow.

Other local expedients.

Or a mixture of glycerine and water in equal parts may be applied by means of a cotton tampon. If you think best, there is no valid objection to adding a few drops of the hydrastis to this preparation. I have sometimes melted simple cerate and applied it directly to the denuded cervix, through the speculum, by means of a camel's hair pencil. Injections of sugar and water are wonderfully efficacious in healing these simple abrasions of the utero-vaginal mucous membrane. The preparation of collodion with castor oil, recently extolled by M. Latour, in his method of treating diseases by isolation, has been of great service to some of my private patients, in whose cases it was applied to the os uteri, in the same manner as recommended for the simple cerate.

The internal remedies most appropriate for the case under consideration are nux vomica and calcarea carbonica. I need not detail their respective indications. If you will study the symptoms carefully, excluding those which are merely sensational and incidental, you will not fail to endorse my prescription. They should be given, for a limited period, night and morning — the nux at night and the calcarea in the morning. Let her report at the end of a week.

PRURITUS OF THE VULVA.

Case.—Mrs. ——, a healthy looking woman, has an infant of three months, which is her third child. She says that when the babe was a month old she began to suffer from an itching of the external genitals. At times this itching is almost insupportable, and she really feels as if she might become insane in consequence of it. She describes it as worse at evening, after being much upon her feet during the day. There is a mucous secretion from the vagina which is sometimes quite copious, but generally scanty, and which she has observed is very apt to dry upon the parts exposed to the air, where it forms into scales that are easily detached by rubbing. Urination is sometimes followed by scalding and burning sensations, which are referred to the vulva rather than to the urethra. Coitus is painful, and apt to be succeeded by a pinkish discharge from the vulvo-vaginal canal. She had this local trouble while nursing both her former children, with the last of which it continued for more than a year. Her skin is fair, and to her knowledge she has never had any eruption. The babe is well, and thrives upon the breast exclusively.

Various causes.

This form of prurigo usually depends upon inflammation of some portion of the mucous membrane lining the vulva. It is incident both to the purulent and the follicular forms of vulvitis, of which pruritus is the most distressing symptom. Among the causes which may induce it are, a lack of cleanliness; the contact of acrid vaginal secretions, as in leucorrhœa, uterine cancer, etc.; masturbation; gonorrhœa; syphilis; vegetative growths; ascarides; indigestion; diabetes; and the use of alcoholic drinks or highly seasoned food. Sometimes it is caused by acrid vaginal discharges poured out during pregnancy, and may result in abortion. Again, it is developed during lactation, and will not cease entirely until the child is weaned. In little girls it may accompany the exanthemata, and disappear with them. In women, it sometimes alternates with a chronic eruption to which they have been subject. In very nervous persons, it may possibly arise from simple hyperæsthesia of the mucous membrane. There may be aphthous ulceration, or perhaps an herpetic or eczematous eruption, or an abrasion at the junction of the mucous membrane with the skin, which shall be sufficient to account for the suffering. Not unfrequently the surface is so heated and inflamed that the mucus secreted is dried upon the parts, and this causes such intolerable itching that, no matter where she is, or what her surroundings, the patient cannot refrain from rubbing or scratching. Another cause of this troublesome affection in certain cases is disease of the uterine cervix. Some attacks of pruritus pudendi have been attributed to a varicose condition of the veins of the vagina. Others are known to arise from the presence either of a peculiar parasite (pediculus pubis), or of the itch insect (acarus scabiei), in the hairy portion of the mons veneris.

Dr. Meigs reports the following case :*

Pruritus from trichiasis. Case.

"I was consulted for a young lady about twenty years of age, who suffered from an intolerable pruritus and uneasiness of the vulva. Her physician had prescribed many and various remedies in vain. He had examined, by inspection, the privities, but could not discover the cause ; which, however, was not dissipated by his application of nitrate of silver and other medicines. When I was called to give my opinion of the case, I was much surprised to find it attributable to a real trichiasis of the vulva. The hairs that grow usually on the derma, and then not very close to the epithelial surface, had sprung from the very margin of the mucous membrane of each labium. They were straight, like eyelashes, and pointed inwards. It was from the tickling and pricking of the points of these hairs that her distress arose. They were all removed by her nurse, with tweezers, and the complaint disappeared."

Clinical history.

The itching, burning or stinging sensation, whichever it may be, is not always constant, but remits and intermits. It may be aggravated by exercise, fatigue, excessive heat of the weather, standing before a fire, by the warmth of the bed, by mental emotion, passional excitement, or urination. It may be worse at evening and at night, thus preventing rest and sleep. Sometimes the patient is compelled to leave her bed and walk about the room in order to obtain the least respite from her suffering. It worries her into a nervous state, rendering her unhappy, petulant and ill. The paroxysms may be so severe as almost to drive her crazy. Sometimes

* Woman : her Diseases and Remedies, etc. Phila., 1859 ; p. 96.

they give rise to local spasm in the form of vaginismus, or in a more general way to an hysterical fit. In the mildest variety the cutaneous surface of the larger labia is the seat of formication, or crawling sensations, which torture the patient exceedingly. In this case she will insist that multitudes of little insects are running over the external generative organs. When the mucous membrane reflected over the clitoris is the seat of the itching, the case develops into one of nymphomania.

Lesions from self-inflicted wounds.

The scratching and rubbing of the parts really affords but little permanent relief, and yet it is impossible for the poor victim to resist such a propensity. In this manner the surface is sometimes so severely wounded that extensive injury is done to the soft tissues. In case there is an eruption, the vesiculæ are broken and the nails may cause extensive abrasions and ulceration. Sometimes the sensation of heat in the parts affected is even worse than the itching.

May precede the menstrual period.

In some women the attack precedes the menstrual flow. The physiological determination of blood to the pelvic viscera, and the irritable condition of the vulvo-vaginal glands and nerves, which usher in the "period," seem sufficient to account for this result. These persons become exceedingly nervous, and suffer greatly at such times. They are on the eve of an hysterical paroxysm, it may be for hours together; fitful, capricious, disheartened, and sometimes almost demoralized. When the flow commences the crisis is soon past, and the pruritus may not return during the month. In such cases the proper menstrual flow is often supplemented by a copious leucorrhœal discharge. The most intractable examples of neuralgic and spasmodic dysmenorrhœa may originate in this form of pruritus. Sometimes the pruritus comes on for a few nights after the cessation of the flow at each period. Or it may be due to menstrual suppression, constituting the prurigo latens of Alibert. The liability to this painful disorder appears to increase with advancing age. Not unfrequently it occurs at the climacteric. A considerable proportion of women suffer more or less from it about the time the menses cease.

Pruritus with dysmenorrhœa and amenorrhœa.

Pruritus at the climacteric.

This itching of the genitals is also one of the contingents of pregnancy. It is more apt to come on after than before the third month, and may either cause abortion, or continue to term. Some women always have it when they are pregnant. Here is a striking instance of general and local pruritus in a pregnant woman, published by M. Maslieurat-Lagémard.*

Pruritus during pregnancy.

"Mrs. ——, aged 32, first became pregnant when twenty-one years old. Prior to the sixth month she suffered but little from the disorders incident to gestation; but after that time, and without any apparent cause, she was attacked with intense pruritus, which extended over the whole body. The legs, thighs and genitals were first seized, but at the eighth month the itching extended even to the palms of the hands and the soles of the feet. The rubbing and scratching, which she could not resist or avoid, caused premature labor, immediately following which the irritation ceased. She became pregnant again, and, as before, continued well until the sixth month. Then the pruritus returned, and continued until the seventh month, when she miscarried. This experience was repeated six times in succession; so that in all she had eight premature labors which were due to excessive pruritus."

Case.

Diseases about and within the uterine cervix are sometimes accompanied by an inveterate pruritus, which may exist for years, and defy all ordinary modes of treatment. It may be due to simple induration, or ulceration of the cervix, endo-metritis, hydatids, polypi, or fibroids. A very painful form of it may arise from inoculation and irritation caused by contact of matters with cauliflower excrescence; and some authors believe that pruritus of the vulva is, under peculiar circumstances, a suspicious sign of uterine cancer in its earliest stages. (?) In other cases, uterine disease is caused by an extension of the inflammation, which is attendant upon the pruritus, from the vulva to the uterine cavity.

Complicated with uterine disease.

As in this case, this troublesome affection may torment the woman only during the nursing period. Under these circumstances, weaning will generally cure it with as much certainty and promptness as did the emptying of the womb in the example just quoted.

Limited to the period of lactation

* Gazette Médicale, 15 Mars, 1848, p. 204.

The danger from pruritus of the vulva is that it may persist until it has so exhausted the nervous energies as to leave the system an easy prey to organic disease. Inveterate cases are likely to be accompanied by digestive disorders of the most serious nature. The prognosis will therefore vary with the clinical history, the cause, the complications, and the duration of the disease, as well as with the temperament, time of life, dyscrasia, and the original strength and vigor of the patient.

Prognosis.

Treatment.—This is local and general. It would be cruel to deny our patient the use of such palliatives as will mitigate her sufferings without in the least interfering with the cure of her complaint. And, since the local expedients to which you will be obliged to resort must vary in different cases, you should possess an ample stock of them in the outset.

First of all is cleanliness, which can be secured by having the parts frequently bathed with suds from castile soap. The honey and juniper tar soaps answer equally well. Pledgets of old, soft linen may be wet either with cold or warm water, as the patient prefers, and applied frequently. Or wheat-bran water may be used in the same way, and, in some cases, injected per vaginum. If there is a vesicular eruption, with a raw surface, or the burning in the urethra and dysuria are very marked, water, or glycerine, or both, may be medicated with the tincture of cantharis, and applied to the vulva by means of compresses. The urtica urens is appropriate to the erythematous form, with a scarlet surface of the mucous membrane, and where there is complaint of burning and stinging as from nettles.

Topical palliatives.

In case of aphthous ulceration, you should not forget the common borax, and the hydrastis, both of which are in excellent repute as palliatives in this form of pruritus. An emulsion of olive oil and lime water is sometimes of excellent service. Or a roll of lint dipped in almond oil may be introduced into the vagina. Colombat recommends a lotion composed of a tablespoonful of cologne water to a teacupful of warm water. Lisfranc prefers a mixture of starch five parts, and camphor one part, to be applied once daily to the inflamed surface, the latter having been washed before the preparation is used. Scanzoni extols a liniment composed of chloroform two parts and almond oil thirty parts. Hewitt prefers them in the proportion of one part of the former to six of the latter. In extreme cases, others prescribe a mixture of melted lard and chloroform. Or the rhigolene, ether, or chloroform spray may be used exceptionally.

If there is considerable local inflammation, I am in the habit of prescribing a poultice of ground slippery elm, or of linseed meal.

For vulvitis, syphilitic or otherwise.

If the case is chronic, and very obstinate, more especially if it is syphilitic, the surface may be painted over with a solution of the nitrate of silver, composed of one grain to the ounce of distilled water. In other inveterate examples the chromic and hydrocyanic acids are permissible and useful.

For pediculi. ascarides, etc.

If the itching is due to the presence of pediculi, a mixture consisting of the ointment of the yellow nitrate of mercury one part, and lard three parts, may be smeared over the pudenda. Or an infusion of tobacco may be applied locally with a view to disgust and destroy the parasite. In trichiasis of the vulva you may follow the treatment prescribed by Dr. Meigs, as quoted above. If the irritation is due to the presence of ascarides in the rectum or vagina, or both, injections of common salt and water, olive oil, or of a decoction of garlic, may be ordered.

Rest, diet, etc.

It is very important to enjoin quiet. The fresh air is, however, requisite. Sexual intercourse should generally, but not invariably, be forbidden. A proper, unstimulating diet should be chosen, and every form of alcoholic drink denied.

Internal remedies.

I will not detain you with detailed indications for remedies that may require to be given internally. Let it suffice that the utmost importance must attach to the special cause and history of each individual case in which you are consulted. For there is no single specific for this affection, any more than there is for hysteria. Natrum muriaticum, sepia, silicea, sulphur, arsenicum, calcarea carb., conium, mercurius, and the various acids, are most frequently given.

LECTURE IX.

OVARIAN NEURALGIA.

GENTLEMEN:

An eminent author has insisted that the ovarian stroma is the sexual center of the female organization. Whether or not this theory is true, it is certain that this spongy structure is erectile, and therefore subject to extreme vicissitudes in respect of its circulation and innervation. For the ovaries are well furnished with blood vessels and nerves. This is a necessary condition of their functional activity which, as in the case of other delicate organs, implies the possibilities of diseased states that shall arise from a derangement in their nutritive and nervous supply.

In health the ovaries are not sensitive. Enclosed in their fibrous capsule (tunica albuginea,) they float out of harm's way. But, under some peculiar or periodical excitement of the generative system, as, for example, in coitus, menstruation, pregnancy, or parturition, they are liable to become irritated, congested, inflamed, or the seat of severe neuralgic pain. And since "women are always about to menstruate, or menstruating, or ceasing to menstruate; or the womb is gravid or going to become so, or it is recovering from the parturient state; these organs have never an even, steady tenor of life." Hence the frequency of ovarian diseases, one of the most interesting and troublesome of which is the theme of my lecture this morning.

Peculiar predisponents of ovarian irritation.

Etiology. — The neuralgic diathesis is the most powerful predisponent of ovarialgia. Women who are subject to neuralgia of the face, head, teeth, and other parts, sometimes suffer severely from this affection. In such persons, if anything is wrong in the pelvic region, the pain is very liable to become neuralgic, in which case the rectum, the uterus, the neck of the bladder, or either of the ovaries, may be the seat

The neuralgic diathesis.

of suffering. In this class of subjects the nervous system may have been originally weak and subject to painful disorders, or that condition has, perhaps, been acquired by habits of life, and the surroundings to which the patient has been subjected. We find examples of this kind among seamstresses, who lead lives of toil and anxiety, and who subsist upon tea, with insufficient and improper food, as well as among those who are buffeted by emotional excitement at the expense of their happiness and general good health. Such persons are almost invariably anæmic or chlorotic.

This neuralgic predisposition may be complicated with a rheumatic diathesis. I have treated several patients for neuralgia of the pelvic organs in whom the suffering was directly chargeable to a metastasis of the disease from some other part of the body. My own observation leads me to conclude that the daughters of rheumatic fathers, especially if the parent was of intemperate habits, are particularly liable to this complication. The rheumatic element may be masked, but it certainly modifies the nature of the attack, and should not be overlooked in its treatment.

The rheumatic diathesis.

So also of hysteria. Very few hysterical women are exempt from neuralgia. Indeed, it is one of the many peculiarities of hysteria, that the slightest causes implicate the nerve filaments and involve suffering. A local congestion which is temporary, incidental, and self-limited, and which in other persons would be an insignificant affair, in women of this temperament will sometimes give rise to extreme suffering of a neuralgic character. It is true that such patients are prone to exaggerate their sufferings, but still the fact remains, that in hysterical women the peripheral nerve filaments are peculiarly sensitive to causes which induce pain.

The hysterical diathesis.

The excitement of the generative system to which this class of persons is especially subject, is a fertile source of ovarian neuralgia. Excessive or fraudulent intercourse; ungratified sexual desire; menstrual derangements; emotional influences, as, for example, too much of theatre-going, of novel-reading, of dancing, or of the worry and wear of fashionable society; carrying too much or too little weight in life, and exemption from proper household cares; may cause such

Sexual excitement.

a determination of blood to the pelvic organs, and especially to the ovaries, as shall induce this form of neuralgia.

The same is true of uterine displacements, organic disease of the ovaries and of the womb, of pregnancy, and of the parturient act. Or it may be caused by nervous shock, by contusions or falls, the taking of long rides or walks, lifting, jumping, singing, running the sewing machine, or, what is worse than any other form of exercise for a woman with intra-pelvic disease of almost any kind, the dressing of her own hair.

Organic disease of uterus and ovaries.

Clinical History.— The attack comes on abruptly, and without premonition or apparent cause. Perhaps she is seized while walking, or upon turning in the bed, upon stepping into her carriage, while sneezing or laughing, or, it may be, after the sexual act.

Mode of attack.

The pain is acute, paroxysmal, and, contrary to the general rule in neuralgia, is increased by the touch and by pressure, whether it is slightly or more firmly applied. According to Churchill, the pain is generally much greater than that resulting from ovaritis. It rarely seizes both ovaries at once, but frequently alternates. It is described as sudden, intense, excruciating, stabbing, cramp-like, and is apt to be accompanied by bending of the body toward the affected side, by fainting, falling, vomiting, hysterical spasms, delirium, or diuresis. Sometimes it radiates, and, in chronic cases (as also in those which occur in pregnancy), it may extend along the corresponding thigh. Usually, however, it is circumscribed and limited to the site of the ovary, which, as you know, varies in different women and at different periods.

Kind and degree of pain.

It is not uncommon for the patient to describe the pain as accompanied by a sensation as if something would burst in that locality. At other times she recognizes a sense of compression, of stricture, or of strangulation. Something upon which she puts the tips of her fingers feels as if tied up tightly. In some cases she cannot lie down, in others to stand is impossible. The pain remits, but does not, as a rule, pass away suddenly. The paroxysm is very liable to recur.

Peculiar sensations.

When it occurs as a contingent of dysmenorrhœa, the pain is "sickening" in character, and peculiarly distressing and exhaustive. In this class of cases, Rigby says, the pain is chiefly confined to a spot about an inch above the middle of Poupart's ligament, frequently extending to the back, and sometimes down the thigh. Ovarian neuralgia is more likely to set in at the very beginning of the period, than after the flow has commenced. It may recur in case the menses come on scantily for a few hours, or a day, and then stop for a little, and finally return more freely. This intermittent form of menstruation is very apt to be accompanied by more or less neuralgia of one or both ovaries, upon the existence of which, indeed, it may be dependent. For the neuralgia may cause the menstrual irregularity, and *vice versa*.

When incident to menstrual disorders.

An engorged state of the ovary is undoubtedly the source of suffering in this disease. From the afflux of blood to it, the substance of the organ becomes swollen. Its fibrous envelope being firm and resistant, limits the expansion of the erectile tissue which it contains, binds it down, compresses it, strangulates it, and intense pain is the direct and inevitable result. Whatever means are capable of relieving the congestion will put an end to the paroxysm.

Cause of the pain.

So likewise the existence of old, inflammatory adhesions between the ovaries and other pelvic viscera, may cause this spasmodic or congestive neuralgia, through a permanent displacement of the organ. Such an attachment may be unnoticed and harmless until the period of pregnancy has arrived, in which it is necessary that the ovary should ascend beside the womb above the superior strait. "If the peritoneal adhesions be slight, they may perhaps get ruptured as the uterus enlarges; the patient will suffer from severe hypogastric pains, especially during the second and third months, and there is sure to be very troublesome sickness."* But if these adhesions, which are sometimes strengthened by fibrous bands and exudations, that have cemented the ovary very firmly, are not broken, the suffering may either persist to term or it may result in abortion.

Peritoneal adhesions.

Diagnosis.—You can diagnosticate ovarialgia from ovaritis by the absence of a chill, fever, or other constitutional symptoms at

* Tanner, on the Signs and Diseases of Pregnancy. Phila., 1868; p. 239.

the outset; by the suddenness of the attack; the intensity of the pain, which is limited to a small extent of surface; by the acuteness and brevity of the paroxysm; the absence of *burning* pain in the affected part; by the fact that it occurs most frequently in nervous, hysterical persons; by the self-limited nature of the disease; and its different modes of termination.

From ovaritis.

The location of the tumor (in case the ovary is very much swollen), the kind of pain complained of, the lack of impulse in the tumor when the patient coughs, its occurrence in one of a neuralgic diathesis, and the impracticability of taxis, would differentiate the worst case of ovarialgia from all forms of enterocele.

From hernia.

In neuralgia of the womb the pain extends over a larger surface, is more marked in the hypogastric than in the iliac regions, never alternates between the two sides of the pelvis or abdomen, is less sudden in the beginning, and less excruciating in degree, seldom follows the course of the sciatic nerves, and is not so apt to leave abruptly as in ovarialgia.

From uterine neuralgia.

Prognosis.—This is generally favorable. No one ever dies directly of ovarian neuralgia, any more than from its more ordinary forms. It may, however, through its persistence and severity, induce such diseases of the ovaries, or of the uterus, or of both, as will ultimately give rise to very serious consequences. Or, in a reflex way, it may light up and perpetuate such sympathetic disorders of the heart, of the lungs or even of the brain, as eventually will terminate disastrously.

Indirect results.

It is not always safe to promise a radical cure. Rheumatic and hysterical complications are tedious and intractable. The same is true of the contingent irregularities of menstruation. In most cases, in brief, it is so difficult to control the patient's habits and surroundings, as well as the emotional and sexual influences to which she is subjected, that we can only hope to afford temporary relief.

Qualify your prognosis.

When it occurs during pregnancy, this painful affection is self-limited, generally disappearing after labor. If, however, the adhesions have prevented the ascent and development of the gravid uterus, there is danger of abortion, in which case the risks of premature delivery are added to those of the neuralgia.

Treatment.—The preventive treatment of this disease is very important. It consists in removing all causes of undue sexual irritation and perturbation; in regulating the kind and degree of exercise to be taken; in changing, if need be, the whole mode of life and habits of the patient, and in curing the diseased conditions upon which this painful affection may depend. Among the items which come under the latter head, none is more prominent and practical than to order such a diet and such general hygienic relations as will improve the quality of the blood. In neuralgia, nutrition is very apt to be impaired. There exists anæmia, or the woman is chlorotic, and while this state of things continues, a cure is impossible. If we would restore those who are ill to their wonted health, it is our first duty to supply the conditions upon which health depends.

Prophylaxis.

Milk is the best standard for blood, and should be used, in one form or another, by this class of patients. The whites of eggs, lean meats, game, salt water food, and vegetables, afford a list from which to select what is palatable and nutritious. The diet should be varied from time to time. If the appetite has failed it may be stimulated by the temporary use of pepsin, as sold in the shops, by the extract of malt, or by the taking of malt liquors in small quantities.

The diet.

If the disease is complicated with rheumatism, great care should be taken to protect against vicissitudes of weather, and especially against taking cold. As a precautionary measure of this kind, I have sometimes directed my patients to wear two or three layers of flannel over the abdominal and hypogastric regions, in the form of an apron applied directly to the integument. A batch of uncarded cotton may be sewed into the clothing and worn in a similar manner. The feet should always be kept dry and warm, but more especially "at the month." Because of the erratic nature of the disease, and its liability to metastasis to the ovary, you should remember that revulsive applications to the seat of rheumatic inflammation, when it is located in other parts of the body, are particularly hazardous in the case of women who are subject to sexual

For the rheumatic complications.

derangements. The same is true of the use of the ointments which are sometimes prescribed for cutaneous eruptions.

During the paroxysm we must institute measures to relieve the suffering as speedily and safely as possible. In every variety of acute painful disorder which is located in the uterine or the ovarian regions, warm applications are more grateful and soothing than such as are either cool or cold. This is especially true in case of intra-pelvic neuralgia, upon which the warmth seems to act as a species of anodyne. Aran's expedient of introducing the speculum, and filling it with powdered ice for the relief of ovarialgia, is too harsh, and might be indirectly injurious.

Palliatives.

Warm applications better than cold.

Acting upon the clinical hint that warmth is better than cold, we may order the application of flannels or towels that have been dipped in hot water, or of dry heat in some available form, directly to the seat of the pain. If the suffering is of traumatic origin, one part of the tincture of arnica may be added to ten of hot water and applied locally. If it is rheumatic, the extract or the tincture of hamamelis, or of aconite, may be used in the same manner. Or the same substances mixed with warm water and glycerine, may be thrown into the rectum or into the vagina. If the attack is incident to dysmenorrhœa, the warm sitz-bath may be serviceable.

Topical expedients.

Sometimes the pain will be made to vanish by the topical application of the strong tincture of the aconite root. Or a very little veratrin dissolved in glycerine, or mixed with simple cerate, may be rubbed in gently. A mixture, consisting of chloroform one drachm, and olive oil and glycerine each one ounce, may be applied to the integument covering the tender ovary, or, better still, introduced into the vagina, by means of a cotton tampon which is saturated with it. A thread should be attached to the tampon to facilitate its removal. It may be allowed to remain for some hours. An injection of the same substances may be thrown into the rectum. You should remember, however, that, owing to contiguity of structure, injections thrown into the rectum for the relief of ovarian pain, are much more useful and prompt in their action in affections of the left than of the right ovary.

In exceptional cases the suffering depends on the presence of dry, hard, fecal matters lodged in the rectum, and to unload the bowel affords immediate relief. In very severe cases of ovarialgia, if the means were at hand, the ether spray might be applied to the iliac region with excellent effect. Unless complicated with hysterical spasms, general anæsthesia is not necessary.

Remove fecal accumulations.

I know that these and kindred expedients are prohibited by some physicians, who insist that they are both unnecessary and harmful. But it is my duty as a teacher to acquaint you with resources that may be useful in emergencies, and which are sometimes permissible on the score of humanity. It is for yourselves, and not for others, to say whether and how often you will employ them.

Of the various internal remedies for ovarialgia, perhaps the valerianate of zinc is most frequently prescribed. It seems especially adapted to the relief of the different forms of neuralgia which are engrafted upon the hysterical constitution. For it obviously has some specific curative relation to the ovaries themselves, and through them, to the whole nervous organization of woman. It will sometimes put an end to the paroxysm at once, but its best effect is in preventing a return of it. It may be given in the third decimal trituration, and repeated from two to four times daily. If the patient has ovarian neuralgia before menstruation, she may anticipate its return and avert the suffering by taking a few doses of this remedy a day or two in advance of the period.

Valerianate of zinc.

Atropine is useful under the same indications for which belladonna is generally given. In very severe attacks it may serve to stop the pain, quiet the nervous perturbation, and promote rest and sleep. The cases to which it is most appropriate are those in which there is a strong tendency to ovarian congestion, with intolerance of light and noise, dilatation of the pupils, and delirium; also, when the ovarialgia is accompanied, as it sometimes is, by vaginismus. When the menstrual return is characterized by downward pressure of the uterus, as if it would be forced out at the vulva, and in consequence the patient is obliged to lie in bed for some days; and when there are incidental paroxysms of acute pain in either ovary; this remedy is almost specific. Two grains of the third

Atropine.

trituration may be dissolved in half a glass of water and a teaspoonful of the solution given every one to three or more hours. Or it may be given in small powders dry upon the tongue. In some cases, however, there is such a susceptibility to the action of atropine, that you will be obliged to substitute it with belladonna in a medium or higher potency.

Colocynth.

Colocynth is applicable to neuralgia in the inguinal region, with boring, tensive, or stitching pains in the ovary, in case the symptoms resemble those of hernia, contractive pain in the stomach, with eructations, nausea, pallor, coolness of the extremities and cold sweat. Also if there is incidental colic, with disposition of the patient to bend herself double.

Other remedies which may be useful are cantharis, coffea, chamomilla, cocculus, cuprum met., ignatia, platina, pulsatilla and sepia. For their special indications I must refer you to the materia medica.

Naja.

Dr. W. H. Holcombe reports* that, while giving naja to a very intelligent patient, a physician's wife, for organic disease of the heart, "she complained that it contained a symptom altogether new to her—a violent, crampy pain in the region of the left ovary." "I met," he says, "a similar case a week afterwards, and gave naja, 3d. It was relieved immediately. I have verified its value several times. Not a month ago I had one of those severe cases of ovarian congestive neuralgia—for that is the best name I can give it. It had resisted chamomilla and hyoscyamus, both at the 6th; generally my first prescription. I was about to prescribe caprum metallicum, 6th, (which is excellent in those cases), when the patient related the curious fact that she had violent palpitation of the heart whenever the ovarian pain came on. I gave naja, 3d, and both symptoms disappeared as if by magic."

Ammonium muriaticam.

My friend, Dr. R. N. Foster, of this city, has confidence in the third decimal trituration of ammonium muriaticum.

Ignatia.

Those members of the class who attended the last meeting of the Chicago Academy of Medicine will recall Dr. Ballard's report of a very interesting case of this disease in a pregnant woman. The affection occurred in

* United States Medical and Surgical Journal, Vol. I, p. 234.

her first pregnancy, and was uncontrollable by the old fashioned means. She went through to term, however, without serious accident. In the second pregnancy the same symptoms came back again, and she suffered extremely. The paroxysms of pain, sometimes in one ovarian region and again in the other, came on almost daily. She was extremely nervous, with headache, and the slightest noise startled her. The doctor prescribed three powders of ignatia, 200th, one to be taken every night. The paroxysms immediately became less severe in degree, and less frequent, some weeks elapsing between them, and she got through safely, with much less suffering than before.

Cimicifuga.

If I may judge from my own observation, the cimicifuga is a good remedy for ovarian neuralgia occurring in rheumatic subjects. It seems also adapted to women of dark hair, eyes and complexion, and to those who are the children of intemperate parents. In this latter class of subjects it is suited to the relief of contingent attacks of hysteria, dysmenorrhœa, intense reflex pains, as, for example, angina pectoris, or the characteristic infra-mammary pain in the left side of the chest.

EXCORIATED NIPPLES.

Case.—Mrs. G.'s third child is but four weeks old. This babe is a fat, hearty boy, while the mother is slender, but of general good health. She reports having passed through her lying-in without any serious illness. She has, however, suffered extremely from sore or excoriated nipples. This trouble began immediately after the appearance of the milk, on the third day after delivery, and has continued until the present time. She says that she could "get on very well, but that each time after nursing the nipple is left raw and bleeding;" and that "when the little fellow lets go his hold, it almost takes her life." She had a similar experience with each of her former children, from which, despite all the means employed, she did not recover until they were weaned, at the age of three months.

This is by no means a trivial case. In private practice you may encounter forty of them for every one like that upon which my brave colleague, the professor of surgery, has just performed a capital operation. And, unless you know how to treat them, each one may give you forty times as much trouble. Although the nipple may be accidentally torn off by the child, you will not be permitted to dispose of this troublesome member by amputation.

Most frequent in primiparæ.

Sore nipples are more frequent in primiparæ than in multiparæ. There are those, however, who, like our patient, suffer from them with each successive pregnancy. The affection sometimes begins during the later months of gestation, but usually not until the child has been "put to the breast" a few times. If the skin covering the nipple is very tender, thin and delicate, the first attempts at nursing may increase its sensitiveness or strip off the epidermis in some places. The more vigorous and voracious the child the greater the danger in this respect. In women with light complexions, and light or red hair, the cuticle is very delicately organized, and easily removed. There is a popular idea that, because they are stronger and more rough in their little manners, boys are more apt than girls to wound the nipple while nursing. There is little doubt but that this painful affection is sometimes due to the removal of the sebaceous matter from about the nipple by the mouth of the infant. In other cases the nipple is bruised by the gums. Or it may arise from a lack of cleanliness, or from not drying the nipple so carefully as should be done after nursiug. Sometimes it may spring from a depraved or cachectic condition of the general system, chargeable to original organization or to the drainage which is consequent upon gestation. Again, it may be caused by an aphthous condition of the child's mouth, whereby it has been inoculated with a poisonous principle. In exceptional cases the child may be syphilitic, and the erosion of the nipple will be found to present some specific peculiarities.

Local and general causes.

Symptoms.

The first symptom complained of is a burning or scalding of the nipple when the child takes hold of it, or upon its removal from the breast. This sensation may be accompanied or followed by pain which is more or less acute. Sometimes the nipple, and again the whole breast, feels as if bruised. Or they may be the seat of acute, lancinating or stinging pains. In some instances the mother can scarcely persuade herself that her nipple has not really been torn off by the child. The torture of nursing the infant is sometimes very great. A fissure or chap in the skin, which is scarcely visible to the naked eye, may be sufficient to cause the most extreme and exquisite suffering. Women of the utmost courage and fortitude are not unfrequently brought to tears by this experience. Occasionally the weak and irresolute, more especially those who desire an excuse for weaning the child, refuse to nurse it after a few trials.

Upon careful examination we may, perhaps, find that a considerable portion of the nipple has really been denuded of its investing cuticle. This excoriation is generally most marked at the free extremity and apex of the organ. It may arise from the warmth and moisture of the child's mouth, which seem as it were, to blister it and to separate the scarf skin from the delicate derm beneath. These abrasions may be either superficial or otherwise, according to the length of time that has passed since they commenced, and the lack of cleanliness or of proper treatment. They sometimes develop into broad ulcers, which are exceedingly vascular and irritable. They are slow to heal, because the reparative material thrown out is apt to be washed away or removed by the child before it is fully organized.

The excoriation.

Not unfrequently the fissures will be found to consist of long, narrow, linear ulcers, which are deep-seated and intractable, and which bleed easily. These ulcers may dip down into the nipple perpendicularly from its summit, or they may take a transverse direction, and finally cut off one-third, one-half, or the whole of the organ. They are exceedingly painful, particularly when exposed to the air, and in case the lips of the fissure, or hair-like ulcer, separate from each other. They may even become fistulous. The symptoms are aggravated by each attempt at nursing. The discharge from the abraded surface, or from the fissure, soon dries upon the nipple and forms a scab, beneath which pus is sometimes collected in considerable quantity. The injury done to the nipple by the nursing process may cause it to bleed so freely as to sicken the child and induce vomiting.

The ulceration.

In exceptional cases this affection may begin with an herpetic eruption about the nipple. The little vesicles are broken, and the almost constant irritation of nursing causes them to develop into ulcers, which finally coalesce and give rise to symptoms such as I have already detailed. At other times it is the outgrowth of a species of scorbutic cachexia, and accompanies the nursing sore mouth.

Perhaps the most serious consequence of excoriated nipples is the danger of mammary abscess, which may result in any case from a lack of determination, or from neglect on the part of the patient and nurse, to have the breasts well and frequently drawn. The milk accumulates, the gland becomes painful, indurated and inflamed from over-distention of its ducts. The suppurative process is soon established, and constitutional and local symptoms of a grave character follow. It is in this manner that the worst examples of mammitis and mammary abscess may be indirectly referable to an erosion or ulceration of the nipple. If the patient is addicted to the wearing of tight dresses, this unfortunate result is all the more likely to follow.

Mammary abscess from sore nipples.

Treatment. — As prevention is better than cure, so we may save trouble by the use of expedients which are designed to prevent the possibility of the nipples becoming sore. They may be "hardened" by applications of a weak lotion of the tincture of arnica, of alcohol and water, of brandy and water, of a linen cloth constantly wet with rum, by a wash consisting of equal parts of the tincture of myrrh and rose water, by bathing them in port wine, in green tea, or in a mixture of three parts of green tea with one of brandy. Or you may direct the use of a cerate of white wax and butter in equal proportions. In the case of primiparæ, simple prophylactics of this kind are especially serviceable in the later months of pregnancy. Care should be taken that the clothing over the breasts is not too warm and tightly fitting. It should be light and thin, especially during the last month of gestation. These precautionary measures are also suited to those who have suffered from sore nipples on previous occasions, and in whom, if possible, it is most desirable to avert such a calamity in the future.

Prophylactics.

Here, as everywhere else in the practice of your profession, you will find great need of discrimination. For although these and other expedients are useful and harmless, when properly applied, they may work mischief if wrongly used. And while too much blame is frequently laid at the door of monthly nurses, it is still true that they do a great

Need of discrimination.

deal of harm by resorting to traditional specifics of whose real properties and powers they are ignorant. An eminent author says: "Most nurses, indeed, possess a catalogue of nostrums — never-failing cures — for chapped or ulcerated nipples; and I think many of the most distressing cases of the kind we meet with are occasioned by these busy characters taking the management on themselves, and, as is usual with the ignorant, relying implicitly on the virtue of their favored *specific* alone, without attending to the necessity either of protecting the nipple, or of duly evacuating the breast."

Watch the nurse.

If there is simple abrasion of the nipple, it may suffice to have it carefully cleansed and then dried with a tuft of soft linen or charpie, as soon as the child is taken from the breast. Then apply a cold mucilage of slippery elm, or, if there is much heat and burning, small cloths wet in cold water. Or the nipple may be dusted with some finely-powdered arrow-root, starch, gum arabic, borax, or white sugar. Or the oil of sweet almonds, arnica oil, simple cerate, or the spermaceti ointment, may cure the case by the exclusion of air and moisture.

For simple abrasion.

If there is aphthous ulceration, borax, hydrastis, baptisia, or one of the mineral acids diluted with cool or cold water, may be applied topically. In some cases simple rose water answers equally well.

For aphthous ulceration.

The nitric, phosphoric, and muriatic acids are also curative in case of fissures, chaps and linear ulcers of the nipple. The organ should be cleansed and dried after nursing, and a weak solution of one of these acids in water and glycerine applied with a camel's hair pencil. Some physicians place great confidence in a lotion composed of an alcoholic solution of gum benzoin and glycerine in equal parts. A domestic expedient of real utility in some cases consists in the application of the oil which may be expressed from the yolk of a hard-boiled egg. Or a species of flexible varnish may be extemporized by rubbing four parts by weight of the yolk of an egg with five parts of glycerine in a mortar, and applying it over the whole nipple.

For the linear ulcers.

Dr. Simpson recommended the topical use of collodion; but this is painful, and seldom answers very well. The mixture of collodion and castor oil extolled by M. Latour might be less severe and more efficacious. Some practitioners prefer the arnicated collodion. Others the cerates of graphites, or calendula. A popular and efficacious remedy in some cases is the mutton marrow. In obstinate, chronic cases, the nitrate of silver in stick or solution carefully applied will stimulate granulation and close the ulcer. Or you may bring the edges of this linear ulcer together and secure them in contact by bits of adhesive plaster properly adjusted. For this purpose the flexible plaster which is spread upon silk is preferable to the old variety.

Cleanse the nipple before nursing again.

If the child nurses directly from the nipple, or, in other words, if a shield is not used, the nipple should always be cleansed after either of the above named applications, before it is again put to the breast. The chief objection to cerates and ointments is the difficulty of removing them under these circumstances.

Choice of nipple shield.

You will find upon the table a dozen kinds of nipple shield. I can not recommend any of them as suited to every case. My plan is to try one and another, if necessary, until I find the one that my patient can use. The more simple the instrument the better. If it has too long a teat it will be very apt to occasion soreness and inflammation in the roof of the child's mouth. It should be kept sweet and clean. In case the breast is so exceedingly sensitive that the mother cannot bear it touched, the shield which is arranged with a flexible tube between the child's mouth and the nipple of the mother answers best. If the milk does not flow very readily through the shield, it may first be drawn a few times by an older child, or very carefully by the nurse. If the child refuses to take hold, a little tact and starvation will mend his manners. The shield should be used on both breasts, and not upon one exclusively, else while one gland is well drawn the other may not be half emptied, and mammary abscess may follow. If the skin of the nipple is very delicate, the shield should be used from the first, and the babe not allowed to take hold of the nipple at all.

Precautions.

Benefits of the shield.

The advantages of this little instrument are that while it secures, if appropriately and carefully used, a thorough evacuation of the breast — preventing the inflammation and suppuration which in many cases would be inevitable without it — it also averts and alleviates suffering.

By preventing the removal of reparative material which is thrown out, as well as by allowing lotions and ointments time to act, and by keeping the nipple from direct contact with the child's mouth, protecting it from the injurious results of suction and friction, it hastens the cure. The child should be nursed regularly, as often as once in three hours during the day.

For local inflammation.

If there is a high degree of local inflammation, soothing applications of cold water or rose water, or, better still, a cold emollient of slippery elm, may be applied. In some cases it is impossible to cure an excoriated or ulcerated nipple while the inflammation in the loose cellular tissue within and about the base of the organ continues. Weaning is a final expedient.

Internal remedies.

Among the internal remedies calcarea carbonica, sepia, sulphur, graphites, rhus tox., chamomilla, silicea, mercurius, alumina, hepar sulphuris, nux vomica and causticum are the more prominent. In selecting the appropriate remedy particular prominence should be given to the patient's antecedents, the peculiar condition of her health during pregnancy, and to acquired predispositions, as well as to the distinctive symptoms of which she complains.

LECTURE X.

URETHRITIS.

GENTLEMEN:

Here is an example of a disease with which you should be familiar:

Case.—Mrs. ——, aged 28, has been ill for fourteen weeks. She is the mother of two children, the youngest of which is one year old. The babe was weaned at six months, since which time she has menstruated regularly. On the eve of the regular "period" she was seized with a strong desire to urinate, but, being "down town on a shopping expedition," she could not conveniently respond. Although suffering great pain in consequence, micturition was deferred for more than an hour, during which interval she rode home, a long distance, in the street-car. But the simple evacuation of the bladder did not end her sufferings. For she still felt an almost irresistible call to urination, which has tormented her at intervals of from ten minutes to an hour ever since. The flow has never been involuntary. If she lies quietly upon her back, the irritation subsides, but the moment she turns upon either side the dysuria comes on again. Although in a less marked degree, standing and sitting produce the same result. She cannot sit in a chair five minutes without the most disagreeable sensations and throbbing, which are referred to the meatus and the course of the urethra. She says the pain is most acute and burning during the flow. This pain is described as always of a burning character. The urine is sometimes cloudy, with a ropy sediment, but usually quite natural in appearance. It has never been bloody or highly discolored. The quantity voided in twenty-four hours is neither excessive nor deficient.

Two years ago she had a similar attack, which continued for three weeks and appeared to subside of itself. Although her attention had not been called to the fact before, she now remembers that it followed a similar imprudence. She is quite positive that it bore no relation to the birth of her first child. This patient has already been under the care of several physicians, at whose prescription she has taken buchu, copaiba, oil of turpentine, and the usual drugs, including the extract of belladonna in large doses.

She has also made use of sitz-baths, suppositories, herb teas, etc., etc., but with only the most temporary relief.

The uterus is prolapsed the moment she assumes the upright position, whether in standing or sitting. With this exception, the womb is normal in every respect. The vagina is not inflamed, neither is it especially sensitive, except along the course of the urethra. Pressure on that canal from above downwards causes the same pain of which she complains when passing water. It also forces the escape of a muco-purulent fluid from the meatus urinarius. The orifice of the urethra is more highly colored and tumefied than the surrounding mucous membrane.

It is a singular fact that most writers upon the diseases of women have said little or nothing of this painful affection. We cannot attribute this oversight to its infrequency, for, in the female subject, urethritis is much more common than stone in the bladder or cystitis, both of which diseases have received a due share of attention at the hands of the gynæcologist. Nor is it an insignificant complaint. For whatever occasions such suffering as our patient has experienced, has a claim upon us for relief.

Urethritis may be acute, sub-acute, or chronic. The two latter are the more frequent. It may arise from taking cold, more especially during the menstrual period, getting the feet and limbs wet, sitting in wet skirts at church, or in the concert room; from the extension of the inflammation in case of vaginitis along the mucous membrane of the urethra, or from the irritation of pruritus in the same canal; vascular tumors of the meatus; polypus of the urethra; from acridity of the urine; the contact of leucorrhœal discharges, or of vitiated semen; from the pressure of a dislocated womb; uterine, ovarian, hernial, or pelvic tumors; cancer; misplaced or illy-adjusted pessaries; horseback riding; mechanical injury during labor, or the induction of abortion by those who are ignorant of anatomy; too forcible or too frequent coitus, especially at the month; also from masturbation, gonorrhœa, syphilitic ulceration, urinary calculus, and indirectly from neglect to respond to the promptings of nature when the bladder should be emptied. A spurious form of this disease is sometimes met with in hysterical women. In the sub-acute variety the attack may recur with each menstrual period.

Causes.

The most prominent symptoms are burning and smarting or

scalding along the course of the urethra, with frequent desire to urinate. In many cases this burning sensation is continuous, being aggravated by the flow of urine. In others it commences when the patient is half, or, perhaps, wholly through with the act of micturition, and continues for some moments after the discharge is completed. The burning and the urging to urinate are increased by motion. Hence, if the patient persists in walking about, or sitting up, these symptoms are aggravated. For this reason, she is generally better at night.

Symptoms.

She may find it possible to lie in a particular position, and in that only, with a relative degree of comfort. Thus, while our patient is easy upon her back, she cannot turn from it upon either side without increasing the difficulty. Sometimes the erect position is intolerable. It is particularly so if the case is complicated with prolapse of the womb, or uterine or other intra-pelvic tumors. The vesical tenesmus is very apt to be increased by the same cause.

Posture chosen.

Usually, the character of the urine is not changed in any particular, except that it is mixed with mucus. The blennorrhagic discharge may be quite profuse or scanty, according to the duration and gravity of the attack. It varies, also, with the individual constitution, scrofulous persons being more apt to have a copious flow of mucus than others. The mucus is mixed with the urine when it is voided, but afterwards separates and settles as a cloudy, ropy material. It is never bloody. In very nervous women, after a paroxysm of strangury, there may occasionally be an abundant flow of pale, limpid urine, such as frequently follows a hysterical fit.

Character of the urine.

When you visit such patients and inquire in general terms concerning their ailments, you will most likely be told that they have disease of the kidneys. For, however intelligent in other matters, most women suppose that anything wrong with urination implies that the kidneys, and not the bladder or urethra, or both, are at fault. A diligent inquiry into the especial symptoms will enable you to discriminate between urethritis and nephritis, for example, and you should not, therefore, be satisfied to prescribe upon the patient's diagnosis.

A domestic fallacy.

Cases of this kind might, perhaps, be confounded with stone in the bladder. The pain at the close of, and after urination, the increased suffering and strangury from moving around during the day, and the frequent, scanty, interrupted flow of urine, are common to both affections. But where the symptoms depend upon urinary calculus, we shall find them modified and supplemented by others which are lacking in urethritis. The pain caused by the contraction of the bladder upon the stone is sometimes acute, but generally of an aching character. And although it may extend along the course of the urethra, it is not accompanied by the burning sensation of which Mrs. —— complains. In stone, the urine is more or less bloody; its chemical reaction varies with the kind of deposit; the microscope detects an excess of some of its earthy constituents, and by "sounding" the bladder we recognize the presence of a foreign body contained within it.

Diagnosis — from stone.

Cystitis is accompanied by more or less marked constitutional symptoms, as chill, fever, anorexia, and rapid loss of strength. The pain, which is referred to the pubic region, is in the first stage acute, lancinating, and extreme in degree when the bladder begins to contract. It is increased by motion, by pressure, and is worse at night during the febrile exacerbation. It may be of a burning character, but is more apt to implicate the rectum than the urethra. There is also a feeling of distension of the bladder. In advanced stages the abdomen becomes tender and tumefied, and in its further development the affection differs entirely from urethritis.

From cystitis.

It is extremely difficult, and sometimes quite impossible, to determine whether a given case of urethritis is or is not complicated with gonorrhœa. If the inflammation is specific, the attack is more likely to be accompanied by marked constitutional symptoms, by more intense suffering when the urine is passed, by a more copious discharge of mucus, and, what is still more characteristic, the more acute symptoms subside spontaneously in from two to four days. But the particular history of the case, and especially the habits of the patient and of her husband, will help you to settle the question as between a benign and a specific inflammation in the urethra. Let me recommend, however, that, whenever it is possible, you shall give all parties concerned the benefit of a doubt, and proceed to the relief of the symptoms which are actually present.

From gonorrhœa.

Treatment.—Perhaps no better opportunity will offer in which to say a word concerning the length of time required for this and similar diseases to recover under proper treatment. In some of our books and journals you will find it reported that a single dose has cured such a patient almost instantly. The inference is that if we prescribe carefully and accurately, the relief will be certain and speedy. The truth it often quite the reverse. Such a case as this, one in which a poor woman has been ill with marked and decided local inflammation for many weeks, must, in the nature of things, convalesce slowly. And so is it with the majority of diseases that the physician is required to treat.

Rapid cures exceptional.

The ill effects of motion are so manifest in urethritis that the first condition prescribed should be rest in the recumbent position. The patient may be allowed to lie on the back, or upon either side, as she prefers, but should not be permitted to stand, sit, or walk about. Riding would be equally injurious. She should as much as possible refrain from doing anything which would increase the pain or the frequency of urination. For this reason, it is best to prescribe sexual abstinence also.

Rest in the recumbent position.

The diet should consist of plain, wholesome food, which is freed from condiments and easily digested. All kinds of wines and liquors are poisonous. Tea may be allowed in moderation. The meals should be taken regularly. Vegetables are better than meats for these patients. If she eats an excess of sugar her sufferings may be greatly increased in consequence. Diluent drinks, as rice water, gum arabic, an infusion of flaxseed or of slippery elm, may mitigate the suffering by rendering the urine less stimulating and acrid.

The diet and drinks.

If the case is at all obstinate or chronic, a careful examination should be made of the meatus urinarius, the urethra, and adjoining organs. If there is a vascular tumor at the orifice, or a polypus in the canal, remove it by the scissors, ligature, or caustic, as you think best. If the uterus is displaced, correct the deviation and cure the remaining symptoms with appropriate internal remedies. If the inflammation is a sequel of vaginitis, or of pruritus of the vulva, treat it as you would have treated the idiopathic affection. And so likewise if it

General indications.

is incident to leucorrhœa or any form of menstrual derangement.

In gonorrhœal urethritis, especially if there is considerable inflammation and heat in the vagina also, I know of no remedy so well adapted to the relief of the acute symptoms as atropine 3d. Besides this we have aconite, cantharis, cannabis sativa, and mercurius, which may be given under appropriate indications.

For gonorrhœal urethritis.

Simple, uncomplicated cases may require cantharis, cannabis, conium, belladonna, nux vomica, calcarea carbonica, hepar sulphuris, or mercurius corrosivus. Mrs. —— will take a dose of cantharis 3d once in three hours.

MEMBRANOUS DYSMENORRHŒA.

I will now invite your attention to the following remarkable case, which is reported by the patient herself:

Case.—I was born in July, 1834, in C——, Ohio. Soon after my birth an eruption made its appearance on the skin, resembling rash, occasioned, it was then thought, by the extreme heat of the season. I passed the usual diseases of children very early in life, and, with the exception of this eruption, which appeared almost every year during the summer months, and generally upon the lower parts of my limbs, I was a vigorous, active child, full of life and spirit, and in apparent perfect health. At the age of fourteen years and five months the menses made their appearance. The first discharge was plentiful, but attended with no pains or inconvenience whatever. One year after they were suppressed about three months—caused by thin shoes, wet feet, and not early acquainting my mother with the fact. I was soon set right with "Cooper's pills." I felt well during the suppression. At sixteen, while at boarding-school, my appetite grew voracious, and I ate immoderately of all kinds of food, pickles, and sweetmeats. The rash had somewhat lessened in its appearance each summer as I grew older. It was, however, upon my body one day when, just after dinner, in passing through a hall to which the outer doors were open, I met a furious gust of wind from an approaching thunder-storm. At the moment I noticed no uncomfortable sensation, but was shortly seized with great difficulty of respiration and extreme prostration, and in less than an hour my life seemed hopeless to those around me. This was the first attack of anything like illness since my babyhood. Two physicians were speedily called, who said, "the rash had suddenly struck inward." Two days before this I remember to have been very nervous, so that I could not go to sleep on retiring, but did not know that anything ailed me. The doctors gave me tumblers full of a mixture of asafœtida; valerian was also given. I do not know what else was administered, as I was only partially conscious. My suffering was almost wholly from the gasping and struggles for breath. The rash never made its appearance again until I was thirty-four years old. I was left weak and sick (*I* think, from the effect of the dosing). It was one or two days before I could be removed home. Very soon my monthly period came on, attended with some pain. My mother told the physician, and he gave me hyoscyamus. My school days ended with my first illness. I was never able to return to school-life again. The remainder of that summer I was weak, and very nervous frequently; had severe palpitation of the heart, and often could scarcely control my limbs and face from twitching violently, which they sometimes did in spite of me. The physicians prescribed for "nervous paroxysms," "constipation," and "general debility." I took quantities of the different preparations of iron and nervines. One medicine was to be dropped, "eighty drops every two or three hours." I knew nothing of modern glass-drop measures, and went entirely through the "dropping" ordered each time as prescribed. During the following eighteen months dyspepsia and nervousness were my prominent troubles; also obstinate constipation, occasionally having some pain at my menstrual periods, which grew somewhat irregular; but I entered into the usual duties of life, and passed for being in pretty good health.

I was married at eighteen. After marriage, nothing about my menstrual periods attracted my attention for three months, when I passed over seven weeks without them. My form grew somewhat fuller, and I craved certain articles of food. I took "Cooper's pills" at my own instigation. When the discharge made its appearance it was attended with great pain, so that I was obliged to go to bed. I felt very sick, and a physician was called — one whom I had never seen. He gave me soothing medicine, but never said what ailed me. He attended me several months, but never inquired about anything but my constipated habit, and the nervous condition of my system. The following monthly period I was able to keep out of bed by taking spirits of camphor, which he gave me, very often through the day. During that year I had severe nervous paroxysms, violent jerking of the limbs and body, especially at night. In a few months I suffered extremely with every menstrual period the first twelve or twenty-four hours.

I then went to C——, to the care of the physician who had attended at my birth, and had known me all my life. He was the first who made vaginal examination. He reported a partial "retroversion of the uterus," and said I had "ovarian tumor." I went through a long series of blisters on my spine and abdomen, purgatives, etc. I was in his care more than a year. As I could not live in the city, I was not constantly with him. I never could myself discover the slightest soreness or enlargement in the ovarian region, and wondered that I could find no evidence of the tumor. About this time I began suffering with what seemed to be rheumatism in my right limb, particularly when on my feet, or standing much. I rarely ever had it when warm or in a reclining posture.

In a year or more I grew weary of going into C——, of blistering and doctoring, and did without professional aid for a year or two. I did better without it than with it, as my general health was better. About this time, I once took chloroform to have a tooth extracted. It was with great difficulty that I was revived from its effects, and for sixteen hours I kept constantly sinking away.

I next went to R——, to a physician. He found "the uterus hardened at the neck and too low in the vagina." He first gave me a violent emetic, used electricity, had my whole body daily rubbed with No. 6, and like stimulating liniments, and put a Banning's body brace upon me. I took a great deal of macrotin, tonics, etc. His treatment, which continued several months, improved my general health more than any I had had. Yet my menstrual flow did not come right. Finally, he one day ran his fingers violently through his hair, and said "he could not see what *did* ail me."

I went home discouraged, and again did without medical aid for two years more. Indigestion, cold feet, rheumatism, attended by the whole train of disorders of the nervous system, had been, and was, my constant experience. I rarely ever had any pain in my head or spine, after the first year of my married life. A naturally gay temperament, a great love of fun, horseback riding (of which I was very fond), carriage driving, travel a part of every year, with never any very laborious household duties, probably kept me from becoming a bedridden invalid.

On removal into the city of C—— I again sought professional treatment. I had then been married six years. Faithful adherence was made to injections of rose-leaf tea, and numerous other local remedies, and a gold pessary was introduced. Finally, after nearly two years of constant treatment, it was satisfactorily discovered that I had "rheumatism of the womb." I was under the care of this physician for six years, and took a great deal of medicine—I think considerable quantities of gum guaiacum in brandy.

The year of 1865 I traveled in Europe, and some in our own country. I have always borne travel well, enjoyed it thoroughly, and fellow-travelers seldom have discovered that I was not in health.

In February, 1868, I removed to Chicago. The cutting winds affected me so that in less than three weeks I dreaded to go out of doors — they seemed to search my very bones. A thirst which could not be satisfied soon set in, and, shortly, a retention of urine, with rheumatism in my whole *right* side. I was very sleepless. The atmosphere seemed too cold for me to breathe, and I was obliged to cover both head and ears to get sleep at all. I found temporary relief in short, repeated visits to Cincinnati and Springfield, Illinois. In May I had several large carbuncles, during which my indigestion and other difficulties were much relieved. About this time I frequently felt sharp pains about my heart, and sometimes a sense of dizziness, which soon left me if I laid down for five minutes. I often would catch my breath in going about in common employments, and drew long, deep sighs in my sleep. I was nervous and wretched — and the monthly period was attended with increased suffering.

In July I went to the sea shore, as had been my custom for several years, and from which I had always returned in much more comfortable health. The weather during the journey was *exceedingly* hot, the warmest known for years. On reaching Philadelphia by a morning train, with scarcely a dry thread upon me from perspiration, I found my body covered with rash or prickly heat, which I had not seen for eighteen years. It did not wholly disappear at once. I had passed through the catamenial period just before leaving home. We reached the sea-side, and the sea-breeze was, as usual, invigorating and refreshing to me. I bathed for one week. I was very fond of swimming, but found the exercise too severe for me, and, this time, could not practice it at all. On retiring one night I found a steady pain in my left breast. I took little notice of it, supposing it to be caused by indigestion, or pleurisy. It often awakened me during the night, but by putting my hand on the spot and warming it, I dropped to sleep. Next morning I folded a flannel several thicknesses and put over it, dressed, and ate my breakfast, as usual. Soon after breakfast I was seized with the pain *most violently*, and seemingly in the region of the heart. In ten minutes I was prostrate. A mustard plaster applied increased my suffering fearfully. Dr. B., of Philadelphia, was summoned, and a young physician was present. Dr. B. at once pronounced the attack "rheumatism of the heart." The pain once suddenly went to the bladder, causing excruciating agony. A very copious discharge of urine soon followed, and the distress was again in the heart. I was relieved by aconite. In two weeks, at Dr. B.'s urgent advice, I was taken to Capon Springs, Hampshire county, Virginia. This spring is celebrated for its use in "the different forms of dyspepsia, and as a remedy in gravel its virtues are said to be unquestionable,' while externally applied in the shape of cold or warm baths, its results "are proved beneficial in rheumatism and diseases of the skin." I spent three weeks here, and my heart was entirely relieved; but, after leaving, I was again attacked, in about a week, in the city of Brooklyn. The medical attendant there never said what he thought my disease was, but "supposed my trouble proceeded from the spine." He was positive there was no disease of the heart.

All the physicians said I must not return to the climate of Chicago, so I went to my relatives in the west, to R——, where I was attended by a physician two months. There was a great deal of soreness to the touch about my heart, with constant, severe pain, and I could not endure a breath of outside atmosphere, though it was only the first of October. He said I had "angina pectoris," and "hydro-pericardium." I had noticed I suffered more with my heart about the time the menses made their appearance—generally a few hours before, and I asked him to find whether there was not something wrong in connection with the uterus, as I had had no attention to that organ for five years. He made examination and told me I "was all right there."

Suppose we recapitulate the chief points in this case, which our patient has detailed in so interesting and truthful a manner. Her first menstruation was prompt, plentiful and painless. One year later, amenorrhœa (suppressio mensium), from cold and wet feet. At sixteen inordinate appetite, the rash declining—sudden and severe illness from repercussion of the eruption, which did not reappear for many years—inveterate and inexplicable nervous symptoms. After marriage, at eighteen, menstruation normal for three months—then seven weeks' interruption—"female pills"—illness. After this, painful menstruation each month—another physician, diagnosis of retroversion with ovarian tumor—blisters—purgatives, etc., for a year—apparent rheumatism in the right limb, worse on standing, relieved by warmth and rest in the reclining posture—was a confirmed invalid at twenty, but disabled only for the first few hours of the "period"—abandoned all treatment for a year or two, and improved in consequence—another doctor; diagnosis, induration of the cervix and prolapsus—emetics, electricity, friction, an abdominal harness, macrotin tonics, etc.,—improvement of general health, but the menstrual disorder unchanged — the doctor at his wits' end — abandoned all treatment for two years more — nervous disorders continue — still another physician — two years treatment and a diagnosis of "rheumatism of the womb" — continue treatment four years more (six in all) — with a faithful trial of Dewees' prescription of guaiacum — 1865 in Europe — 1868 removed to Chicago — prairie winds in spring unfavorable — critical and salutary boils — increased cardiac trouble — rheumatism of right side — monthly symptoms worse — goes to the sea-shore in July — after a copious perspiration the eruption, which had not been seen for eighteen years, makes its appearance — cardiac paroxysms at night and next day — alternation of rheumatic pain in the heart and bladder — relief from aconite — the mineral springs improve the heart symptoms — one more doctor and another diagnosis.

The additional particulars, of clinical interest, which were given me when I took charge of this case, are the following:

About five months after her marriage she commenced passing membranous shreds, and since then has never escaped more than two consecutive "periods" without them. The size and firmness of the shreds vary at different times, but they are not larger, nor is the suffering relatively greater at the next period, after passing one month without them. The degree of pain and discomfort vary with the presence or absence of the membrane, and also with the amount of exercise taken at the time the flow commences. If she lies in bed for a day or so, there is little relative suffering. Although she had frequently spoken to her physicians of these membranes, only one had concerned himself about them, and he had decided, in an off-hand way, that they were the result of a miscarriage. None of them ever made any inquiry with respect to the character of these products, and until I procured this first specimen for microscopical examination, no one, except the patient and her husband, had ever seen them.

Upon careful inquiry, I learned that she suffered at times, usually some hours in advance of the flow, from a circumscribed pain in the right ovarian region. She could cover the spot with the tips of her three fingers. The pain would radiate somewhat, and extend thence along the limb. It was invariably worse in damp weather and after exercise.

While the cardiac symptoms were more or less constant, they were greatly aggravated at the month. Indeed, her sufferings at this time were extreme and alarming. She had discovered that aconite 2nd would relieve this distress in a very few minutes, but disliked to take it on account of unpleasant symptoms, which almost invariably followed some hours after. The chest had been most carefully wrapped in flannels. The slightest change in her clothing or exposure resulted in her taking cold and in an increase of suffering. Daily and prolonged friction, with stimulating liniments, had been resorted to in order to keep the blood in motion. The spine was exceedingly sensitive to pressure throughout its whole extent, for the relief of which porous plasters had been worn almost constantly for months.

I found the uterus so prolapsed that, unless it was supported by a sponge, pessary or tampon, which she had worn habitually for years past, she could not stand or walk. With this deviation of the womb there was more or less of strangury, which at times annoyed her exceedingly. She has never borne any children.

This case presents some striking practical facts. It illustrates that one physician, and sometimes a number of them in turn, may be deceived concerning the nature of the disease which they have been called upon to treat. It shows how the reflex and secondary phenomena dependent upon uterine disorder may mislead the practitioner; and how apt the most experienced in our ranks are to overlook the most important symptoms, while at the same time they put great stress and emphasis upon such as are merely incidental.

Membranous dysmenorrhœa is a rare affection, and, when it does exist, is very apt, as in this case, to have continued for some years before being recognized. In exceptional cases, it occurs in young girls, but is usually met with in married women. In the majority of instances it begins soon after marriage, when it is accompanied by such slight symptoms as to be deemed of little consequence. Under these circumstances, it is usually regarded as the sequence of an early abortion.

Rare—may be overlooked.

We have to confess that the special pathology of this disease is not very well known. Dewees and others have taught that it occurs most frequently in women of a rheumatic diathesis. Some authorities insist that the membranous formation, which is its chief characteristic, is always the product of conception. But this cannot be true, for it may occur in the virgin, and also in those who have for many months abstained from sexual intercourse. It is the commonly received opinion that, while in its beginning it may date from a

Causes.

miscarriage, the continuance of the complaint is not necessarily connected with conception.

Others hold that the membranous product results from uterine inflammation. Upon this theory a recent author proposes to style the disease "endometritis epithelialis." But it is not of the exfoliation of the epithelium merely that we are speaking. That may, and often does, occur in healthy menstruation. Oldham and Tilt refer the exfoliation of this membrane to the morbid influence exerted upon the lining membrane of the womb by disease of one or both of the ovaries. In rare instances, it may originate in syphilis. Sometimes it is related to a cutaneous eruption which has been repelled from the surface, with the appearance of which its symptoms seem to alternate.

Here are two excellent specimens of the membrane which this patient has expelled with the menstrual flow. Let us examine into its anatomical peculiarities. The old authors thought it to be a kind of croupous deposit upon the uterine surface. They talked wisely, as some surgeons do in our day, of the spontaneous organization of coagulable lymph into a pseudo-membrane. Dewees even suggested that these membranes might be formed from the lymph contained in the menstrual blood.

Anatomical peculiarities of the membrane.

If we compare this membrane with the decidua vera in the early weeks of pregnancy, we shall discover an exact correspondence. It is triangular, smooth within, and rough and villous on the outer surface. If the entire cast has come away, or if we can place the shreds together properly, we shall find the three orifices corresponding with the internal extremities of the Fallopian tubes, and the os internum of the uterine cervix. Moreover, here are numerous little openings through which the utricular glands have discharged their product. The microscope proves these membranes to be identical in structure. And their histological elements are precisely the same as those of the uterine mucous membrane also.

Identical with decidua vera.

It is undoubtedly true, therefore, that the decidua menstrualis, as Virchow named it, is not a new or heterologous membrane which is formed and expelled the womb at each menstrual period, but the altered lining of that cavity, which has been cast off by a species of physiological moulting.

Inflammation is accidental.

Now, inflammation is not a factor in the organization of the decidua menstrualis, any more than in that of the decidua vera, or the outer envelop of the embryo. It is, indeed, incidental to both these processes, but it is not necessary to either of them.

Oldham's theory of ovarian influence

There is, therefore, something plausible in the theory of Oldham, that ovarian influence has much to do with the frequent exfoliation of the uterine mucous membrane in this class of subjects. In case of conception, this influence undoubtedly initiates those changes which finally develop the decidua vera before the fecundated ovum has dropped into the uterine cavity. And do you not perceive that a slight perversion of function in the ovaries may induce a similar physiological change in the uterine textures as a contingent of menstruation? In the former case, the egg is retained throughout the period of gestation, and finally extruded at term. In the latter, it must escape, with its accompanying flow, as soon as practicable. In both, the deciduous wrapper is sooner or later expelled.

Its clinical confirmation.

This view has its confirmation in such clinical facts as the following: When the "period" sets in, the ovaries are often found to be swollen, tender, and the seat of discomfort. In a majority of cases there is considerable pain in one ovarian region (usually the left), which persists until after the escape of the flow, and of the shreds also. Grailly Hewitt is quite emphatic on this point and its significance:* "There is often pain in one or other ovarian region; and it appears reasonable to conclude that in some way or other this pain is connected with the formation of the membrane. The intimate functional relation between the ovaries and the uterus lends support to the view that in a morbid condition of the ovary — a functional perversion, so to speak, of its influence over the uterus — we have an explanation of this abnormal occurrence."

Clinical history.

The single pathognomonic symptom of this disease is the discharge at the menstrual period of such a membrane as is shown you in this specimen. Sometimes, although rarely, it comes away in the form of a sac, or complete cast of the uterine cavity, in which case it may be mis-

* The Diagnosis and Treatment of Diseases of Women; London, 1863; p. 479.

taken for a mole. Usually, however, it is in shreds and pieces, which vary in size from that of your thumb nail to two or three square inches. These pieces may be so regularly formed that you can place them together in such a manner as to be certain from the triangular shape of the mass, as well as from other characteristics, that the womb has been stripped of its lining membrane throughout. In some cases a very considerable quantity of this menstrual decidua is thrown of.

Shape and size of the membrane.

It may happen that this membrane will be seen but once in the same patient. Or it may be observed each month regularly in others. Sometimes it appears at alternate months, and again only once in three months. In the case which I have just detailed, my patient did not for many years pass more than two consecutive "periods" without their being present. And this under every variety of climate and external circumstance.

Regularity of its appearance.

The subjective symptoms vary in different cases. Beginning usually with a delay in the appearance of the accustomed menstrual flow, the suffering is analogous to that in an early abortus, and in other varieties of dysmenorrhœa. Subsequently it will be modified by the condition and susceptibility of the patient, as well as by the size of the membrane to be extruded, and the ease of dilatation of the cervical canal through which it must pass. Some women suffer as severely as they would in labor at term. As I have already said, the ovarian pain is seldom lacking. One of my patients finds her suffering greatly mitigated by lying in bed for one or two days when the "period" arrives. And the patient whose case is under review has remarked that, when she ate very lightly, the menstrual suffering was very much lessened. In her experience, a hasty meal taken immediately before the catamenial flow occasions extreme suffering. Scanzoni reports that two of his patients "could always say, with perfect certainty, one or two weeks before the return of the courses, whether or not they would pass membranes. Every time that this was the case they experienced for one or two weeks previously, a sharp, pinching pain in the umbilical region."

Its expulsion.

The quantity of blood discharged in such cases is in excess of that proper to healthy menstruation. This can be readily explained as the consequence of detaching the lining membrane of the womb from a sub-mucous surface which is unusually vascular. It corresponds in every way with the hæmorrhage incident to abortion prior to the formation of the placenta. Sometimes the flow is profuse and alarming, but as a rule it is held in check by the contractile efforts of the womb to dislodge and expel the membrane. When this has escaped, it usually, but not always, ceases. Where some small shreds are retained, there is danger of subsequent loss of blood. In women of an hæmorrhagic diathesis, the flow may degenerate into a passive hæmorrhage and continue during the inter-menstrual period. In case the decidua menstrualis is not cast off, but remains until the next month, as sometimes happens, the flow may be scanty in amount at one period and copious at another.

The "flow" proper.

The reflex nervous symptoms which are present in this form of dysmenorrhœa vary in different persons. In some the stomach is the focal point of disorder, and a most intractable vomiting results. Our patient has suffered from this symptom for nearly a fortnight at a time. In others, the greatest care is requisite to avoid severe fits of indigestion. A majority of these patients are habitually costive.

Reflex gastric symptoms.

If she is of a rheumatic diathesis, the cardiac symptoms may be so pronounced and so clamorous as to lead to the belief that the heart is the real seat of the difficulty. It was this state of things which induced my predecessors in the management of Mrs. ——'s case to form an incorrect diagnosis. In the frequent recurrence and severity of her paroxysms of dyspnœa, the palpitation, cardiac pain, oppression and perturbation, there were evidences of functional derangement, but of nothing more serious. The doctors must have drawn on their imagination for the physical signs of organic disease of the heart. At least, I have examined her repeatedly, and most carefully, without being able to discover any lesion of the valves, of the pericardium, the endocardium, or of the parietes of the heart. Moreover, as soon as she was put upon the remedy which was appropriate for the relief of the menstrual disorder, the cardiac symptoms vanished.

Reflex cardiac symptoms.

You should bear in mind that the remote symptomatic affections of the heart, and of other organs, which are dependent upon uterine disease of whatever variety, are invariably aggravated at the month. Indeed, in most cases, they intermit and return as regularly as the menses themselves. Independently, therefore, of the presence of the decidua menstrualis, this one circumstance would have led any one of you to infer that in this case the heart symptoms were reflex, and not idiopathic. It is true, however, that organic disease of the heart may finally result from such an indirect cause, when that cause is in almost constant operation for many years. But such cases are exceptional.

Practical deductions.

As in other forms of dysmenorrhœa so in this, uterine displacements, more especially prolapsus and retroversion, are very apt to result. In some cases the most obstinate and distressing anteversion has been caused by membranous dysmenorrhœa. Either and all of these deviations increase the difficulty and embarrass the treatment. Fibroids, polypi, metro-peritonitis, endo-metritis, and endo-cervicitis, are also coincident diseases.

Consequent uterine affections.

You would diagnosticate a case of membranous dysmenorrhœa from one of abortion, by the regular return of the monthly period, by the membrane usually coming away in shreds, or if it were entire, by the sac containing no rudiment of an embryo or of other membranes enclosed within it, and by the perforated, sieve-like appearance of the membrane itself. These symptoms, however, are not positive, for the patient might abort exactly at the first month; or, because the ovum is sometimes dissolved, the sac might be empty. But it would be quite extraordinary and unprecedented for one to abort each month regularly.

Diagnosis — from abortion.

The only danger is from concomitant disorders. The patient might possibly die from hæmorrhage, but that would be very rare. A continuous and copious loss of blood might so undermine the general health as ultimately to endanger life. Or real organic disease of the heart, lungs or stomach, or even of the brain or spinal cord, might finally develop and destroy it. In the case of patients who are approaching the climacteric, your diagnosis should be guarded. It is very probable that, could they be seen at an early date in the history of the

Prognosis.

disease, most cases would be curable. Sterility is an inevitable, but not always an incurable, consequence of membranous dysmenorrhœa.

Treatment. — The proper management of this disease will draw largely on your skill, your professional knowledge and experience, your tact, your deliberation, and your patience. You will have to consider the modifying influences of the rheumatic diathesis, of the abortive tendency, the ovarian disease, the repelled eruption, the reflex complications, and even of secondary disease in the uterus itself. There is no specific treatment which is suited to all cases of membranous dysmenorrhœa alike. An exclusive idea of its therapeutics would certainly mislead you.

General therapeutics.

Some cases of this disease are undoubtedly rheumatic, while others are not. The susceptibility of our patient to the damp, chilling prairie winds in the spring, the fugitive pains in her chest and right limb, the cardiac symptoms, and the relief afforded to all these by removal to a milder and more equable climate, betray the rheumatic complication. These and similar symptoms in one who was predisposed to rheumatism, would suggest such remedies as aconite, bryonia, rhus tox., nux vomica, mercurius and macrotin. Care should also be taken to protect the patient against the harmful influence of exposure to storms, or sudden and extreme vicissitudes of weather. She should be warmly clad, and in a measure insulated by flannel or silk wrappings. Above all things, the night air is especially injurious to this class of subjects.

Special therapeutics.

For rheumatic complications.

In a few women, the tendency to a periodical exfoliation of the uterine mucous membrane constitutes a species of dyscrasia. If these persons conceive, they are very likely to abort; and if they do not become pregnant, they are fit subjects for the disease in question. This abortive habit is a powerful predisponent of membranous dysmenorrhœa. Most of the hints which are applicable to the prevention of threatened abortion are equally appropriate here. I need not pause to detail them.

For the abortive dyscrasia.

It may happen, in exceptional cases, that the character and history of a repelled eruption will point out the proper remedy.

When this patient placed herself in charge of her last physician, she was put upon sulphur 30th, with prompt and evident relief of all her symptoms. This was prescribed on account of the chronic nature of her disease, and its manifest relation to the eruption which had been repelled. A few doses of apis mellifica 3d were then given for the ovarian pains, the urinary trouble and the cardiac symptoms, and she was finally ordered calcarea carbonica 12th, which she is now taking.

In case of repelled eruption.

In so far as the reflex symptoms are concerned, there are but very few of them that are distinctive, suggestive, or reliable. They are quite too sensational to be trustworthy. You cannot depend upon them as indicating the suitable remedy, any more than upon a majority of similar symptoms in hysteria.

Reflex symptoms irrelevant.

The ovarian lesion and its symptoms are more significant. For, in most cases, if we can recognize and remove them, we may hope to cure the menstrual disorder. Apis mellifica, calcarea carbonica, platina, belladonna, colocynth, lachesis, thuja, kali jodatum, mercurius, or hamamelis, may be appropriately and successfully employed.

For the ovarian symptoms.

Since we understand the origin and structure of the decidua menstrualis, the stereotyped advice to employ such remedies for the cure of this disease as are given in pseudo-membranous croup and diphtheria, would be of very doubtful service. For other reasons than those usually given, it is possible that in some cases the bichromate of potassa, mercurius jodatus, cantharis, ammonium causticum, or even the chloride of lime, might prove serviceable. In a case of this disease, Dr. Mandl,*, however, applied the kali chlor. directly to the uterine mucous membrane, at short intervals, for the space of ten months. The effect was to interrupt the formation of the decidual product while he continued the application, but as soon as he desisted, it was formed and expelled as before.

An antiquated prescription.

There is no evidence that local applications to the uterine sur-

* Wiener Med. Wochenschrift, No. 1, 1869.

face have ever accomplished any more in this disease than in the case just cited. The good they do is temporary, and even this is more than counterbalanced by the risk attending their application; for you may take all the precautions prescribed, and yet, as a rule, they are not safe or advisable.

Local applications are of temporary benefit.

Marriage has sometimes been prescribed as a remedy for this disease, but it is an unwarrantable expedient, and is very likely to aggravate the complaint. Conception may cure it, provided the patient can go to term. It may be indispensable to the cure that she should live absque marito. Or we may prescribe that intercourse shall take place only at long intervals.

Other expedients.

Very decided benefit may sometimes be derived from the employment of the sponge-tent, with a view to dilate and remove any obstruction of the cervix which prevents the free escape of the menstrual blood. This would cause the womb to disgorge, unload its capillaries, relieve the hyperæmia, avert an excessive hypertrophy of the mucous membrane, and possibly prevent its exfoliation. Moreover — and it is by no means an inconsiderable thing — this dilatation greatly mitigates the sufferings of the patient. I applied the tent repeatedly, and with excellent effect, in the case of which I have now spoken to you at such considerable length.

The sponge-tent.

LECTURE XI.

MENSTRUAL RETENTION A CAUSE OF UTERINE DISPLACEMENTS.

GENTLEMEN:

Dr. Rigby to the contrary notwithstanding, it is undoubtedly true that many examples of uterine displacement are referable to other causes than external violence, morbid growths, and the parturient act. Among these causes there is one which has been almost entirely overlooked. I allude to an habitual delay or retention of the menses.

Retention may increase the weight of the womb.

A patient has dysmenorrhœa. As a condition of functional activity, the uterine tissues are surcharged with blood, which moves sluggishly through them. The uterine mucous membrane has shed or secreted the menstrual product into its cavity; but this product cannot pass through the internal os uteri and the canal of the cervix. In order to empty the womb of what should escape without suffering or delay, the reflex phenomena of labor are requisite. The increase in the blood-supply, the torpidity of its circulation, and the retention of the menses within the womb, add to its volume and weight so as to drag down and displace it.

Whether the dysmenorrhœa be congestive, obstructive, ovarian, spasmodic, or membranous, the consequence is a stasis of blood, and incidental suffering and disease. The proper balance between supply and waste, whether as respects structural repair or secretory demand, is lost. Textural changes in the inferior segment of the womb and in the cervix are almost certain to follow. The infiltration of the tissue may result in induration, hypertrophy, neoplastic growths, or unnatural adhesions.

In such a case the displacement is, perhaps, active and temporary. It may alternate with almost perfect health, and return with each menstrual cycle, to be relieved by the flow. It is not unusual for patients to complain of symptoms that are due especially to prolapsus or anteversion, whenever they menstruate. Many women learn from experience that much of the suffering incident to dysmenorrhœa may be relieved by raising the hips and lowering the head. One of my patients told me that for years she had derived more comfort at such times from placing her feet upon the high foot-board of her bed, and dropping the head very low, than from anything she had ever taken internally or used locally as a palliative.

Displacements at the month.

More frequently, however, and for reasons already specified, the luxation becomes chronic. The monthly period recurs so soon that the patient has not recovered from one attack before another is precipitated upon her. It is like attempting to cure an acute gastritis while the patient continues to eat regularly and heartily of indigestible food.

May become chronic, and why.

Nor is the mere increase of weight in the womb the sole cause of the uterine deviations which are incident to dysmenorrhœa. The more decided and powerful the expulsive pains (which are designed to force the flow), the greater the liability to displacement; just as in labor at term the uterus descends in ratio with the strength and persistence of its contractile effort, and may even escape the vulva without first being delivered of its contents. And this is a veritable labor. There are the same contingents of structural change in the uterus, and of relative displacement of the organ, that attend upon abortion and full term delivery. The difference is one of degree, and not of kind.

Expulsive effort of the uterus.

Amenorrhœa (suppressio mensium) sometimes results in uterine displacement. This is especially true of those cases in which certain kinds of exposure or exercise have arrested the flow at the moment it was due. If a woman sets out for a sea voyage, or a voyage by rail, the day before her menses should appear, she will be very apt to skip one period, and perhaps more. Or, if the flow comes, she may experience greater suffering than usual. If it be too scanty, or too profuse, she may be very ill. As an indi-

Uterine displacements from temporary suppression.

rect consequence, she will be likely to suffer from some form of uterine flexion or dislocation.

There is no question but that many cases of this kind are due to such slight and apparently trivial causes. It may be as harmful and injudicious for some women to leave home on the eve of menstruation as it would be for others to go to church or to a concert when in momentary expectation of childbirth. I have known a rough ride in the carriage or upon horseback, taken at this particular period, to cause a decided prolapse of the womb. And in the nature of things, there is no reason why it might not frequently happen. According to Wright, "a displacement of the uterus is just as much an absolute fact as the occurrence of a hernial protrusion," and hernia has certainly resulted from a similar cause.

Carelessness at the month.

I do not wish to be understood as teaching that all, or even a majority of cases of uterine displacement are chargeable to menstrual obstruction or derangement. I only insist that this class of causes and their manifest consequences shall not be overlooked. The truth is that our writers and practitioners are accustomed to magnify the importance of hygiene as applied to gestation, while they make but little account of that proper to menstruation. In so far as uterine deviations are concerned, we are prone to discriminate loosely in favor of those sequelæ which may follow the parturition of the embryo and fœtus, and to discard all such as are consequent upon that of the menstrual product.

Treatment.—If this view is correct, the inference is obvious. The cure of this kind of displacement must hinge upon the relief afforded to, and the regularity of, the menstrual process. If the dislocation, of whatever variety, depends either upon dysmenorrhœa, or simple retention of the menses, the first thing to be done is to remedy the catamenial disorder. To treat the case simply as a diaplacement, and to expect to cure it by any universal expedient whatever, whether local or internal, will be unsatisfactory and unsuccessful. Emmenagogues would only increase the difficulty. And so also would astringents. The pessary would be of no more service in such a case than a hernial truss. Indeed, it might prove as harmful in a displacement arising from this cause as it has been beneficial in others.

The indication is to cure the menstrual disorder.

This theory explains the wonderful efficacy of some of our remedies, when prescribed for the relief of uterine luxations. Through their manifest and well known relation to the menstrual function, we have learned to rely upon them for the cure of those displacements of the womb that are consequent upon certain derangements of that function. In other words the key to their curative range and adaptability is found in their power to remove the condition upon which the disorder of place depends. From the provings alone we might never have learned what we already know empirically, logically and physiologically, of the power of certain remedies indirectly to influence the position and relations of this very important organ.

Modus operandi of some remedies for prolapsus, etc.

There is an excellent and harmless auxiliary which can be used in some of these cases to great advantage. I allude to the sponge tent, which by removing the mechanical cause of the retention, may relieve the difficulty and help to cure the displacement. I am not aware that others have recommended this instrument in any form of uterine luxation. But it is a temporary, non-medicinal, unobjectionable expedient, which can be employed without risk, and in such a manner as to secure the free exit of the menstrual fluid as soon as it is poured into the uterine cavity. It certainly does not interfere with the action of internal remedies, nor will it, if properly applied, give rise to any lesion of the cervix. It promotes the painless and gradual dilatation of the internal os, obviates suffering, and averts the reflex symptoms of which the patient is so apt to complain. It does not lift the womb directly, but ministers to its reposition by unloading its vessels, so that it can retract. It should be introduced from twelve to twenty-four hours in advance of the menstrual period. At this time the internal os is "off-guard," and the operation is less painful and more successful. It should be allowed to remain in for from four to eight or ten hours according to circumstances. When it is removed, the patient should keep to the bed or sofa, and not be allowed to stand upon her feet for some hours, or even, perhaps, for days.

The sponge tent a useful auxiliary.

It is a singular and significant fact that cases of dysmenorrhœa which merge into menorrhagia are rarely followed by uterine deviations of any kind. It is only when the absolute loss of blood causes extreme atony of all the utero-vaginal tissues that such a result is witnessed.

UTERINE COLIC.

Case. — Mrs. —— sent for me in haste, on account of her sudden illness. She had reached home from a long journey, and in perfect health, only an hour before. After a general bath, she took a vaginal injection of cool water, and, almost immediately, felt a sharp, spasmodic pain in the region of the womb. This pain increased in severity, and, before my arrival, became almost insupportable. It would remit, and then return with redoubled violence. I found her pale, with a cool surface, an anxious, imploring expression of countenance, and a slight nausea. She was midway in the inter-menstrual period, and had not eaten anything unusual, or, indeed, anything whatever, for some hours.

A clinical lecture without a practical lesson would resemble a sermon without a moral one. There is a point in this case which you should carry home with you. It is this, that there are certain conditions of the womb and other pelvic viscera in which the shock of an otherwise harmless injection thrown into the vagina may work mischief. Whatever determines the blood to these organs increases the risk of using such an expedient suddenly, and, as it were, without proper warning and delay. A woman has been at work with a sewing machine for some hours consecutively. Having finished her task, she takes a bath, and directly afterwards a vaginal enema. Almost immediately she is seized with symptoms resembling those from which my patient suffered. Or a similar result may follow a ride on horseback, or in the carriage, a game of croquet, standing for an hour or two at an evening party, too long a walk, a protracted lesson at the piano, or, as in this case, a fatiguing journey, all of which acts predispose to irritable conditions of the uterus. Under these circumstances there is an exalted sensibility of the organ, and it may happen that a single injection of cool water brought into contact with it suddenly will act as an exciting cause of pain and disease.

Vaginal injections sometimes injurious.

The same is true of cool or cold injections per vaginam before the menstrual flow has entirely ceased. And likewise also of similar injections taken immediately after coitus, with a view to prevent impregnation. At such periods the capillary system of the whole generative intestine is surcharged with blood. If we wait a little, this physiological afflux is removed, the erection of the organs subsides, and the proper vascularity is restored. But if we shock the delicate structures in the manner of which I have spoken, we must expect that, sooner or later, they will become diseased in consequence.

Symptoms.

In uterine colic the pain usually intermits. Sometimes the paroxysm returns with almost as much regularity as the after-pains which torment multiparæ, and which it is said to resemble. Or it may remit and not leave entirely between the more aggravated periods. The suffering is referred directly to the uterine region, although it sometimes radiates into the sacrum, and again into one or both groins. It is characteristic of this pain that it may be in a measure and sometimes entirely relieved by pressure. The attack commences and terminates abruptly, and is not preceded or accompanied by any particular constitutional symptoms, as chill or fever. There is more or less of tympanites, which develops very rapidly and disappears as suddenly. There is usually considerable intestinal flatulence, distension and pressure. This bloating of the abdomen has all the characteristics of hysterical tympanites. Nausea is a frequent symptom in severe cases.

Duration of the attack.

The attack may continue for a few minutes only, or may extend through some hours, or even days. If it depends, as it sometimes does, upon uterine displacement, it may not subside until the organ is restored. If it is due to the presence of coagula, or other foreign bodies in utero, it will only cease with their expulsion. In this case the pains resemble cramps, are expulsive, and labor-like.

Incident to dysmenorrhœa.

Women who are subject to dysmenorrhœa are likely to have a mild form of uterine colic upon slight provocation. Such persons may be seized with it while walking in the street, and be obliged to sit down or bend themselves almost double for a few moments, until the paroxysm passes off. Or the pain may be so severe as to cause fainting and great alarm.

Incident to hysteria.

Emotional causes often give rise to it in hysterical persons. With this class of patients a fit of anger or jealousy may bring on the attack at almost any time. Or it may precede menstruation and worry the patient for some hours or days in advance of the flow. Although usually amiable, she will become petulant, is disgusted with and distrustful of humanity in general, and of the male sex in particular. Sometimes she is in a mellow or pathetic mood, or she has a fitful religious melancholy, or, what is still worse, is possessed with the insane idea to work, to set her room to rights, and the plants, the birds, the books, the pictures, stoves, chairs and furniture must be squared up and cleaned up instanter. She must do an immense amount of work in a short time, and only in so doing can avoid this tormenting species of colic and ill feeling in the uterine region. After which, when the flow sets in, she is exhausted, fitful, capricious, cross, tempestuous, drums on the piano by the hour, or writes explosive letters to her husband, or friends, and regulates everything with the utmost irregularity.

May precede menstruation.

Extraordinary fatigue of body or mind may induce it. Intellectual, cultivated women, are more prone to it than others. Seamstresses, young ladies in boarding-schools, actresses, and those whose minds are harassed with family cares, or who are victims of the social fret and friction which wear out so many valuable lives, suffer much from this painful disorder.

Most frequent among intellectual women.

Not unfrequently it arises from incompatibility in the marriage relation. Circumstances which develop a loathing of the sexual act, are very apt to produce it. It may originate either from immoderate indulgence, or from being deprived of accustomed intercourse. I have known it to be caused by drinking ice-water while menstruating.

Uterine colic is also incident to the neuralgic diathesis. It may alternate, or be complicated with ovarian neuralgia, hysteralgia, and even with rheumatism of the womb. In women who are thus predisposed, whatever causes an irritable state of the uterus may bring on an attack of the colic. This form of the disease is very apt to seize upon nervous and delicate patients during the period of pregnancy.

In neuralgic subjects.

Treatment.— Proper hygienic precautions will doubtless suggest themselves to your minds. You should warn the patient of the possible consequences of vaginal injections at improper times. And also of the ill effects of rude and violent exercise, whether of body

Hygienic and prophylactic.

or mind. If she is intelligent — and your merits will commend you to this class of patients especially — explain the modus operandi of those very common causes of disease and suffering among women. One good, logical reason will have better and more lasting effect upon her than any amount of scolding and fault-finding. A good prophylactic is to have the patient wear an extra layer of flannel, silk, or cotton batting over the abdomen habitually.

Various palliatives have been recommended to put an end to the paroxysm. Among the more ordinary and available of these is the application of towels or flannels that have been dipped in hot water, mustard water, hot brandy and water, and the like. In some cases, a sinapism will cause the pain to vanish in a very few minutes. Bags of hot salt, or of dry bran heated thoroughly, are especially useful in case of menstrual colic, and of uterine colic following abortion. In hysterical subjects, the ether spray may be thrown upon the hypogastrium. In inveterate cases, the vapor of chloroform has been injected into the vagina. Dr. Simpson advised a similar application of carbonic acid gas. When complicated, as it sometimes is, with vaginismus, I am in the habit of prescribing a vaginal injection consisting of chloroform one drachm, olive oil and glycerine each two ounces. Or the same may be applied by means of a cotton tampon. If the attack is incident to delayed menstruation, the warm sitz-bath may afford the desired relief.

Palliatives.

In the majority of cases, belladonna or atropine answers every purpose. This is especially true if the attack has been caused by the shock from vaginal injections taken at improper times. If the case is manifestly neuralgic, and more particularly if it is complicated with ovarialgia, the valerianate of zinc may be indicated.

Internal remedies.

Other remedies are colocynth, ignatia, caulophyllin, cocculus, chamomilla, nux vomica, pulsatilla, sabina, and secale cornutum.

POST-PARTUM ULCERATION OF THE WOMB.

Although ulceration of the womb is not usually classed among the sequelæ of labor, there is little doubt but that it sometimes occurs in this connection.

Case. — Mrs. ——, aged 28, has an infant five months old. She nurses the child, which is thrifty, and lives exclusively upon the breast. The mother is not well. She has not menstruated since her confinement. She complains of aching in the loins, weariness on very slight exertion, pain in the left iliac region, with inability to lie upon her left side, malaise, anorexia, frequent headache, occasional strangury, and a leucorrhœa which at times weakens her very much and increases the old pain in the back. These symptoms began during her lying-in, and have continued until now.

An examination with a speculum discloses a simple suppurating ulcer within and around the external os uteri.

When uterine ulceration occurs in women who have but recently been confined, it is very apt to be overlooked. The patient may have escaped the perils of childbirth, but for some unknown reason she has a lingering convalescence. At first there may have been a considerable degree of puerperal inflammation, and following this a state of things analogous to what Trousseau styles "colliquative suppuration." Lactation, is, perhaps, normal, and the other functions are intact, but she is extremely weak and reduced, and rallies but slowly. A month or two may have passed before she is able to make an excursion to the dining-room, or the parlor, and three, or even six months before she can take a drive. Meanwhile she has lost her accustomed elasticity, and life is become a burden. She drags around, impelled by circumstances, and the probabilities are that her ill health will be charged to some other cause than the ulceration, which dates from the birth of her child.

Likely to be overlooked.

In such a case the lesion of the os is undoubtedly a result of the inflammatory process. After delivery the uterine tissues readily become inflamed. This inflammation is often, but not always, of such a low grade and type as to develop into ulceration. And once the ulcerative metamorphosis is begun, it is likely to be overlooked and perpetuated. It is altogether probable that pressure upon the cervix, and traumatic injuries thereof during the labor, may indirectly occasion such symptoms as those of which our patient complains.

A sequel of inflammation.

If there were anything distinctive in these symptoms, they would be more easily and generally recognized. But, in a given case, we cannot know positively that a lesion of the cervix exists without ocular examination. Here the speculum is as requisite a means of diagnosis as if the disease were idiopathic, and did not follow parturition.

There are two general causes for this species of uterine ulceration, or, rather, for ulceration of the cervix, occurring in women at this particular period. The first is the drain upon the mother's blood during gestation; and the second, a similar drain through the mammary glands while she is nursing. By impairing the quality of the blood, and thus lowering the grade of vitality, these causes increase the risk of post-partum inflammation. And in such depraved states of the system there is but a short step from inflammation to ulceration of the uterine neck. The same remark applies to ulceration as a sequel of abortion, more especially after the fourth month.

Impaired quality of the blood.

Treatment. — The hint which I have just given you concerning the relation between the depraved and impoverished condition of the blood and the symptoms complained of, is of great practical significance. Acting upon it, you would prescribe the proper hygienic regulations. If you are satisfied that there is too much of waste and expense to the mother's organism in the quantity of milk that she furnishes, it is better to feed the child with something else than to bankrupt the mother's strength in this manner. Weaning is a last resort. It is not necessary, except in extreme cases, and where the quality of the milk is such that the child is finally poisoned by it.

Weaning the child.

The diet should be as nourishing as possible. Allow milk, lean meats, eggs, game, fruits, and good bread and butter, instead of the sick-room teas, slops and kindred abominations. Fresh air and sunlight should also be ingredients in the prescription. But let me caution you to remember that walking may be very harmful, in case of uterine ulceration, and for this reason, the womb being pendulous when the patient walks, the denuded cervix is brought into contact with different portions of the vaginal mucous membrane. Friction irritates it, and excites the local circulation to such a degree as greatly to increase the suffering, and to extend the lesion. Moreover, the blood gravitates into the pelvic organs, and the consequent congestion more than counterbalances the good effect of the out-door air and exercise.

The diet.

Walking.

Riding is less objectionable, but I have observed that many patients with uterine ulceration complain seriously of the street-cars, the stopping and starting, as well as the roughness of which, worry them more than riding in the stages on the avenue, or in a private conveyance, if it be carefully driven. You would not send such patients to ride in a rough country wagon, neither upon horseback.

Riding.

Compared with ordinary cases of uterine ulceration, the post-partum variety may be more easily and promptly cured. The explanation of this fact is to be found in the exemption of the menstrual return, which so much retards the cure under different circumstances. Here is no periodical determination of blood to the womb. In lieu thereof we have a physiological afflux of blood to the mammary glands, which is really derivative in its influence upon the intra-pelvic organs. For this reason, the proper treatment should not be deferred, else the menses will re-appear, and the cure be very much delayed in consequence.

Cure comparatively easy, and why.

It sometimes happens that the too early return of the menses in one who is nursing is an evidence of debility and of waning strength. It may signify that the mother's force and vitality are fast ebbing away. Much will depend upon a proper interpretation of the symptoms in such a case, and upon the line of treatment which you adopt.

Menstruation during lactation.

There are those who insist upon the necessity of cauterization in every form of uterine ulceration. They cannot divest themselves of the idea that such lesions are removed from the sphere of influence of internal remedies. They argue, and with some show of reason, that there is a lack of responsiveness on the part of the tissues which compose the uterine cervix to the best selected constitutional treatment. Some even go so far as to insist that no such ulcer can be healed except by topical applications, among the best of which are the various escharotics.

Indiscriminate and exclusive local treatment.

But many physicians are in the habit of treating ulceration of the mucous membrane and of the integument by means of internal remedies exclusively. The various forms of stomatitis, ulcerated sore throat, chronic laryngitis, and bronchitis, typhoid fever, chronic enteritis, typhlitis and dysentery, yield to this method of medication. If in any of the three former affections they consent to apply the caustic, it is an exceptional case; while, in the latter, it would be altogether impracticable to do so.

Only *specific* ulceration needs specific local treatment.

A large proportion of cases of external ulcer need nothing more topically than to be protected from the irritating influence of the atmosphere by some bland and harmless application. In some cases we may facilitate the healing process in them by the local use of the same remedy that is given internally; but, excepting in specific ulcers, not one in a thousand of them needs cauterization. So in ulceration of the os uteri — when there is no specific reason, either in the nature of the lesion, or in its cause and symptoms, why some specific remedy, as for example the nitrate of silver, or iodine, or what not, should be applied locally, your good sense and judgment would dictate their prohibition.

Arguments pro and con.

It has been argued in advocacy of the indiscriminate local treatment of uterine induration and ulceration, that a spontaneous cure thereof was impossible, because of the frequent return and concomitants of the menstrual flow, the dependent position of the uterus, and the evil consequences of sexual excitement. But it does not follow that, because these cases do not get well of themselves, therefore they all need to be cauterized. It is bad practice to prescribe at wholesale.

Interdiction of coitus.

In the case before you the menstrual aggravation is not present. The peculiar position of the womb does not so strongly predispose to its vascular derangement, or to the perpetuation of a chronic lesion unless the woman menstruates, or its tissues are undergoing the changes which are proper to gestation. In serious cases of ulceration of the womb, the worst consequences may follow a frequent repetition of the sexual act. Such a patient should live apart from her husband. A large share of the benefit attributed to the local treatment of uterine ulceration by caustics of all kinds should really be ascribed to the necessary interruption of the marital intercourse, which is thus rendered impossible. The same is true, but in a qualified sense, of the advantage claimed for change of air, etc., by those who leave their homes and husbands behind them, to seek for treatment elsewhere.

You will not understand me as objecting to every variety of local application in simple ulceration of the os uteri. Such an extreme view would be as untenable as that which holds that such means, and only such, are absolutely requisite and curative. There is no valid objection to the topical employment of diluted glycerine, with or without the calendula, of sweet oil, or of the oleaginous collodion in the case of this poor woman. Either of these substances will be grateful to the diseased part, will serve to protect it from the injurious effects produced by contact of the vaginal mucus and the leucorrhœal discharge, and will also stimulate the reparative process whereby the lesion can be healed. The calendula is especially useful where the purulent or muco-purulent flow, as in this case, is very considerable. It may be used as a vaginal injection morning and evening.

Allowable local treatment.

The internal remedies that may be required will vary with the symptoms presented in each individual case. Chief among them are calendula, calcarea carb, arsenicum, sepia and sulphur.

LECTURE XII.

STOMATITIS MATERNA: NURSING SORE MOUTH.

GENTLEMEN:

This is one of the most interesting, as well as vexatious diseases with which we are acquainted. It is interesting because of its limited history and prevalence, its peculiar pathology, its mortality under the old regime, and the imperfect development of its therapeutics; vexatious, because of its multiplied forms and complications, and its intractable nature, if not modified and remedied by appropriate means.

Nature.—Concerning the essential nature of this malady, various opinions have been, and are still, entertained by the profession at large. The most plausible of these, we apprehend, is that which refers its phenomena to a scorbutic cachexia. It has been convenient for the majority of medical men to attribute its origin to miasmatic influences; to a diminution of the red corpuscles of the blood; to scrofula; to menstrual irregularities, antecedent to conception; to a depraved and insufficient nourishment, and the like; but the best writers incline to the opinion that this catalogue embraces only the crude outline of its causes and consequences, while it leaves the radical nature of the malady itself an open question.

Theories of its origin.

That it is of scorbutic origin is evident, from the following considerations:

First; its causes are such as tend to derangements of nutrition and assimilation.

Second; it is invariably accompanied by anæmia.

Third; except in degree of violence, many of its symptoms are identical with those of the scurvy.

Fourth; the same dietetic regulations are requisite to cure the one as the other. Both demand a pabulum largely composed of vegetables, and of vegetable acids especially.

Fifth; they are alike mortal under treatment by excessive and improper medication, as by mercurials, quinine, etc.; and this fatality is induced by an identical process of disintegration of the tissues, in which their elements are forced to remain, without elimination, as abnormal constituents of the blood.

Sixth, those remedies which are most valuable in stomatitis materna, are also such as are most successfully employed against scorbutus.

Peculiarities.—The stomatitis materna has the following characteristics; It is peculiar to females, and of those to women during the term of utero-gestation, or at some period of lactation. A few writers, indeed, claim to have witnessed examples of this disease in males; but as a rule, one would as readily anticipate attacks of "morning sickness," among the latter sex (rare cases of which do indeed occur), as of this particular variety of stomatitis; and in what follows, we are therefore to declare, and to keep in view the essential characteristics aforenamed.

Limited to gestation and lactation.

Symptoms.—These may be properly classed into local and general.

The local symptoms of the stomatitis materna are not subject to a regular order of development, but vary with each particular example of the disease. Their more usual approach, however, is as follows: The patient calls attention to a burning or scalding sensation in the mouth, which sensation is greatly aggravated by the taking of warm, or even of cold drinks, and by efforts to masticate her food. Upon inspection, the physician remarks a fiery, red appearance of the mouth, which redness is found to exist in patches, or diffused more or less continuously over the whole buccal surface. Sometimes this eruption is isolated, presenting the appearance of ulcerated tubercula of the size of a pea, less or more. Again the aforesaid patches attain the diameter of a quarter of a dollar, when they may degenerate into ragged and indolent ulcers, thus constituting the worst examples of the disease which are to be met with, and which frequently spring from chronic neglect, or from that still more deplorable cause—a dyscrasia induced by drugs that have been ignorantly prescribed for their removal.

Peculiar lesion.

With this local inflammation, whether it be diffused or isolated, deep-seated or superficial, there are other symptoms which are equally characteristic. Among these there will be found a marked pallor of the surface, resembling chlorosis; a sad and dejected expression of the countenance; soft, flabby muscles, while the rotundity of the form remains as in health; anorexia, pyrosis, and other disorders of digestion; a profuse flow of saliva; the tongue is red and smooth; cutting and colicky pains from the simplest ingesta; alternations of constipation and diarrhœa; strangury, with strong and scalding urine, which is acid to test paper; palpitation, especially troublesome at night; the secretions are generally normal, the skin soft, but without any sensible perspiration; and, if during lactation, a decided sympathy between the child and its parent, whereby it is discovered to have inherited thus early, some of her more immediate and palpable frailties.

Incidental symptoms.

Chronic cases are likely to be accompanied by a diarrhœa which is chargeable to an extension of the specific inflammation to the middle and inferior portions of the alimentary mucous membrane. This symptom is frequently a very perplexing one, as well on account of the increased emaciation and debility which it occasions the general system, as because of its intractable nature, as shown in its alternating with the mouth symptoms, being better when they are worse, and vice versa.

In these examples, it is not unusual to discover that all the mucous membranes lining the different interior surfaces of the body partake of this inflammation. Thus the inner coats of the larynx, the trachea, and of the lungs, of the pharynx, œsophagus, and of the whole alimentary tract, as well as of the vagina and urethra, are sometimes found to be separately or universally involved. Hence result great disturbances of function, nutrition, etc.; for the destruction of the epithelial scales which marks the invasion of this disease upon local surfaces, interferes very materially with the healthy condition and requirements of those organs which are indirectly but more seriously implicated.

The foregoing symptoms are liable to so frequent modification, both in the order of their succession and in their severity, that authors have fancifully described some three to five distinct varieties of the nursing sore-mouth, for which classification, practically speaking, there would appear to be no real necessity. We shall, however, consider a few of them separately.

Of the buccal symptoms: These are the primary and more palpable symptoms of the stomatitis materna. There is very little question, however, but that these local phenomena are symptomatic of a more profound disturbance of the general organism; and that, properly speaking, we are to regard them as the certain evidence of some such original disorder. Examples are not wanting in which this disease is believed to have pursued a latent course in the system, during which interval, for a greater or less period of time prior to the development of these symptoms, it has sapped the strength and impaired the functional processes of the economy.

A constitutional disease.

Indeed there is every reason to believe that those cases of digestive and assimilative disorder, incident to utero-gestation, which distress and harass the patient exceedingly while carrying the fœtus, and which, subsequent to her confinement, will not unfrequently result in a manifestation of the above local symptoms, are to be referred solely to the existence of a latent stomatitis from the beginning. These examples are perhaps as infrequent as they are invincible, but in the practical experience of those physicians whose opinions are of value, the remark will hold good that it is only through a close and careful study that we may come to appreciate the worth of this class of symptoms, as affording us an index at once to their pathology and treatment.

The peculiar characters which such symptoms present are found to vary with the severity and duration of the complaint. In very mild cases the eruption assumes more of an erythematous appearance, being diffused in patches over the sides of the tongue and of the cheeks. Or it may consist of common vesicles, resembling the aphthæ adultorum of some writers, which vesicles ultimately degenerate into more or less troublesome centers of infection, each showing at its base a hardened and whitish colored ring. These indurations terminate either by cicatrization or ulceration. To this form of the complaint the name of follicular stomatitis has been given, for the reason that the peculiar eruption finds its more frequent seat in the mucous follicles of the mouth.

In bad cases, when these vesicles burst, they develop into ulcers, which are either superficial or deep-seated. If the system has been very much depraved, and the vitality runs low, these ulcers may be very numerous and of large size. You will find them located on the sides or upon the

The local ulceration.

upper surface of the tongue, upon its frænum, on the frænum of the lower lip, on the gums, the cheeks, or the roof of the mouth, and even in the throat and fauces. They are painful in proportion to the extent of the raw surface which is exposed, and to the depth of the ulceration. In exceptional instances these ulcerations have dipped down to the bone beneath.

Capricious nature of the lesion.

It is not unusual for these characteristic lesions to disappear suddenly, leaving the patient in apparent health. After a brief interval, however, they reappear, and may thus keep coming and going for weeks, or even for months. In the most serious cases this sudden metastasis increases the danger, by implicating other and more vital organs.

Incidental gastric disorder.

Symptoms of gastric or alimentary disorder almost always accompany those peculiar to this variety of sore-mouth. They may precede, follow or alternate with the buccal symptoms, but are rarely altogether absent. I have seldom treated a case of this form of stomatitis, during either pregnancy or lactation, which was not accompanied by epigastric uneasiness, anorexia, or pyrosis. Instances in which this disease runs its course without a more or less decided implication of the stomach and bowels are believed to be very rare.

In this respect the stomatitis materna resembles the aphthæ of infants which, as you are aware, is almost invariably accompanied by intestinal derangement, more especially indigestion and diarrhœa.

Causes of the digestive derangement.

The concurrent digestive disorder in this variety of sore-mouth has been attributed to various causes, among which are the imperfect mastication of food; an improper and unwholesome diet; the actual transfer, or the continuation, of the local lesion to the gastric and enteric mucous membrane; to a depraved nutrition from other causes, and to glandular disease either in the intestine or the mesentery, or both.

Diarrhœa.

Among the numerous contingencies of pregnancy and parturition there are few which are more troublesome than an inveterate diarrhœa. This is especially true in patients of a scrofulous or tuberculous diathesis. And it is this class of subjects which is most liable to be seized with it after labor. When complicated with stomatitis the diarrhœa may either anticipate or follow the symptoms already enumerated. More frequently, however, it alternates with them — a fact which implies a metastasis of the peculiar disorder from the oral to the intestinal mucous membrane.

Disordered digestion and assimilation are, therefore, almost certain to exist in well-marked cases of stomatitis materna. Not unfrequently they are the source of well-grounded apprehension, and, if ever so slight, they will occasion you no little anxiety. You should bear in mind, however, that the coincident diarrhœa is but a symptom, and that its essential pathology is the same as that of the buccal erythema, eruption, and ulceration.

Renal and vesical symptoms.

Beside local suffering in the mouth, the patient may complain also of a troublesome strangury, with smarting or scalding sensations during, or immediately after urinating. Occasionally these symptoms precede those already enumerated. Sooner or later they are almost certain to be present, and when they are not mentioned voluntarily, you will learn, upon inquiry, that they really exist.

The urine is most commonly acid in its reaction — a symptom reputed by some authorities to be pathognomonic of this variety of stomatitis. Its specific gravity will vary from 1024 to 1030.

The anæmia.

For the most part, the general symptoms are such as imply a debility which may be extreme. If the disease has existed for any considerable time, the patient is usually anæmic. She is pallid and exhausted, and the face appears puffy and bloated. Her complexion is less waxy and clear than in chlorosis, but has a sallow and cadaverous shade in it, which is not common in other diseases.

These symptoms are likely to be accompanied by an irritative fever which may remit regularly and finally develop into a real hectic. It is said that primiparæ are more liable than multiparæ to this form of stomatitis. With certain women it appears to be constitutional, and always recurs during pregnancy or lying-in. The milk furnished by the breast may be either deficient or excessive in quantity. Not unfrequently it is of such quality as to poison the child and render it sickly and short-lived.

Wherever it may be located, authorities are not agreed as to whether the anæmia in this disease is the cause or the consequence of the local inflammation and ulceration. The simple fact that it is limited to the periods of gestation and lactation, when the blood is being drained of certain elements for the support of the young, and that, as a rule, it ceases as soon as the child is born, or weaned, suggests that the anæmia must have preceded the local lesion. And such is the case. The woman may have been in ill-health for a considerable time before the sore mouth commenced. This primary impairment of the quality of the blood explains the greater liability of young, scrofulous, weakly and sickly persons, as well as of those whose systems have been reduced by frequent child-bearing, to the disease under consideration. It also affords a reason for the more general prevalence and malignity of this disease in miasmatic districts, and in those localities and seasons in which there is a scarcity of fruits and vegetables, and where, as a consequence, the stomatitis degenerates into a species of "land scurvy."

Is it cause or effect?

We can not otherwise explain the migratory character of the disease, its tendency to invade the pharynx, the œsophagus, and the gastro-intestinal tract, the respiratory apparatus, the nasal passage, the Eustachian tube, and even the genito-urinary outlet. In the order of its occurrence therefore, the anæmia is doubtless the first visible sign of the impaired nutrition upon which the stomatitis really depends, and without which it can not exist.

This form of stomatitis may commence in the early, the middle, or the latter months of gestation, and persist to term or even later. Or it may date from delivery, from the first month of nursing, or perhaps later and continue for an indefinite period. In very rare cases it exists in the form of pruritus of the vulva during pregnancy, and after child-birth develops into stomatitis proper.

Onset of the disease.

Diagnosis. — The diagnosis is not difficult. The sex of the subject and the peculiar circumstances in which she is found — either pregnant, or in one or another of the stages of recovery from her confinement,—with the local symptoms already detailed, will enable you to diagnosticate it readily. It is only when this disease is obscure and runs a latent course, being limited to the gastric, alimentary, or urinary

It may be latent.

mucous membranes, that you would be likely to overlook it, or fail to distinguish it from other similar and serious affections.

Prognosis.—The prognosis will vary with the original strength of the patient's constitution; her age, habits and surroundings; the co-existence of tuberculosis of the lungs, or of the mesenteric glands; the period of the commencement, and the duration of the disorder; the type and persistence of the accompanying fever; the seat, nature and extent of the local lesion; the anæmia and the emaciation.

Qualifying circumstances.

If, prior to becoming pregnant, the patient was robust and healthy, and had no cachexy, either hereditary or acquired, the probabilities are in favor of her recovery. This result is the more certain if she is young, of good habits, and lives in a healthy neighborhood. A tendency to phthisis in any of its forms is always a grave complication. If the stomatitis commences in the early months of gestation, it can seldom be cured before delivery, and other things equal, the longer its duration prior to labor the greater the danger. In rare cases it results in abortion, after which it ceases spontaneously.

If the accompanying fever is either typhoid or hectic in its type and character, you will need to qualify your prognosis. And so also if the disease has become chronic, with deep-seated ulceration in the intestines, the stomach, or the larynx and trachea. The occurrence of passive, or repeated, or excessive hæmorrhage from the mucous surface implies great danger. The more the blood is impoverished and vitiated, and the greater the emaciation and the muscular and nervous exhaustion, the fewer the chances of a speedy and certain recovery. It is sometimes quite impossible to eradicate this disease in the case of women who have had it in several successive pregnancies. Although recovery frequently follows the weaning of the child, yet even this expedient sometimes fails. The danger is increased by excessive or prolonged medication.

Treatment.—The first thing to be done is to select a suitable diet. This consists of a proper admixture of vegetable and animal food, for you will observe that in many cases the patient has lived almost exclusively upon meat. In frontier settlements, people sometimes eat little or nothing excepting bread and bacon. In such communities the

The diet.

women suffer from an aggravated form of the nursing sore-mouth, which is closely allied to scorbutus, and which may sometimes be cured by merely regulating the diet. Even in towns ana cities similar cases are not infrequent.

The taking of solids is usually so painful that food must be given either in the semi-solid or fluid form. If, however, she can eat it, rare roast beef or mutton, or broiled meats which are juicy and nutritious, may be prescribed with good effect. She may also have milk, eggs, oysters, game, plain custards, animal jellies, cracked wheat, oatmeal, or, if she prefers, a little codfish with cream. Salt food may be permitted as an appetizer, but should be used sparingly. Potatoes, carrots, tomatoes, baked apples, and other fruits and vegetables, if fresh and fully ripe, are not only permissible but indispensable. Cures have been effected by allowing the patient to drink freely of butter-milk.

Acidulated drinks.

Other acidulated drinks are almost specific. Lemonade, orangeade, and jelly-water, are most available. They may be taken either warm or cold, as the patient prefers, and are not contra-indicated in most cases of indigestion and diarrhœa. Nor will they antidote the proper remedies. The best criterion, in their selection, is to consult the patient's preference, or craving, if she has any. The same is true with respect to the diet. As a rule, you may let her have whatever she longs for in the way of food or drink, providing it is not wholly indigestible or absolutely poisonous. The malt liquors and cod-liver oil have also been added to the bill of fare.

Rule for choosing them.

Expedients for arresting this disease.

The expedients devised to check this disease, and to hold it in abeyance, and which are sometimes successful, are the induction of premature labor, the weaning of the child, and a change of climate.

Premature labor.

The induction of premature labor is justifiable only in those extreme cases of stomatitis in which it is morally certain that the patient must die unless pregnancy is terminated and the womb emptied of its contents. Fortunately such an extremity is almost never reached prior to the seventh month of pregnancy, after which the child is viable. In a resort to this expedient under such circumstances there is no warrant for the performance of criminal abortion, which implies and includes the intentional sacrifice of the fœtus.

Because taking the child from the breast of the mother who has stomatitis will sometimes be of immediate and lasting benefit to her, physicians have inferred that weaning was the best remedy. The custom with some is to prescribe it indiscriminately. So soon as they discover the slightest inflammation and exfoliation of the oral mucous membrane, further nursing is prohibited. But weaning will not always mitigate or arrest this disease. Nor is it necessary to resort to this expedient in a majority of the cases that come under our care. Unless it is manifest that the mother is pretty nearly bankrupt in strength and nutritive resource, that she is drawing her life away to keep her child alive, that she is so anæmic and emaciated as to be totally unfit both on her own and the infant's account to nurse it any longer, we prefer not to interrupt this very important function.

Weaning the child.

A change of climate, especially if the patient leaves a miasmatic district, will sometimes cause the symptoms of this disease to disappear promptly and permanently. In exceptional cases a removal of a few miles only will work almost as marked a change in her feelings as it does in certain cases of asthma and of intermittent fever. This expedient is particularly applicable if the stomatitis is complicated with chronic bowel affections. Railway travel is indicated if there is an inveterate diarrhœa, and residence in an equable climate for those mothers who are consumptive. Hysterical subjects, with the nursing sore-mouth, may sometimes be sent away from home with the greatest relief to themselves and all concerned.

Change of climate.

The medical treatment of this disorder is constitutional and local. Of internal remedies, the various acids are in the best repute. The nitric acid has been given in the lower and higher potencies, under almost every variety of indications, and often empirically, with good results. The sulphuric and muriatic acids are equally useful. I remember a case in which two prominent physicians had treated a lady for stomatitis materna for two whole months. She grew worse and worse. Finally they told her that she must wean her infant, and that after doing so she could not recover her health under at least one year. I made her but

The medical treatment.

The various acids.

three visits, ordered a nutritious diet, and prescribed sulphuric acid in the third decimal dilution to be taken four times daily. She continued the remedy for the space of a fortnight. A radical cure followed, without weaning the child, or the employment of any local application whatever. My practice is to put twenty-five drops of the second or third attenuation of either of these acids in half a glass of water, of which two teaspoonfuls are to be taken once in from three to six hours.

Case.

Arsenicum is generally suitable for cases of this form of stomatitis which are to be met with in malarious districts. If there is burning in the mouth, with frequent desire for cold drinks; if the water which the patient drinks habitually is stagnant or impregnated with decomposing matter of various kinds; if there is great prostration of strength, anorexia, with chronic disorder of digestion and painless diarrhœa; if the system has been poisoned with quinine in large doses, or if the accompanying symptoms are analogous to those of typhoid fever, it may prove of excellent service. The same indications will call for natrum muriaticum. Dr. Murch was in the habit in these cases of alternating the arsenicum with small doses of Belloc's charcoal. If the disease is complicated with glandular disease of a scrofulous or syphilitic character, the arsenicum jodatum might be preferable. Dr. D. T. Brown* has witnessed the best effects from preceding the employment of arsenicum with a few doses of carbo vegetabilis. Dr. W. C. Barker extols the use of "arsenicum 6th in alternation with sulphur 6th, repeated once in four hours, in those cases of nursing sore-mouth which are characterized by a very slight and almost imperceptible odor of the breath, with considerable prostration of the general strength." Dr. I. S. P. Lord vouches for the superior efficacy of arsenicum and natrum muriaticum in the 30th, in preference to other attenuations.

Arsenicum album.

The form of this disease to which mercurius is best adapted is that in which the ulceration of the tissues is very marked. The ulcers are corroding, the breath offensive, the secretion of saliva profuse, in short, the symptoms are those of the stomatitis ulcerosa of the old writers. If

Mercurius.

* Vide Transactions of American Institute of Hom., for 1860, p. 78.

there is no syphilitic taint, the mercurius corrosivus is preferable, otherwise the mercurius jodatus, or even the mercurius solubilis, may be selected.

Calcarea carbonica.

Where disorders of digestion in pregnant or lying-in women are due to a latent stomatitis, and particularly in patients who are predisposed to scrofula or phthisis, the calcarea carbonica may be of excellent service. The symptoms which indicate it are dryness of the mouth and tongue, with a sense of roughness and stinging; a dry, bitter, sour, or metallic taste; great aversion to boiled food and to meats in particular; inclination to salt diet, or to such indigestible articles as pickles, dirt, chalk, slate-pencils, etc.; nausea, with acid eructations; vomiting of ingesta; profuse colliquative diarrhœa, with undigested stools; a sudden metastasis of the eruption from the mouth to the alimentary mucous membrane; and acidity of the urine, with burning in the urethra during micturition. There are some examples of this disease which it would be very difficult, if not indeed impossible, to cure without this remedy.

Ammonium carb.

Dr. Helmuth reports* that ammonium carbonicum cured a case of long standing in which there was great prostration, hollow cough, and burning in the tongue—the whole buccal cavity being filled with vesicles and ulcerated depressions, and the tongue swollen, stiff, and very sensitive to cold air and drinks.

Baryta carbonica.

He also cites the case of a young lady cured by the use of baryta carbonica, for which remedy the chief indication was the absolute and complete anorexia.

Natrum muriaticum.

"In an emaciated female who had suffered severely from the disease, and had been troubled for a long period with ague, natrum muriaticum and arsenicum, in repeated doses of the 6th attenuation, effected a cure in twenty-one days."

Veronica beccabunga.

In the report to the American Institute, from which I have already quoted, my friend, Dr. N. F. Prentice, says: "Formerly I had a great deal of trouble in the treatment of this disease, and of sore mouth in children, but during the last three or four years I have used the veronica

*U. S. Journal of Hom., Vol. I, p. 413.

(empirically it is true, for I have but a very few provings of it,) almost exclusively, and with universal success. I have been in the habit of giving it internally in the first decimal attenuation, and of applying it locally to the mouth in the proportion of ten to thirty drops in two fluid-ounces of soft water. When they are indicated, I use other remedies in alternation with veronica."

Dr. J. Davies has succeeded in some obstinate cases by the application of a trituration of the rhus toxicodendron, and an internal use of the attenuations of the same remedy. He triturates the berries of this plant with saccharum lactis, in the proportion of one berry to ten grains of the sugar, and applies the powder, moistened, through the medium of a thin linen cloth.

Rhus toxicodendron.

Other remedies which are sometimes serviceable are belladonna, causticum, china, nux vomica, sulphur, hepar sulphuris, ferrum and staphisagria.

Topical applications of various kinds are grateful and beneficial. The most common and harmless consist of lotions, washes and gargles, composed of borax, or borax and honey, sage and borax, a mixture of equal parts of borax and sugar in a pulverized state, tincture of myrrh, an infusion of the golden seal, or of cayenne pepper, butternut oil, or glycerine. Some physicians recommend the chlorate of potassa to be dissolved in glycerine and applied locally. Others prefer a very weak solution of the carbolic acid. And yet others are in the habit of prescribing the topical use of hydrastin in water, or glycerine, or both. In cases where the buccal and faucial mucous membrane is badly ulcerated and the breath is fetid and offensive, a drachm of the mother tincture of baptisia may be added to four fluid-ounces of water and applied locally. Or Bretonneau's mixture of one part of hydrochloric acid and three parts of honey may be used instead. Dr. Barker has the greatest confidence in frequent rinsings of the mouth with simple cold water. There are those who, in exceptional cases, think it necessary to touch the ulcers with a pencil of the nitrate of silver. I prefer calendula, or hydrastin. Tannin and other astringents are harsh and revulsive, and may do more harm than good.

The local treatment.

LECTURE XIII.

PUERPERAL CONVULSIONS.

GENTLEMEN:

I propose to-day to offer you some remarks on puerperal convulsions. I will first read you the history of a case which has been kindly furnished by my friend, Dr. L. H. Holbrook of this city:

Case. — Mrs. K——, primipara, aged 26 years, of leuco-phlegmatic temperament; seven months advanced in pregnancy; had been troubled with pains in the left hip and leg, with some enlargement of the limb; pains were relieved by rhus tox. 3rd, and pulsatilla 3rd, and still more decidedly by rhus tox. 200th.

Jan. 6th. — She ate hickory nuts at an evening entertainment.

Jan. 7th. — Ate baked beans for dinner, and quite freely of fried ham for supper.

Jan. 8th. — At 12:30 A. M., was attacked with pain in the lower part of abdomen, more like colic than labor pains. At 5 A. M., I was called and found that she had had two movements of the bowels, and had twice vomited bilious matter. In view of her errors in diet I gave pulsatilla 3rd, which was followed by slight improvement. I left her at 7 A. M., on chamomilla 3rd and nux vomica 3rd, in solution, a teaspoonful to be taken every half hour alternately.

11 A. M. The pain is lessened, but she is very much nauseated. Gave a single dose of ipecac, 3rd, and continued former prescription. At 5 P. M., administered an injection per anum, containing one drachm of opium 1st. At 6 P. M., pain nearly all gone; vomiting still troublesome. At this hour left her, feeling confident that she would recover without implication of the uterus. About 7 P. M., she said that she felt strangely, and was immediately convulsed. Digital examination was now made. Found the head of the child presenting at the superior strait; the os uteri not dilated or tense, but soft and patulous; no expulsive pains. Gave of atropine, 2nd decimal, in water, a teaspoonful every half hour. This was followed by apparent benefit, as the intervals between the spasms were lengthened. The paroxysm commenced by first

the eyes, then the head turning towards the left side; this was followed by muscular tremor and a jerking motion of all the limbs. She then subsided into a state of stupor, with stertorous breathing, until the next paroxysm came on, when the same symptoms would be repeated.

Jan. 9th. — 5 A. M. Prof. R. Ludlam was called in council. A careful examination, per vaginam, disclosed the os uteri in the same condition as already described. There was an entire absence of uterine contraction. We decided that operative interference was contra-indicated. Gave ignatia every half hour. She also received an enema of sulphuric ether and milk.

11 A. M. The interval between the fits is lengthened, but it is characterized by great restlessness and constant motion of all the limbs. Has passed urine involuntarily several times. Fœtal heart-sounds heard distinctly. At 3 P. M. the bag of waters ruptured suddenly, and upon examination found the head pressing hard upon the perineum. At 4 P. M. she was delivered, during a convulsion, of a dead fœtus. After delivery only two convulsions occurred, but the jactitation and constant motion of the limbs continued.

8 P. M. At the suggestion of my friend, Dr. Kellogg, camphor was given for the restlessness. I decided upon its use, although it had been freely administered by olfaction during the first spasm, without any positive benefit. Five drops of the tincture of camphor were dropped upon a little sugar, then dissolved in half a glass of water, and a teaspoonful given every half hour. Marked improvement soon followed. Gradually the motion lessened, and at 12 M. she was quiet and sleeping.

Jan. 10th. — 9 A. m. My patient begins to manifest signs of returning consciousness. Camphor was used continually through the day, with intercurrent remedies.

Jan. 11. — Has rested well during the night. Partial recognition of friends; answers questions correctly, but is oblivious of what has passed. Tongue and lips very dry, red and swollen, notwithstanding our efforts to protect them, she had injured them somewhat during the spasms. Continue the camphor; mouth moistened with slippery elm water; barley water for drink.

Jan. 12th. — Was called at 1 A. M.; patient possessed with the idea that she will not get well, and talks about dying. Discontinued camphor and gave aconite 3rd every two hours. At 4 P. M., marked improvement of mental faculties, although her peculiar fancy is still troublesome. Has passed urine copiously, which deposits a brick dust sediment. The past is yet a blank to her; does not remember that she has been pregnant even, but thinks another, a friend of hers, was in that condition.

Jan. 13th. — The mind much clearer; has concluded to get

well; remembers the marriage of her sister, which occurred a few months ago; has troublesome hæmorrhoids; never had them before.

Jan. 14th.—Sleeps well; improvement gradual and constant; she begins to ask questions about her illness.

Jan. 20th.—Mind quite clear; inquired about her baby, and when informed of her loss was affected to tears. Ignatia 3rd every three hours.

Jan. 22d.—Continued improvement; appetite good; she sat up three hours yesterday; has some headache in consequence of seeing too much company. There has been no secretion of milk.

Of all the contingencies of parturition perhaps none is so alarming and serious as puerperal convulsions. Fortunately, however, they are among the rarest complications and sequelæ of labor. Cazeaux gives a table of 38,306 deliveries by English obstetricians, in which only 79, or one in 485, had convulsions. In a thousand labors superintended by him at La Clinique, Velpeau did not observe a single case. In 10,387 cases of labor, Dr. Joseph Clarke met with 19 cases of convulsions; Dr. F. H. Ramsbotham, in 68,435 deliveries, had 67 cases, or less than one in a thousand; Dr. Collins in 16,414 labors, encountered 30 cases of convulsions. As with preternatural labors in general, their very infrequency affords a powerful argument for the careful study of the pathology and treatment of puerperal convulsions.

Relative frequency

These convulsions have been divided by obstetrical authorities into the epileptic, the hysterical, and the apoplectic. There is good reason, however, for considering the true puerperal eclampsia an affection which is quite distinct from, although it is not unfrequently complicated with, epilepsy, hysteria, apoplexy, and sometimes with chorea, catalepsy and tetanus.

Varieties and complications.

Only a very small proportion of women who have puerperal convulsions are predisposed to, or have ever had epilepsy. In those who have been subject to epilepsy prior to conception, the pregnant state is more likely to arrest than to increase the frequency and severity of the paroxysms. Dr. Tyler Smith reports that in 51 pregnancies occurring in 15 epileptic subjects, only two had puerperal convulsions, while only one of all Dr. Churchill's patients afflicted

Exemption of epileptic subjects.

with epilepsy had them. The manner of approach of the fit, the absence of the "aura epileptica," its frequent recurrence, its various causes, its relation to the uterine contractions and sympathies, and its clinical history throughout, prove that the epileptiform symptoms present in the convulsions of child-bed are mere contingencies thereof, which may modify, but are not essential to, and do not explain the real nature of the disease.

Hysterical convulsions.

The hysterical convulsions are more liable to occur in the earlier than during the later months of pregnancy. They scarcely deserve the title of convulsions, and their consequences are not often directly serious. Patients of a well-marked hysterical constitution are perhaps more strongly predisposed than others to puerperal convulsions. The local and limited spasmodic phenomena that sometimes accompany or follow labor in nervous and highly excitable women, are purely hysterical. In brief, hysteria, like apoplexy, catalepsy or tetanus, "may occur in the puerperal state, either as the principal disease, or as a termination or complication of eclampsia."

Date of commencement.

Clinical History. — The attack may set in at any period of pregnancy, during labor, immediately subsequent to the delivery of the child and the secundines, or some hours, days, or even weeks after parturition. Of 59 cases reported by Ramsbotham, 17 commenced before labor, 28 during its progress, and 14 after its termination. In the experience of Braun and Weiger 24 per cent. set in before the commencement of uterine pains, 54 per cent. during labor, and 24 per cent. after the birth of the child.

During gestation.

Depaul cites a case of puerperal convulsions which occurred in the fourth month of gestation; Perfect two cases before quickening; Meigs one at five months; Empson one at the tenth day after delivery; Ramsbotham one at the sixteenth day, and Sever, Hardy, Braun, Simpson and Devilliers report examples commencing as late as the sixth week. It is believed that convulsions incident to the pregnant state are more likely to occur at and after, than before the seventh month.

Influence of delivery.

When they take place during labor, the convulsions are apt to terminate with delivery. In some cases they continue for a period but recur at longer intervals, after the uterus has been emptied. More rarely, however, they do not seem changed either in degree or frequency by the conclusion of labor. Braun says that the fits completely cease after the evacuation of the womb in 37 per cent., become weaker in 31 per cent., and in only 32 per cent. continue of the same severity.

Coming on of the fit.

Convulsions are most likely to commence when, having escaped the os uteri, the presenting part occupies the vagina, lies upon the perineum, or is about to protrude at the vulva. There are, however, exceptions to this rule, in which rigidity of the anterior lip of the os may prevent the passage of the head, and convulsions begin before it has emerged from the uterus. A highly irritable and sensitive condition of the soft parts renders the more nervous and delicate women liable to attacks of convulsions during labor. This state being always more marked in those who are in labor for the first time, it follows that such patients are more subject to convulsions than those who have already borne children. More than two-thirds of all the cases of puerperal eclampsia occur in primiparæ. Of thirty cases of this disease noted by Dr. Collins, 29 occurred in women for the first time in child-bed; and of those reported by Dr. Merriman the same was true of 36 out of 48.

Most frequent in birth of male children and in head presentations.

In the great majority of examples of this disorder, excepting of course where there are twins, the child is of the male sex. Of 28 cases cited by Dr. Collins, in 17 the offspring was a male. So also, in nearly all cases of puerperal eclampsia we have head presentations. In the Dublin Lying-in Hospital only a single case of convulsions coincident with malposition occurred in 48,397 labors. The only variety of preternatural labor, due to false position or presentation, to which convulsions are incident, is placenta prævia.

Liability of recurrence in subsequent pregnancies.

It is not certain that because a woman has had puerperal convulsions in her first labor, she will therefore have them subsequently. Nor will one attack exempt her entirely. There are exceptional instances in which the pregnant, parturient, and lying-in states may always be accompanied by them. An example of this kind is reported in the Proceedings of the London Obstetrical Society (Vol. I, p. 108), in which abortion with convulsions occurred six times successively in the same patient. Lumpe relates a case in which convulsions were experienced in the first, second, and fifth deliveries; Dr. I. S. P. Lord one in which a woman had convulsions in three, and Litzmann another in which a like result followed in nine successive pregnancies.

Premonitory symptoms.

The fit may set in abruptly, or there may be premonitory symptoms which vary in individual cases. Excessive restlessness, irritability, rigors, flushed face, headache, malaise, delirium, imperfect vision, amaurosis with dilated pupils and staring expression, rumbling noises in the ears, hypochondriasis, vomiting, a slow pulse which rises very quickly when the paroxysm has commenced, and twitching of the muscles of the face and extremities, are among the prodromi of this dangerous affection. An intent·look of the patient at the ceiling or corner of the room upwards, and the following as of an object by the eye is a threatening symptom.

Dropsy a precursory symptom.

In the majority of cases, however, there will have been observed by the modern and more intelligent physician, a tendency to anasarcous swellings in various parts of the body. This symptom, first observed by Hamilton and Demanet more than sixty years ago, may sometimes be remarked many weeks before "term," and, although it is not always followed by convulsions, is really to be interpreted as a foretoken of *convulsibility*. This dropsical puffiness may be limited to the upper extremities and the face, but is more frequently seated in the lower limbs, the ankles, the feet, and even in the labia majora. In exceptional cases, it nearly or quite disappears towards the end of gestation, so that its significance is sometimes over-looked, by one who sees his patient for the first time during the parturient act.

The convulsive stage.

As the fit approaches, the eyelids wink incessantly, the eyes are rolled upwards and fixed, the pupils dilated, the features are changed, the facial muscles jerk and twitch spasmodically, the angle of the mouth is drawn to the side corresponding with the unnatural position of the eyeballs, the head rotates slowly in the same direction, and the muscles of the neck, arms, trunk, and legs are successively convulsed. The throat, the larynx, the pharynx, the diaphragm, and other respiratory muscles are also seized, and respiration becomes interrupted, irregular, tumultuous, or altogether suspended.

There is stridulous expiration with hasty inspiration. In consequence of these latter spasms there is asphyxia, with discoloration of the surface and turgidity of the skin, neck, features, eyes, and tongue. The anal and vesical sphincters may be affected, and involuntary passages of fæces and urine follow. In some cases the uterus is suddenly emptied of its contents. The hands are clenched, and occasionally the arms thrown wildly about. I have read of an example in which the head of the humerus was luxated from this cause. The muscles of the jaw are spasmodically contracted and the teeth closed firmly and suddenly, in consequence of which the tongue, mouth, and cheeks may be badly bitten. The salivary glands secrete an unusual quantity of saliva, which is discolored by blood from the wound caused by the sudden closure of the jaws. M. Finney cites a case in which the lower jaw was dislocated during a convulsion. Denman observed that the forcible expiration of the breath through the teeth, which are firmly set, produces a hissing sound that is quite pathognomonic. Sometimes this is the first symptom noted in an attack.

Peculiarities of.

There are several items of interest connected with the natural history of convulsions. I can only name a few of them in this connection. The progress of the spasmodic action from above downwards is peculiar and significant. In all the cases treated by me, the head has been turned to the *right* side. Meigs has remarked that the spasms affect first the extensor and then the flexor muscles of the extremities, and that this is followed by a rigidity of both.

The brain symptoms.

Although, if long continued or frequently repeated, the interruption of respiration and consequent asphyxia may result in fatal effusion into the cerebro-spinal cavity, yet the discoloration of the blood and complete insensibility induced thereby are to be regarded as a species of critical anæsthesia, which is designed to put an end to the paroxysms. When the fit is over the patient may sleep quietly, or it may be followed by stertorous breathing. Where the convulsions have not persisted for a considerable time, and are neither very frequent nor severe, there is a gradual return of consciousness. Otherwise the patient becomes comatose and finally quite insensible to external impressions. In plethoric subjects who are predisposed to apoplexy, this symptom is observed at an earlier period of the disease, and is of much more serious import. The more rapid the paroxysms, if truly eclamptic, the more sudden and complete the loss of consciousness.

The pulse.

Litzmann has remarked that at the onset of the convulsion the pulse is slow and then rises very quickly to 120 or 150 in the minute. It also becomes smaller and quicker as the intervals between the convulsions are lessened.

Duration and repetition of the paroxysm.

The duration of the fit, of which I have given but a brief outline, varies from one to five or more minutes. If they take place during labor, they are likely to recur with the regularity of the uterine contractions. Sometimes, although rarely, the convulsions commence before the pains. Wegscheider reports a case in which the fits began forty-eight hours in advance of labor. In post-partum convulsions, even in primiparæ, I have observed that they usually return with each "after-pain," and, if all goes on well, they diminish in frequency as these tormenting sequelæ of labor disappear. They may continue, at longer or shorter intervals, for from a few hours to several days. The patient may have but one fit, or she may survive, or succumb to thirty, forty, or even a hundred of them. As a rule, if the mother has more than three or four severe convulsions prior to delivery, the child or children will be still-born. Where they occur subsequently to labor, the milk and lochia are suppressed.

Predisposing causes.

Etiology. — The causes are predisposing and exciting. Among the former are the hysterical constitution, and all those influences and habits of life which develop it, whether directly or indirectly. A tendency to apoplexy, epilepsy, anæmia, or renal disease, also predisposes to an attack of puerperal eclampsia. The same is true of an hereditary liability to spasmodic affections generally. Puerperal convulsions are more frequently met with in cities and larger towns than in rural districts.

Exciting causes.

The exciting causes are numerous and varied. Eminent authorities have observed that convulsions in child-bed are in a sense gregarious. In 2,000 deliveries, of which Cazeaux had charge at the Hotel Dieu, and the College de la Faculté there were but three cases of convulsions, while in his service at La Clinique during only four months there were seven cases of this kind. Ramsbotham remarked the same fact, and also the occurrence of several cases during warm weather, when the clouds were charged with electric fluid. In private practice I once had two patients, who were in no wise related or acquainted, seized with puerperal eclampsia during the same week — a coincidence by no means grateful or desirable.

Certain emotional states may predispose to, or precipitate an attack. In one of my patients, a primipara, the post-partum seizure was induced by mental agitation of the mother, lest scandal might come of the fact that her child was born at somewhat less than nine months after marriage. Fear and dread of the fit is a powerful exciting cause. In rare cases, where the parts are in a state of hyperæsthesia, or the patient is more than ordinarily averse to the necessary examination, the "touch" may bring on the first paroxysm. Excess of joy and demonstration over the birth of the child, especially if the labor has been brief and rapid, fright and anger, shame, misery, disgust, or the meeting between husband and wife during or subsequent to delivery, may have the same effect. The eating of improper food in the later months of gestation has been known to induce convulsions. Mr. Owen Davis reports a case of this kind occurring at the eighth month, that was caused by eating mussels. In advanced pregnancy shellfish are, for this reason, objectionable articles of diet. In Dr. Holbrook's case the improper diet of the patient probably caused the convulsions. Great exhaustion from excess of fatigue, protracted labor, or profuse hæmorrhage, will, in some cases, occasion puerperal convulsions.

But the causes I have enumerated are not in themselves sufficient in all cases to account for the production of this frightful disease. Concerning the conditions and circumstances that are necessary and adequate to this result, authorities are not agreed. There are three several theories on this subject, which, for the sake of perspicuity, we shall style (1) the mechanical, (2) the nervous, and (3) the toxæmic.

The *mechanical* hypothesis attributes the symptoms of puerperal eclampsia to pressure of the gravid uterus upon the larger vessels, and consequent derangement of the circulation both in the abdomen, the lower limbs, and also in the head and upper extremities. Not only is the proper distribution of the blood directly interfered with by this means, but its quality is impaired, and it becomes less nourishing and more noxious to all the tissues with which it is brought into contact. The nerve-centers being especially susceptible, are the more likely to suffer from this cause, and nervous and convulsive phenomena are the natural and necessary consequences. This view is supported by the fact that convulsions occur more frequently in those whose abdominal parietes and tissues have not been developed and relaxed by a previous pregnancy; that the liability to them, and the danger from them, increases as the uterus is more largely developed, and, also, that they are so often arrested by emptying the womb of its contents and securing its involution.

The mechanical origin of puerperal convulsions.

Those who hold to the *nervous* origin of puerperal convulsions may be divided into two classes. The first of these recognizes in the pregnant state a peculiarly impressible condition of the nervous system in which slight causes, not ordinarily harmful, may engender the most fearful consequences. This morbid "irritability," or convulsibility, constitutes, according to this view, a powerful predisponent of convulsions. With respect to its mode of operation, no very definite idea appears to be entertained, but a vague notion prevails that, in some manner, at this particular period, the nervous apparatus is easily deranged in its action, and that spasmodic and convulsive movements are thereby induced.

The nervous origin of puerperal convulsions.

The celebrated Marshall Hall proposed the rationale adopted by the second class. This theory holds that morbid complications and modifications of reflex action through the spinal cord are quite sufficient to explain all the phenomena belonging to this and to other varieties of eclampsia. The development of the womb during the whole period of gestation, but especially after the fourth month, involves very considerable changes in its nervous, as well as in its sanguineous circulation. Its afferent conductors may convey such impressions to the spinal center as are not capable of being reflected upon and appropriated by the generative system. These impressions, or so-called currents, which are abnormal in quality,

Reflex causes.

and perhaps in degree also, are made to take a new direction. Other and remote muscles are thereby implicated, and convulsive symptoms result. So also of mammary, ovarian, and other varieties of excitation of the peripheral nervous filaments, which indirectly produce the same results.

If the fit sets in during labor, the pressure of the presenting part, the forcible dilatation of the os uteri, an unyielding perineum, the contact of the finger of the accoucheur, or of instruments when the forceps are attempted to be applied, or of the hand in the operation of version, may be the exciting cause of impressions that are telegraphed to the spinal center, and thence to the medulla oblongata, to be reflected upon the muscles successively convulsed during the paroxysm.

Post-partum seizures may result from the presence of clots, or of placental fragments retained in the womb, an incomplete folding of the organ upon itself, or from actual displacement thereof. Either of these irritants applied to the sentient extremities of the nerves may thus indirectly originate and perpetuate the convulsive attack. As in the case cited at the beginning of this lecture, the fit may derange, or supersede the proper uterine contractions. Labor may be arrested, and life jeopardized, by the mal-appropriation of the very forces designed to consummate and insure them.

The toxæmic theory.

The *toxœmic* theory refers the symptoms of this affection to the presence of one or more poisonous principles retained in the blood. Their correspondence to those of uræmia led to the inference that they might be identical in origin. The defective elimination of urea by the kidneys, the presence of albumen in the urine, and the œdema, which sometimes occur at an advanced period of gestation, imply a state of convulsibility, or of liability to convulsions. The non-elimination of urea from the blood is believed, by Braun and others, to be the chief cause of the phenomena presented in puerperal eclampsia.

The albuminuria.

The history of the renal complication in this disease is singularly interesting and suggestive. The presence of albumen in the urine in almost every example of puerperal convulsions is something more than a mere coincidence. According to Blot, the average proportion of albumen in the urine in albuminuria without eclampsia is 33 per cent., while in the eclamptic it may be 74 per cent. There are, doubtless, many cases of albuminuria in pregnant women that are not accompanied or followed by convulsions, but the converse of this proposition is not true. As an accidental ingredient of the urine, a considerable proportion of albumen implies a great drain upon the nutritive resources of the economy. It also signifies that the elimination of urea is less thoroughly performed than it should be by the kidneys. Viewed as a premonitory symptom of puerperal eclampsia, albuminuria is of the utmost significance. The œdema of the inferior extremities, the ascites, and dropsy of the amnion, which are not complicated with albuminous urine, containing fibrine cylinders, are not followed by uræmic eclampsia in the parturient state.

Whether we regard the albuminuria as resulting in a majority of cases from acute desquamative nephritis, which, in this instance, will subside when delivery is accomplished; or if we recognize it as a neurosis—a functional derangement of the kidneys dependent upon nervous causes, the meaning and the hint are equally obvious. So also, if it be true that kiesteine is separated from the blood by the kidneys, and mistaken for albumen, as Simpson and Bedford have suggested. It is not so much that the renal function suffers, as that idiopathically, or symptomatically, the nervous system is implicated.

Whether it be the urea, the carbonate of ammonia, or some other primary, secondary, or tertiary product of the depurating process, that is dammed up in the circulation and works all this mischief, we may perhaps never know. That some post-organic material is responsible therefor is evident. That it is urea is very probable, and it is to the action of this noxious principle that the cerebro-spinal centers are especially susceptible. Frerichs, Bichat, Courten and Gaspard did indeed inject filtered urine, and even a solution of urea, into the veins of animals without ill effect. And there can be no question that in some cases of granular or fatty degeneration, of dropsy and extensive disorganization of the kidney in the human subject, the patient has shown a remarkable exemption from nervous and convulsive symptoms. These are facts of curious interest and real clinical import, but they do not prove that the pregnant state may not render the patient peculiarly susceptible to the toxical effect of a substance that should have been eliminated. Uræmia appears greatly to augment the hysterical excitability of pregnant women, and to predispose them to convulsions. Simpson believed that "this diseased condition of the blood produces a preternatural excess of irritability or polarity of the nervous system, and more especially of the spinal system of nerves," in consequence of which they are more easily affected by the exciting causes that indirectly occasion convulsions.

Uræmia increases the convulsibility.

It is evident, from the foregoing remarks, that an exclusive view of the etiology of puerperal convulsions is not to be entertained by the enlightened and experienced physician. Mechanical impediments to a free circulation of the blood, and pressure of the uterus upon the vagina, the rectum, the bladder, or the stomach and renal vessels, may undoubtedly produce them. The same is true of a state of hyperæsthesia of the general or local nervous system, and of causes which derange the distribution of nervous influence through the excito-motory system. Yet other attacks may be due to uræmic intoxication and poisoning, of which the albuminuria, œdema, and general infiltration of the cellular tissue in successive portions of the body are the first and more prominent symptoms.

An exclusive view is apt to mislead.

I venture the suggestion that a single and significant physiological fact has been overlooked by obstetrical writers who have treated of this subject. Although not clearly recognized and taught, it is, nevertheless, true that *certain of the bodily tissues are especially susceptible to the irritation of their own post-organic products.* This view is confirmed in the effects of cholesterine upon the nervous system in a large class of diseases dependent upon hepatic derangement. Urea results from the destructive metamorphosis of the muscle tissue. The kidneys are designed for its secretion. When, by reason of its non-elimination, its proportion in the blood is greatly increased, the muscular system is likely to suffer. Cramps, spasms, and convulsive movements are the natural result of the irritation of this noxious agent, not only in the nerve-centers, but in the muscle-cells themselves. Grant that these cells have an inherent power of contractility, a point conceded by some modern physiologists, and we can readily conceive that the direct contact of urea

Physiological deductions.

might produce the most mischievous consequences. It is for this reason, I apprehend, that in some cases the convulsions induced are decidedly tetanic, and in others cataleptic. Nor would the idea, advanced by Frerichs, that the urea is decomposed into the carbonate of ammonia, alter the fact, or change the inference with respect to the mode of its operation. Tessier, Piberet, Rilliet, Barthez, Picard, and others, have remarked the absence of lesions of the nerve-centers in those who have died of uræmia.

Pathological Anatomy.—The *post mortem* record of this disease is not complete. The lesions noted in other organs than the kidneys are incidental, and not pathognomonic. Changes in the structure and vascularity of the brain vary with the apoplectic character of the attack. The same is true of serous and sanguineous effusion within the ventricles or between the meninges of the brain and spinal cord. Sometimes there is a bloodless appearance of the brain, with diminished consistence or *ramollissement* of the cerebral mass. In most instances the heart is empty and flaccid. The pleuræ and pericardium may be the seat of effusion. The lungs are sometimes pale, or œdematous, and even emphysematous. There may be traces of abdominal and uterine inflammation.

Bright's disease as a concomitant.

In 1843 Dr. Simpson noted the first case of granular disease of the kidney, on *post mortem* inspection after the death of a patient from puerperal eclampsia. Numerous well-authenticated cases, selected since that period, establish the relative frequency of Bright's disease of this organ as a coincident affection. Braun is cognizant of more than thirty cases, and Hasse, Hohl, Blot, Cohen, Simpson, and other authorities swell the list of those who confirm this observation. The renal lesions, revealed by the scalpel in cases of uræmic convulsions, are those proper to one of the three stages of Bright's degeneration of the kidney. In the first there is congestion of the organ, slight hæmorrhagic effusion, the epithelium is not changed, but the uriniferous tubes are filled with coagulated or fluid exudation, in which are fibrin cylinders, discoverable with the microscope. In the second the kidney is increased in weight, is more friable, fatty, soft, and milky. This is the stage of exudation. In the third stage the organ is shrunken, diminished in bulk and weight, indented, tuberculated, and of a dirty yellow color on its surface. The urinary tubules are completely denuded of epithelium. This latter condition is peculiar to the chronic form of Bright's disease, and is seldom witnessed in those who have died of puerperal convulsions.

Much discussion has resulted concerning the origin of these evident symptoms of Bright's disease, revealed by autopsy in this form of eclampsia. Scanzoni is the champion for the theory that, when they do exist, they are to be regarded as among the consequences, rather than the causes, of the convulsive attack. But Brücke declares that "the occurrence of uræmia depends not so much on the *intensity* of the textural changes as on the *extent* of the morbid exudation of the kidneys. Christison has also shown that 'coma and convulsions may come on in the very earliest stages of Bright's disease, and that then, indeed, they advance more rapidly than when the degeneration is more advanced. He also mentions their occurrence independently of any dropsical effusion, and their occasionally coming on shortly after dropsy has been dispelled.'" The transient duration of the albuminuria, in most cases of puerperal convulsions, proves that the lesion of the kidney is not necessarily very deep-seated. The presence of fibrin cylinders, and of fatty casts, in the albuminous urine, and in the renal tubes on *post mortem* examination in the field of the microscope, is evidence that structural changes have begun, which, but for the termination of pregnancy, would probably in every case result in granular degeneration of the kidney. Simpson is of opinion that "albuminuria, with convulsions, etc., occurring in any labor later than the first, generally results from fixed granular disease of the kidney, and does not disappear after delivery."

Diagnosis.— Puerperal convulsions are so likely to be complicated with hysteria, apoplexy, or epilepsy, and their nature, severity and treatment are so modified thereby, that their differential diagnosis is very important.

The hysterical form.

The hysterical convulsion partakes more of the nature of a spasm than of a convulsion; the muscular contractions are neither marked nor regular in the order of their coming; the muscles of the trunk and extremities are affected to a greater degree than those of the face; not unfrequently there is opisthotonos; there is no frothing at the mouth, or biting of the tongue; no stertorous breathing, or hissing respiration; no anæsthesia, with turgidity of the features and blueness of the skin; no marked increase in the frequency of the pulse after the beginning of the paroxysm; no gradually-increasing coma; no albuminuria before the fit, and, if it is present afterwards, no tubular casts, fatty, waxy, fibrinous, or epithelial; no regularity in the recurrence or duration of the paroxysm, which often ends with an emotional outbreak in the form of sobbing, sighing, weeping, or laughing, or with the eructation of flatus. It is no doubt true that many cases of hysterical convulsion have been mistaken for puerperal eclampsia.

The apoplectic form.

From the outset the apoplectic convulsion will be recognized as dependent upon intra-cranial effusion and compression. Consciousness is suspended; sensibility is lost; the coma comes on suddenly, and is profound with stertorous breathing; the convulsions are slight, and afford no reliable criterion of the gravity of the attack, the muscles becoming flaccid and powerless.

The epileptiform variety.

We have already detailed the diagnosis between the true epileptic convulsion and puerperal eclampsia. In epilepsy, as in hysteria, the renal symptoms are essentially different from those proper to puerperal convulsions. The presence of albumen in the urine, with cylindrical casts, has never been observed as a sequel to the epileptic paroxysm. Epileptics may have Bright's disease, and during gestation, labor, or child-birth, be seized with uræmic eclampsia; but this is a mere coincidence. The frequent connection between the epileptic convulsions and imperfect eliminatory action of the kidneys, however, led Dr. Todd to designate a variety of this disease as renal epilepsy (epilepsia renalis). The antecedent and coexisting symptoms, in a given case, would enable one to decide between epilepsy with renal complication, and puerperal eclampsia dependent upon uræmia.

LECTURE XIV.

PUERPERAL CONVULSIONS. — CONTINUED.

Gentlemen:

We will resume the subject of our last lecture.

Prognosis. — Out of 328 cases of puerperal eclampsia tabulated by Churchill, 70 mothers were lost, or about 1 in 4½. Wieger records that of 65 women seized with convulsions at different periods of pregnancy, 25 died. Of 48 cases reported by Dr. Merriman, 37 recovered; and of 30 reported by Dr. Collins, only 5 died. Of the latter, three of the fatal cases were complicated with laceration of the vagina, one with twins, and one with peritonitis. Braun is of the opinion that 30 per cent. have proved fatal to the mother. These tables display varied results and are defective for the reason that no distinction is made between the several forms and complications of the convulsions incident to parturition. The relative mortality which in Hunter's time amounted to one-half, and has already been so considerably reduced, will doubtless be still farther lessened by a more discriminating diagnosis and rational treatment.

Mortality from.

The prognosis is favorable in proportion with the predominance of hysterical and epileptiform symptoms, especially if the convulsions have not been preceded by albuminuria and anasarca, and if they continue synchronous with the uterine contractions, subsiding when the womb is emptied of its contents. Hysterical eclampsia will, other things equal, recover under almost any treatment, providing it is not too severe. In this form the attack is self-limited.

Favorable symptoms.

Women sometimes have spasms and convulsions during pregnancy, and afterwards escape them at "term." I had a case of this kind a month ago, in which my patient had had severe convulsions every four weeks from the fourth to the eighth month. When the proper time arrived,

Case.

her labor commenced and was finished without any convulsive symptoms. Nor did she have anything of the kind subsequently.

Unfavorable symptoms.

The earlier the advent of apoplectic symptoms, the more profound the inter-paroxysmal coma, and the implication of the brain, the greater the danger. This variety of the disease may terminate very abruptly, or a single fit may throw the patient into a state of coma to which she shall succumb when one or more days have elapsed. If one pupil is dilated and the other contracted, it signifies a dangerous lesion of the brain on the side opposite the dilated pupil. It is safer to base our prognosis upon the condition of the patient between the paroxysms, than to judge by the severity of the fits only. Drowsiness and obliviousness between the fits, where there is no coma, are less fatal symptoms. Mania after coma is less dangerous than low delirium, which latter is a symptom of puerperal pyæmia. Stertorous breathing is a more dangerous sign than sibilant respiration. Excessive rigors, which are in reality a species of convulsion, if frequently repeated, imply great danger. The same is true of syncope, collapse of features, and the coldness of the extremities induced by excessive exhaustion from protracted labor or hæmorrhage. Davis says explicitly that: — "Convulsions complicated with profuse hæmorrhage, and *a fortiori* if the loss of blood shall have been very great, should be considered as harbingers of a rapidly approaching death, the convulsions in that case being a part and parcel of the dying state;" — and Braun, "anæmic convulsions are justly regarded as a symptom of the last agony."

Serious complications.

In convulsions occurring in twin deliveries, and in cases of placenta prævia, the prognosis is generally unfavorable. Where, during the later months of pregnancy, albuminuria with infiltration of the cellular tissue has existed, and the urine is nearly or quite suppressed, it implies a complication from which the patient is not likely to recover. If the renal affection is of long standing, and has already passed into the third stage of Bright's disease, recovery is still more doubtful. If the fits occur at longer intervals, if the amount of urine voided is increased, and of albumen diminished, the patient may get well after a somewhat lingering convalescence. Until the albumen has disappeared from the urine, however, there is a liability to a sudden return of the convulsions, even when some days or weeks have elapsed since the last fit. "After from six to ten days, if the child-bed patient continues to go on well, there is generally no trace of albumen to be discovered. If during child-bed the albuminuria continue for weeks, it arises either from the admixture of pus from an acute catarrh of the bladder, or from nephritis metastatica, or from a far advanced destruction of the kidneys being present, and the Bright's disease being chronic."

Forebodings before delivery.

Where violent mental emotions, especially if they are depressing in character, have been at work, and the patient has been possessed with the idea that she is about to die of convulsions in child-bed, recovery is exceptional. But, as in the case cited at the commencement of the last lecture, if the fear of death follows the cessation of the convulsions, it is a less serious symptom. The alarm of bystanders is a source of great danger to those patients who are very impressible.

Are præ- or post-partum convulsions the more dangerous?

Authorities are divided as to the relative danger in convulsions coming on before, during, or after delivery. Ramsbotham is of opinion that "convulsions coming on after labor, if the patient has not suffered an attack before, are not so dangerous as those which arise during pregnancy and labor." Dugés is of the same mind, and Churchill regards the post-partum variety nearly as manageable as those which occur during gestation. Churchill's worst examples are those in which the convulsions commence while labor is progressing and continue afterwards. In my opinion the most dangerous cases are those in which the convulsions begin with little or no premonition shortly after the birth of the child. When from twelve to twenty-four or more hours have elapsed after delivery, and convulsions ensue, they are almost always of an hysterical character, and therefore less dangerous. The only exception is in case of convulsions from an attack of acute nephritis from cold during the first fortnight of the lying-in. It is said that post-partum convulsions are most likely to make their advent towards evening, or in the early part of the night.

Braun sums up the progress of this disease as follows: "The dangers of eclampsia are greatly increased by complications with diseases of the heart and lungs, rupture of the uterus, etc. The

16

prognosis in other kinds of eclampsia is the same as when pregnancy has not occurred. Cholæmic, apoplectic, toxic, and anæmic eclampsiæ are very often fatal; hysteric and epileptic attacks and chorea, almost never so."

The danger from exposure to any of the zymotic diseases, as for example erysipelas or diphtheria, during the lying-in period, is referable to the depraved and poisoned condition of the blood, which renders the organism more susceptible to the action of specific disease-producing agencies.

The mortality of the children, in cases of convulsions occurring in the mother, is proportionally large. What the ratio is I am unable to say. In præ-partum convulsions perhaps one-third of the children are lost. The danger to the offspring is more imminent in case the fits commence before labor has really set in. Under these circumstances the paroxysms may be very numerous before delivery is effected, whether artificially or naturally, and it is an exceptional case for the fœtus in utero to survive any considerable number of them. The same is true where "the waters" have discharged prematurely, or where for any other cause, as for example, a considerable disproportion between the size of the fœtal head and the pelvic brim or outlet, on account of hydrocephalus, or deformity of the pelvis, mal-presentation, rigidity of the soft parts, uterine inertia, or profuse flooding, a prompt delivery is rendered impossible. Many of these little innocents are sacrificed to the obstetric expedients of version, the mal-adjustment of the forceps, and the more barbarous and unwarrantable resort to the perforator and crotchet. Given in such an extremity, ergot has doubtless slain its thousands.

The danger to the child.

Concerning the actual cause of death in children under these circumstances, where they are not the victims of "meddlesome midwifery," there are differences of opinion. It has been attribted to an interruption of the circulation in the maternal side of the placenta, to the sudden shock from the paroxysm experienced by the mother and communicated to the fœtus, and to poisoning of the blood contained in the fœtal vessels. In some cases life is abruptly destroyed, while in others it gradually becomes extinct. Not unfrequently the child is born in an asphyxiated state, from which it may be rescued by appropriate

The cause of its death.

means. If they survive, such children are apt to be weakly and delicate, frail and nervous, and are not in general long-lived. Exceptionally they are subject to spasms and convulsions from the moment of birth. When the mother dies in convulsions during parturition, the child's life can very rarely be saved, for the Cæsarean section discloses that it is already lost.

According to Braun: "If after numerous uræmic convulsive fits, the child is born alive, a large quantity of urea is found in the blood taken from the umbilical cord; but if it is born dead, we can immediately after birth, demonstrate the presence of carbonate of ammonia in the blood."

Sequelæ. — However gradually affected, recovery from this disease is perfect. The exceptional cases are those in which some pre-existing disorder has been aggravated thereby, or in which the harmful consequences of the shock to the nervous system, or of mal-treatment are perpetuated. A very common sequence of the attack is a species of obliviousness to what has passed, and of continued indifference towards the child, the father, and all her domestic interests and relations. Sometimes this mental aberration is of a less passive nature, and positive mania sets in. Under these circumstances she would destroy the infant, denounce the husband, and deny that labor has been completed. This form of mania is temporary, self-limited, and generally recovers of itself, providing the physician is sufficiently sane and determined to keep her from being sent to a lunatic asylum. The mental faculties are often weakened and impaired for a considerable time.

Secondary mental disorders.

Paralysis is sometimes a sequel of the apoplectic form of puerperal convulsions, but it never follows true and uncomplicated puerperal eclampsia. The hysterical type may be succeeded by various derangements in the functions of calorification and sensibility. In rare cases the extremities become flexed and immovable, as in catalepsy, a condition which passes away after a few weeks have elapsed.

Paralysis.

Although Denman and other authors insist that puerperal peritonitis is a frequent sequel of puerperal eclampsia, the idea is not confirmed by modern and more extended experience. Indeed there appears to be a greater liability to pulmonary than to puerperal disease

Peritoneal and pulmonary diseases.

of any kind. The pectoral affections that sometimes result are, the rapid development of phthisis, œdema and emphysema.

In rare cases vision may be impaired. Amaurosis, which is a frequent concomitant of albuminuria, sometimes continues for weeks or even months after an attack of puerperal convulsions. Unless consequent upon granular disorganization of the kidneys, or structural changes in the optic nerve itself, it is not a very serious affection. It sometimes disappears entirely after recovery from the convulsive attack, and returns at or after a subsequent labor, even when there are no convulsions. Ingleby cites a case of this kind in which a patient "had common puerperal convulsions in her first pregnancy; and who in a subsequent accouchement, was attacked with complete amaurosis, which continued during the whole period of her labor. Vision was gradually restored."

Amaurosis.

Treatment. — It is conceded that the relative frequency of puerperal convulsions depends upon circumstances which, if he is skillful and faithful, are largely under the control of the physician. In threatening convulsions during pregnancy, child-birth, or the lying-in, it is of the greatest importance to regulate the surroundings of the patient. You will be obliged to exercise great tact in adapting yourselves to their several peculiarities. For it will not do to treat all alike. You can amuse one, while you must threaten another. You will have to be decided, emphatic, and sometimes even peremptory. The more emotional they are, the greater the need of their attention being diverted from themselves. Keep them busy with *you.* Do not let them brood over contingencies. They must be kept saying something, or hearing something, cheerful. If there are long-faced attendants, you had better banish them. One good, trusty nurse is sufficient.

Preventive Treatment.

Tact.

The room should be shaded from too strong a light, and the lamp or gas-light not permitted to shine directly in the patient's eyes. Let there be no shadows on the wall. Shut out the noise. Open the windows for fresh air. Prescribe the removal of all ligatures from about the body and extremities, for corsets, garters, etc., impede the circulation, and may do positive harm. Caution her against a

Remove possible exciting causes.

sudden check of perspiration, lest there be an additional embarrassment of the renal function; against falls, sudden shocks, sleigh-riding, racing, over-anxiety about domestic affairs, worry about finance and the future, or about her children, if she has any.

Be careful of her diet, for indigestible food, or food which is too rich, may excite intestinal irritation, and provoke convulsions in adults in the same manner that it does in children. The case which formed the commencement of my last lecture is an illustration of this fact. The diet should be plain, simple, and unstimulating.

Prescribe cheerful society.

The patient should enjoy the society of one or more cheerful, sensible friends, who, no matter what happens, will not frighten her out of her wits by their own conduct and counsel. For, if a woman who is predisposed to this form of convulsions, observes her own bad feelings reflected in the faces and actions of others, she will forthwith take alarm, and all your efforts at prophylaxis may fail.

The physician's manner.

So also of your own manner and conduct in her presence. If you are fussy or frightened, lacking in self-reliance and resource, the worst possible consequences may come of it. While, on the other hand, if you are calm and self-possessed, if you show yourself thoroughly conversant with this state of convulsibility and all that concerns it, you may and frequently will succeed in averting the danger. Under these circumstances, it is of the highest importance to recognize the different shades of mental constitution in your patients, and to adapt yourselves to them.

Early recognition of prodromi.

You should cultivate a tact in the recognition and removal of obscure and shadowy symptoms. These are the signals of impending danger, and they appear in every case of this disease. If she complains of insomnia, do not neglect its cure. Fresh air and exercise, in her room and out of it, proper food and society, going to rest at regular hours, the avoidance of excitement and conviviality, as well as of too close sewing, or reading and study, will often suffice to cure the habit of sleeplessness, which might otherwise result in an attack of convulsions, either at or before term. Among the remedies suited to the relief of this state, the more prominent are coffea, bella-

For the insomnia.

donna, caulophyllin, ignatia, opium, moschus, aconite, and hyoscyamus. One of my patients, at the eighth month, complained that she had become exceedingly nervous and had had no good sleep for weeks. I learned that six weeks before, by the advice of a friend, she had quit drinking coffee, of which she was inordinately fond, and which had never disagreed with her. I prescribed that she should take a good cup of coffee morning and evening. She was cured at once.

For cerebral symptoms.

If she complains of headache, to which she has or has not been subject before, and it persists, give it your attention as one of the possible precursors of eclampsia. Congestive headache, with flushed face, dilated pupils, photophobia, intolerance of noise, incoherency of speech, and confusion of the mental faculties, are a class of symptoms which need watching, and should be remedied. Belladonna, aconite, glonoine, gelseminum, bryonia, nux vomica, or other similar medicines may be indicated. Their timely use may avert the development of the convulsive disorder and, so to speak, tide the patient over the difficulty.

For local suffering elsewhere.

Local pains elsewhere are equally significant. Convulsions may follow colic, gastralgia, nephralgia, pleurisy, or a sudden accession of rheumatic inflammation of the joints. Occurring in a pregnant woman, after the fourth month especially, these affections should be remedied as promptly and carefully as possible.

Incipient paralysis.

The same is true of a species of local anæsthesia, or paralysis of the sensory nerve filaments, in different portions of the body, characterized by numbness and tingling, or absolute insensibility, of the affected parts.

For the dropsical symptoms.

Although there are exceptional cases in which dropsy occurring in pregnant women is not followed by puerperal convulsions, yet the rule is quite the reverse. Hence you will be on your guard whenever it occurs, and more especially if the œdema began in the face and upper extremities. For in most cases of dropsy, whether incident to gestation or not, if the infiltration begins in this manner, we take it as a hint of renal disease or embarrassment of some kind. So your patient may have had a latent form of Bright's disease, which has been aggravated by her condition, or she may be suffering for the first time from an attack of acute desquamative nephritis, from congestion of the kidney, or from uræmia, due to direct pressure of the gravid uterus upon one or both the ureters, the earliest token of which may be seen in the puffy and bloated face and eyelids. If you act upon this suggestion you may avert the threatened eclampsia — always providing the degeneration of the kidneys has not gone too far already, and that the pressure upon the ureters does not cause a complete retention and resorption of the urine.

Albuminuria can not take place without more or less congestion of the kidney. The more acute the symptoms the better the indication for aconite, belladonna, or nux vomica. When the albuminuria has existed for some weeks, mercurius corrosivus or arsenicum alb. are remarkably efficacious. Or apis mellifica, colchicum, hyoscyamus, and merc. jodatus may be required.

For the albuminuria.

In this connection I should remind you that the patient must not be permitted habitually to lie upon her back. The reasons are obvious.

The patient's posture.

But, suppose your patient is just on the eve of a convulsive paroxysm. Is there no way of immediately controlling the symptoms? My friend, Dr. L. E. Ober, once told me that it was his practice, in cases of this kind, to instruct the women to look him directly and constantly in the eye, while he returned the gaze as steadily, after the manner of mesmerizers. To my certain knowledge this is an admirable expedient, provided you are healthy yourself, calm, cool, collected and confident. If, however, the bodily and mental conditions of the operator are not favorable, he may do more harm than good, and he had better let it alone.

An available expedient.

Caution.

If labor has already begun and convulsions threaten, you may sometimes ward them off by urging her to "bear down," or to encourage the pains. If the expulsive effort is slackened, the pains may "scatter." While they are confined to the womb, the excess of nerve force finds vent through a proper channel. If they are "misplaced," she will be more liable to go into convulsions.

Encouragement.

"If at all anxious or worried, she should be reassured, not by a tiresome repetition of the hackneyed rallying cry, 'courage, courage, cheer up, cheer up,' but by a calm cheerful address to her judgment, which has far more power to inspire her with confidence in us and in the issue." *

Palliative treatment.

No matter what the period of pregnancy, if all these preventive means shall have failed, or if the fits have already commenced before your arrival, your first duty will be to lessen the severity of the symptoms, and if possible to prevent their return.

An old rule and a good one.

"Until labor actually begins," says Gooch, "we have nothing to do with the uterus, but solely to attend to the convulsions." This is especially true of convulsions occurring before the seventh month. For prior to that time the fit is less likely to depend upon uterine irritation and development than it is at a later period. It is for this reason that we often succeed in arresting these convulsions without the womb being emptied of its contents, and are sometimes so fortunate as to carry these patients to term without untoward consequences. The more decidedly hysterical the attack, especially if it comes at the menstrual cycle, the less the danger of miscarriage as a contingent of convulsions.

The induction of labor.

But since, in every case, and whatever may have been the exciting cause, the eclampsia usually persists until delivery is effected, and generally ceases as soon as the fœtus is expelled, it may become a question whether or not you should hasten this result by the induction of premature labor. The general opinion of the profession is opposed to this expedient, and there can be no doubt that great harm has sometimes been done by an indiscriminate resort to it, under the impression that, in the case of a pregnant woman especially, nothing could be worse than the existence and continuance of convulsions.

Caution.

In general, and especially before the child is viable, it will be safe to follow Gooch's advice, and let the uterus alone. For nature usually evacuates the womb spontaneously, if the fits do not otherwise abate in violence, or cease altogether. And although it may consume a little more time to await her slow movements than it would to

* Puerperal Convulsions, by Prof. J. C. Sanders; Trans. Am. Inst. of Hom., June, 1867.

despatch the offending ovum *secundum artem*, still the patient will get on better afterwards and you will be better satisfied not to have interfered. If the os is not patulous, or the cervix uteri sufficiently softened, it will be better to follow Dr. Holbrook's example, and await the result.

When if ever justifiable.

As "term" approaches, the convulsions are more serious and alarming than in the earlier months of gestation. The degree of uterine irritation is necessarily increased. But, as a critical means of relief, the induction of labor is much less difficult and dangerous. The cervix uteri does not present so great an obstacle, and its forced expansion, by manual or instrumental aid, will neither wound the tissues nor shock the general system so severely. Hence I conclude that if the induction of premature labor is ever justifiable as a palliative in puerperal convulsions, it is where the fits are becoming so frequent and severe as really to threaten the life of the patient by apoplectic effusion or otherwise; where the symptoms have not been relieved by appropriate remedies; and where the neck of the womb is so dilatable that its resistance could be very readily overcome. These cases are comparatively rare, but they do sometimes occur, and we should not therefore entirely repudiate this expedient. For it may prevent "the loss of time where the loss of minutes is the loss of life."

Ways and means.

The means of inducing labor in these exceptional cases are, the introduction of the sponge tent, the warm douche, manual dilatation, and the use of Barnes' dilators.

Note the progress of labor.

In advising you to "let the womb alone," where the convulsive patient is not supposed to be in labor, I do not wish to be understood as saying that an examination by the "touch" is ever unnecessary. On the contrary, you should resort to it in every case of the kind, and, if the fits continue, repeat the examination from time to time, in order to ascertain if the parturient process is really going on, and how far it is advanced. Otherwise, and before you are aware of it, the labor may be finished. One of my medical friends had a case of puerperal convulsions at seven and a half months, in which, although the patient had apparently had nothing like a labor pain, the child was found

Case.

dead in the bed with the funis wound about the neck. Apply the hand upon the abdomen occasionally, and to the vulva, and if you are obliged to leave the house before the convulsions have ceased, explain to the nurse, or some responsible person, that it is quite possible that the child may be born during your absence.

Rupturing the membranes -- the forceps.

In case the bag of waters is very large, we can sometimes stop the paroxysm by rupturing the membranes and evacuating the liquor amnii. Fortunately in most cases, the presentation is favorable for the employment of the forceps. They should, however, be carefully applied, more especially in primiparæ.

Emptying the bladder -- Case.

Dr. Vines reports* the case of a patient, a primipara, aged twenty-eight years, who, at the eighth month, was suddenly seized with convulsions. "On examining the abdomen, the lower part was found greatly distended, and retention of urine was suspected. The catheter was passed and five and a half pints of urine withdrawn. Great improvement of the symptoms followed. There was no return of the convulsions after this evacuation of the bladder." Copious diuresis may sometimes be induced by giving a few doses of aconite, hyoscyamus, or apis mellifica.

Fæcal accumulation; clots.

The eccentric cause of the convulsions may be the accumulation of fæcal matter in the rectum, or of clots within the uterine cervix and vagina after delivery. The removal of these foreign substances will sometimes afford prompt relief.

The use of cold water.

If the fit is hysterical, it is said that you may palliate it, and perhaps prevent its return, by an enema of ice-water thrown into the rectum. The dashing of cold water upon the head and face is rude and uncivilized. The face and forehead may be bathed with it, or cloths wrung out of iced water may be applied to the head and to the back of the neck. In a case of puerperal eclampsia the celebrated Denman succeeded in keeping off the fits until delivery was completed, by sprinkling cold water on the face on every accession of pain. Another expedient is to apply bags or bladders of pounded ice to the head, or the spine, or both. This is too harsh. The feet should be kept warm.

* Braithwaite's Retrospect of Practical Medicine and Surgery, Part XII, p. 293.

LECTURE XV.

PUERPERAL CONVULSIONS. — CONTINUED.

GENTLEMEN:

Those of you who were present at the meeting of the Academy of Medicine last evening do not need to be told that physicians are not agreed upon the employment of anæsthetics in the treatment of puerperal convulsions. While the majority would use them indiscriminately, others would be more cautious; some prefer the sulphuric ether to chloroform, and yet others could not be induced to prescribe either of them.

Anæsthetics.

I believe, however, the general impression is that, as in surgery, so in midwifery, the sulphuric ether is less harmful and more safe than chloroform. But I apprehend that in the employment of anæsthetics in puerperal eclampsia we should exercise the greatest care and judgment. For it is not a mere question of lessening the spasm of the muscular fiber and putting an end to the paroxysm, else it could be more easily settled. We must decide whether the attack is hysterical, epileptiform, or apoplectic. If it is hysterical, the patient will not be in any considerable danger of serious congestion of the brain or spinal cord. She may indeed pass into a state of pseudo-narcotism, but will not become absolutely comatose. Now, although chloroform produces an evident hyperæmia of the nerve centers, and might do positive harm if the case were tending toward effusion, with or without a clot, there can be no very serious objection to it in simple hysterical convulsions. It is in this form of eclampsia that it has been given with almost uniform success, and has achieved such a reputation.

Need of discrimination.

Chloroform — hysterical convulsions.

But suppose the fit is epileptiform. The more frequent its

recurrence, and the greater its severity, the more profound the inter-paroxysmal coma. The case becomes more and more serious. The chief danger is from the possible extravasation of blood, or of serum. Whatever means would multiply the chances of this result should properly be withheld. It is under these circumstances that opiates are prohibited. And why? Because they would be likely to overwhelm the brain and spinal cord with an increased determination of blood to them. If we desired to develop such a case into one of real apoplexy, we should give opium in substance or one of its salts. And since chloroform acts in a very similar manner, to blunt and suspend the perceptive faculties by a congestion of certain portions of the cerebro-spinal center, it may really be just as harmful a narcotic in this variety of eclampsia. There can be little doubt that thousands of lives might have been spared if this view of the modus operandi and possible effect of chloroform, to increase the danger while it lessens the spasm temporarily, had been taken and acted upon before.

Contra-indicated in certain cases.

Why?

If we could attenuate the chloroform and give it internally as we do opium, it might prove not only a harmless, but a very useful agent. The parallel which Dr. O. H. Mann drew in his paper read before the Academy a short time ago, between the symptoms observed in his cases of puerperal convulsions and those of a patient under the influence of chloroform, preparatory to a surgical operation, was very striking and suggestive.

Practical reflections.

In a medical convention, I once heard a physician say that chloroform was "as harmless as cold water," that it would cure any case of puerperal convulsions, providing you gave enough of it, and that its failure in this disease should be attributed to timidity on the part of the physician who administered it. Such unqualified dicta are sensational and mischievous. A young physician who was present was captivated with the idea. A fortnight later, he had an opportunity of putting it into practice. He afterwards called upon me and frankly stated his experience and his convictions. He had given chloroform of an excellent quality to an almost unlimited extent, in a case of

Danger and folly of dogmatizing.

Case.

post-partum convulsions. At first it lessened the severity of the paroxysms, but after some hours had no apparent effect in controlling them, and his patient died of apoplexy. He recalled my lecture upon this subject when he was a member of the college class, and thanked me for the advice *never to administer chloroform in a case of puerperal convulsions if there is a manifest tendency to apoplectic effusion, but more especially if that effusion already exists.*

A good rule.

If you can not determine beforehand, in a given case, whether the anæsthetic would be beneficial, it may be well to let the patient inhale a little of it, by way of experiment. If its effects are such as they should be, you can continue its administration, otherwise it may be withdrawn. Sometimes we fail with chloroform, and afterwards succeed with sulphuric ether.

Feel your way.

Dr. W. H. Holcombe, of New Orleans, reports* the following interesting case of a stout young negro woman who had had convulsions in her first labor, but who had escaped them in her second labor:

Chloroform per anum — Case.

"Twenty days after her confinement I was called in great urgency to see her. The overseer reported that she had been doing well up to that morning, although he had noticed considerable swelling of the face and legs for two or three days previous. In the afternoon she complained of a very severe headache, and toward sunset went suddenly into a violent spasm. I saw her about eleven P. M. She had had nine convulsive paroxysms, and was perfectly comatose. There was stertorous breathing, and great and alarming tracheal rattle. Whilst I was examining her she became convulsed. The muscles of the face were twitched with inconceivable rapidity, the limbs participating in the contortions; respiration was entirely suspended, and the whole bed shook with the violence of the movements. It lasted about one minute, when relaxation took place, followed by increased tracheal rattle and very labored respiration. Bloody, ropy mucus had to be extracted with the finger from the mouth. She was in a state of profound coma, and deglutition was impossible.

"Having no confidence whatever in the lancet in such cases, although the pulse was full and corded in the interval, or in cold

* North American Journal of Hom., Vol. IX, p. 277.

douches, or sinapisms, or anything else which is calculated to increase reflex action, I determined to administer chloroform by the rectum. * * * * I can not imagine that she could have survived another convulsion, so thoroughly asphyxiated was she by the last one. The paralysis of the medulla oblongata, the great respiratory ganglion, or 'vital knot,' appeared almost complete. I dissolved two tablespoonfuls of brown sugar in about a gill of lukewarm water, added a tablespoonful of chloroform, drew it up once or twice into the tube, forcibly ejecting again, so as to disseminate the chloroform throughout the mass of water, and then injected the whole into the rectum, causing it to be forcibly retained by a napkin pressed between the nates.

"No more convulsions occurred; the remedy had acted like a charm. She relaxed into an apoplectic stupor, which became less and less stertorous by degrees, until in two or three hours, the respiration and pulse were natural. She did not speak for nine hours, and then only in monosyllables. She did not recover consciousness in full for twenty-four or thirty hours after the last paroxysm. In three days all signs of œdema had disappeared, and thenceforward the patient made a rapid recovery. She remembered nothing which had occurred since the headache of the first day.

* * * * "I think it was eminently fortunate that I used the chloroform by injection into the rectum and not by inhalation, and I strongly recommend my professional friends to try that mode in the future, and for this reason: In puerperal convulsions the aerating function of the lungs is greatly impeded, and it is very desirable that as much oxygen as possible may enter with each inspiration. The patient's life depends upon it. Any aeriform substance taken into the lungs, however valuable in a medical point of view, must mechanically occupy space which had better be pervaded by atmospheric air. The chloroform injected into the rectum exerts its specific action on the nervous system just as well (perhaps, indeed, better, for the nerves of organic life no doubt preserve their sensibility long after that of the nerves of animal life is apparently obliterated by the convulsive paroxysm), and the oxygenating power of the air is preserved as far as possible."

Practical inferences.

Of late frequent allusion is made in the medical journals to the power of veratrum viride to arrest and control the fits in puerperal eclampsia. If the half that has been claimed for it in this respect is true, it should sometimes be a valuable remedy. I have had no experience with it, but will cite you quite a marked case communicated to me some months ago by my friend, Dr. W. H. Burt:

Veratrum viride.

"In the case of a plethoric young woman, a primipara, the cause was doubtless *psychical.* The husband became intoxicated and was discharged from the only position he could fill, the very day his wife was confined. The labor was natural, but a little tedious, the waters having escaped the day before. She was delivered at 4 A.M., and no lady ever did better than she until 4 P.M., when her husband came home greatly excited and told her all his troubles. At 9 P.M., I was sent for in great haste. Found my patient sitting up in bed, pressing the sides of her head with her hands and exclaiming, 'My head is so full it will burst.' For two hours I gave her belladonna 2d, every half hour. Then she went into a violent convulsion. The face became livid, the pupils dilated; she frothed at the mouth, and passed into a profound coma, from which it was impossible to arouse her. I gave opium 2d for two hours, and afterwards the same remedy in the third dilution, letting her inhale chloroform meanwhile. In spite of my efforts, continued from ten in the evening until seven in the morning, the fits were at no time more than fifteen minutes apart. Most of the time, indeed, they recurred every five minutes. Hyoscyamus was also tried, but without effect.

Case.

"At 8 A.M. I commenced giving eight drops of the fluid extract of the veratrum viride, repeated every half hour. After the third dose vomiting set in. She had but three paroxysms after commencing the remedy. Drop doses were then given at intervals of two hours. She became rational the second day, and made a good recovery."

Concerning the employment of the lancet for the purpose of lessening the severity of the fit, and of doing away with the possible consequences to the brain and spinal cord, authorities are not agreed. There are those who would bleed in all cases whatsoever, and, on the other hand, those who could not be induced to try it at all. It is possible that

Venesection.

the reaction against the use of this expedient, *in exceptional cases*, may have gone too far. As a means of mechanical relief to the surcharged vessels of the brain it may, perhaps, be more direct and available than any other. For it is really no argument against its employment to say that the indiscriminate abstraction of blood in puerperal diseases has slain its thousands. I have no experience of my own to relate, but will cite you the following cases communicated to me by the late Dr. Geo. W. Perrine, of Milwaukee:

Case.

"Mrs. ——, a young woman, primipara, of rather full habit, was seized with convulsions four hours after delivery. Nothing had occurred to attract attention during labor except that she was more quiet than usual, and that, although she evidently suffered a great deal, she made but little outcry. During the first convulsion the pulse was not remarkably strong, but its strength increased so decidedly that after the third fit I bled her about twelve ounces. The pulse became less strong, the convulsions ceased and did not return for several hours. I went home, but was summoned to her again, to find that the fits had returned. I bled her again, this time from both arms, the blood being thick and dark, but had not drawn more than half as much blood as before, when the muscles became relaxed, the face pale, and the convulsions ceased entirely. After about six hours consciousness was restored. She was oblivious to all that had passed since the first paroxysm. By the employment of proper means she had a rapid convalescence."

Case.

"About three months after this, my friend, Dr. J. S. Douglas, had a case of convulsions during labor. The patient was young and very robust. The fits recurred with each labor pain. When I first saw her she had had several of them; was wholly unconscious; the face was swollen, flushed, and of a purplish hue; the eye-balls protruded; the pulse was slow, full and strong; the respiration stertorous, with frothing at the mouth during expiration. On consultation, it was determined that I should bleed her. I took about twenty ounces, when her pulse lowered, the turgidity and leaden color of the face subsided, the convulsions ceased entirely, and she made a safe and speedy recovery."

Domestic expedients—Mustard.

I have witnessed good results from the domestic expedient of applying sinapisms to the calves of the legs. In two cases of convulsions, occurring at the sixth month, they served to stop the fits entirely, even when the most appropriate internal remedies had failed.

In case the congestive tendency is very marked, dry cupping may sometimes afford temporary relief. It has the merit of being harmless, and is always available. In the hysterical form, camphor given by inhalation or internally, sometimes acts like a charm.

Dry cupping — Camphor.

You should in no case fail to examine into the condition of the os uteri and the perineum. If the former is rigid or exceedingly sensitive, measures addressed to its relaxation and paralysis may prevent or put an end to the eclampsia. It may answer to give the patient a few doses of belladonna, or of gelseminum, or, if you prefer, to dilate the unyielding cervix with your index finger, or by the local application of sweet oil, or of the extract of belladonna, mixed with equal parts of lard, or by the vapor of chloroform directly applied, or by warm water injected into the bowels, or a constant stream of warm water, thrown from an Essex or a similar syringe into the vagina. Sweet oil, or lard, or the belladonna ointment may be applied and rubbed into the perineum, if necessary, but you should remember that too much manipulation, more especially too firm pressure of the hand upon it, may serve to increase the severity and frequency of the fits. A good rule in making applications designed to relax the perineum is to place them in contact with the mucous surface of the part. By the same rule, if you apply the belladonna ointment to the inner instead of the outer surface of the uterine neck, it appears to act more promptly and efficiently.

For rigidity of the os uteri and perineum.

If labor is progressing, the soft parts are dilated or dilatable, and the presentation and position of the fœtus are favorable, it would be best to finish the delivery as speedily as possible, in the hope that, the uterus being emptied, the fits would not return. In general, the forceps are not to be applied in case there is any considerable spasm and rigidity of the os uteri. This is the rule; but there are exceptions to this rule also. For example, you may have a case in which the anterior lip of the uterine cervix is so unyielding as to interrupt labor and perpetuate the convulsions. The forceps are contra-indicated, and the convulsions may continue indefinitely. Let me tell you how I managed a case of this kind:

Rule for use of the forceps.

Exceptions.

17

Case. — On April 14, 1864, at eight A.M., Mrs. ——, primipara, was seized, while dressing for breakfast, with a severe labor pain, in consequence of which "the waters" escaped suddenly. She was placed upon the bed, and with the next pain, which came on within five minutes, she went into a convulsion. When I arrived she had had three paroxysms, and they continued to recur with each pain. The "touch" revealed the os high up towards the promontory of the sacrum. It was dilated to the size of a shilling, and its anterior lip was thick, hard and unyielding.

At eleven A.M., the symptoms had not changed materially. The fits were repeated as often as once in from five to seven minutes, and she remained comatose in the intervals. Prescribed belladonna 3d, to be repeated every fifteen minutes, and resolved to await further dilatation.

At three P.M., my colleague, Prof. A. E. Small, was called in counsel. When the patient was placed upon her back in bed, only the anterior lip of the cervix could be felt, but when upon the side, we were able to recognize the vertex in the vicinity of the sacro-vertebral angle. The os uteri was now about the size of a quarter of a dollar. The convulsions and coma continued as before. We concluded that it would not be safe or expedient to attempt the use of the forceps. Continued the belladonna at intervals of half an hour. Chloric ether to be inhaled at the commencement of each paroxysm.

Met again at eight P.M. Very slight change. The os uteri dilated to the size of a silver dollar, and the soft parts dry, hot and tumefied. The anterior lip, however, was as prominent, rigid and unyielding as in the morning. She was totally unconscious, and the convulsions quite as severe and frequent. An attempt was made to apply the forceps, the patient lying upon the back with her hips to the edge of the bed; but it was unsuccessful. This expedient was therefore abandoned until further dilatation should take place, and my friend, the Doctor, left me for the night at nine o'clock.

On subsequent reflection, I resolved that something must be done forthwith; for I feared that either the cervix uteri might be torn off, as has sometimes happened, or my patient's life sacrificed to protracted delay on my part. Since it was impossible to apply the forceps with the patient in the usual obstetric position, I determined to try and adjust them while she was lying upon the left side, with the limbs flexed, in the position recommended by the old English authors. In a little while I had the satisfaction of passing both blades of the instrument quite within the cervix and locking them properly. By careful manipulation, I soon delivered her. The child was still-born. For twenty-four hours the fits came, at longer intervals, and finally ceased altogether. Consciousness was not restored until the fourth day. She made a good recovery.

Three years later this woman had a living child at term, with less than half a dozen pains, without any convulsions or other untoward symptoms. Indeed, her labor was so brief that all was over before I could reach her bedside.

You may even be justified exceptionally, for example, in case of extreme rigidity, with long-continued and dangerous convulsions, in attempting the application of the forceps within the cervix uteri before it is sufficiently expanded to permit the head to pass. But before doing so, you should be very certain that your patient has reached "term," that the "waters have broken," that the head is below the superior strait, that you have a presentation of the vertex, and that she is actually in labor. Here is a case in point:

Applying the forceps within the cervix.

On the 24th of March, 1868, at seven P.M., my friend, Dr. E. Kniepcke, of this city, was called to visit Mrs. ——, aged 28, who was in labor with her first child. She had already been in labor for three days and nights. Four physicians and as many midwives had been successively in attendance. In order to put a stop to her pains and to the convulsions also, the last of those who had preceded Dr. K. had given the patient, by actual weight, one and a half grains of morphine! The amniotic liquor had escaped with the first pains.

Case.

For twelve hours the fits had recurred as frequently as once in five minutes. The os uteri was rigid, hard, and of about the size of a half-dollar. So much of the uterus as the basin could contain was prolapsed into the pelvic cavity.

I saw the patient at Dr. K.'s request, at half-past nine P.M. She was in a semi-conscious state between the pains and the convulsions, which were synchronous. The margin of the os uteri was thick, well defined all around, and cartilaginous to the touch. It rested on the perineum. The soft parts were hot, dry, and very much swollen. In reality the os uteri felt like an ivory ring of an inch and a half in diameter, and half an inch in thickness, placed directly around the presenting vertex. These symptoms were verified by our private pupils, Messrs. Dorion and Poppe.

We applied the extract of belladonna, mixed with lard, to the rigid cervix most thoroughly, and then determined to attempt the use of the forceps. By my direction, the patient's hips were brought to the edge of the bed, and she was placed in position as in ordinary forceps cases. Chloroform was then administered by

Dr. K., to the extent of complete anæsthesia. Having warmed a Naegele's forceps, and anointed the back, or external, surface of both blades *with the belladonna ointment*, I proceeded by careful and continued manipulation to introduce the right-hand blade. When it was finally applied, this brought the os uteri into the shape of a button-hole, and filled it completely. It was only by persevering effort, stretching the orifice with the blade on the one side and the finger on the other, that it was made possible to insinuate the second blade at all.

The instrument was finally adjusted in the direction of the occipito-mental diameter of the child's head, and the delivery accomplished. The utmost precaution being taken, the soft parts sustained no injury, and the woman recovered without any unusual symptoms, having survived the prolonged suffering and the eclampsia, not to speak of the morphine, six doctors, two medical students, and four midwives.

At the recurrence of the fit, a thick piece of india rubber, or of soft wood, should be placed between the teeth, in order to protect the patient's tongue. She should not be held forcibly or firmly to the bed, but simply prevented from throwing herself upon the floor or otherwise inflicting bodily injury. Too much constraint might increase the difficulty, and would do no good. If she has an antipathy to the nurse, the husband, or any one in the room, you had better send them out. And do not let bystanders give vent in her hearing to exclamations of fright and horror at the contortions of which they are witnesses.

Curative Treatment.—Having faithfully carried out the directions that I have given you, the application of remedies to the treatment of puerperal convulsions is very much narrowed down and simplified. If you bear in mind that its hysterical, epileptiform, and apoplectic complications and terminations are the chief peculiarities of this disorder, you will have the key to its special therapeutics. For, whatever may be said to the contrary, one or more of these three incidental ailments will, in every case of puerperal eclampsia, give rise to the symptoms that you are to treat medicinally. There is no remedy for the disease *per se*, and no specific for either of its different varieties and modifications.

If the predominant symptoms are *hysterical*, a careful study of them will be likely to show that one of the following remedies is indicated: belladonna, ignatia, hyoscyamus, camphora, chamomilla, moschus, pulsatilla, stramonium, coffea, or gelseminum.

If they are *epileptiform*, under the appropriate indications, which you have learned from my colleague, the Professor of Materia Medica, you may prescribe cuprum, nux vomica, nux moschata, gelseminum, secale cornutum, colchicum, ignatia, or stramonium.

If they are *apoplectic*, aconite, belladonna, veratrum viride, bryonia, opium, or glonoine.

A fallacious dogma.

It has been claimed that some particular remedies are especially efficacious in certain potencies, as, for example, belladonna in the twelfth or thirtieth attenuations, and stramonium in the two hundredth, when they are prescribed in the treatment of puerperal convulsions. Let me caution you, however, against the one-sided view that would commit you to the exclusive use of these or the lower potencies. Opinions of this kind, when they are based upon the experience of individual practitioners merely, as they always are, are more suggestive than satisfactory; for, in truth, no single obstetrician has treated a sufficient number of cases of this disease to warrant him in asserting that such is the fact, or in laying down such a rule for the guidance of others.

How to give the remedy.

It is sometimes so difficult for these patients to swallow the medicine in a liquid form that you will do well to prepare it for them in the form of powders or pellets. By this means it can be given dry upon the tongue. Whatever fluids are administered should be introduced into the mouth very slowly and cautiously, else they may strangle the patient, and thus cause an unnecessary repetition of the fit.

In the subsequent treatment, it is very important to keep the patient well nourished; to avoid unnecessary excitement; to have the breasts well drawn, either by the child or artificially; not to permit the lochia to cease suddenly; to keep the bowels and bladder free from excessive accumulation; and, if there are symptoms of amaurosis, to protect the eyes from too strong light.

LECTURE XVI.

MENSTRUAL HEADACHE.

GENTLEMEN:

Having heard a good report of our Clinique, this poor woman presents herself for treatment.

Case.—Mrs. ——, aged 40, began to menstruate when she was only twelve years old. About that time she commenced to have periodical attacks of headache, which, she says, have always returned just before or just after the "courses." She is the mother of three children. With the exception of the time in which she was pregnant and while nursing her children, in each case, and also when, for some unknown reason, the menses were suppressed for twelve months at another time, she has never failed in twenty-eight years to have this headache every four weeks. The arrest of the catamenia took place two years ago, and afforded a complete immunity from these attacks. When the flow was first restored it was slightly irregular in its return, but the headache came on again, and since that time it has been more severe in degree than ever before.

The pain is located in the temples, and across the frontal region, is aggravated by light, but not by noise. It occasionally, although very rarely, happens that a paroxysm is caused by over-fatigue and anxiety. During the attack she sometimes has slight nausea, there is occasional vomiting, weakness, a feeling of inability to stand or walk, and a very decided anorexia. She has consulted many physicians, but without benefit.

These few symptoms convey no very adequate idea of the suffering involved in the monthly martyrdom to which our patient has been subjected for more than a quarter of a century. The case is by no means a rare one. There are those who have had this painful affection during their whole menstrual life. And, strange to say, it frequently happens that this particular variety of headache is

Chief symptoms frequently overlooked.

often improperly diagnosticated and treated. I have seen patients who have been under the professional care of a number of physicians for this complaint, and although the monthly periodicity of their symptoms was as marked as in the case before us, no reference had been made to it at all.

The especial significance of the different kinds of headache that are incident to the sexual diseases of women is not as thoroughly understood by the profession as it should be. I can not hope to remedy this defect in their special pathology, but I desire to offer a few practical hints that are founded upon clinical experience.

Nearly, if not quite all, these forms of cephalalgia are of reflex origin. The only prominent exception to this rule occurs in case of the impairment of the quality of the blood, as in chlorosis, chloro-anæmia, the debility following abortion, menorrhagia, uterine leucorrhœa, or too prolonged lactation. The "menstrual headache," as it is termed, is almost always dependent upon ovarian irritation or inflammation. Hence the relation of the paroxysm to the return of the menstrual cycle. It comes regularly each month. It may either anticipate, accompany, or follow the discharge. The pain is most frequently located in the crown of the head, or it may be in one or both temples, in the orbital region, or even in the back of the head. It may or may not be accompanied by the "clavus hystericus." In chronic cases, it is sometimes described as "crushing, as if there were great weight upon the vertex." This is an intractable and persistent symptom, especially in women who are passing through the climacteric period. More frequently, perhaps, the pain is said to be "burning" in character, and circumscribed in extent.

Reflex headache.

It is quite common for women with this kind of headache to complain of "strange" sensations in the head, or of "forgetfulness;" or they will tell you that "half the time they do not know what they are about." Sometimes, during the paroxysm, they will threaten to "go crazy," and, *nolens volens*, may put the threat into temporary execution. This is the form of headache with which those who are subject to difficult and delayed menstruation are most afflicted. Those who are of the hysterical or the neuralgic diathesis are particularly liable to it. When it occurs as a concomitant of uterine

Peculiar symptoms.

ulceration, I think you may refer the lesion of the cervix and the headache to some primary disease in one or both of the ovaries.

Headache from uterine displacement and leucorrhœa.

Attacks of headache which are incident to uterine displacements and to leucorrhœa, resemble what is vulgarly styled "sick headache." In this form of the disorder, the paroxysms recur without regularity and without any special reference to menstruation. In those who are susceptible, over-fatigue, want of proper rest, or of food, or an excess of mental excitement, may induce it. Here the gastric function is prominently and principally implicated. Incidentally, the most curious symptoms may attend it. One of my private patients described the feeling in her head as "a sort of wriggling, as from the movement of long worms, such as are found in vinegar." It is not unusual for such persons to complain of a sensation "as if the head had been scalped, and the brain left exposed."

Case.

I once knew a woman to be confined to her room for fifteen consecutive weeks with a spurious typhoid fever. In her case, this headache returned every fifteenth day with the regularity of an ague. Her description of the paroxysm led me to infer that there was a possible dislocation of the uterus, although it had never been suggested to my patient by her previous medical attendant. I found that the womb had settled down upon the perineum. As soon as it was restored, the periodical headache vanished and her fever did not return. If we except the expedient of setting fire to the house, nothing will place some of these patients upon their feet so speedily as to restore the womb to its proper position, and to keep it there.

Cause of menstrual headache.

There is a prevalent idea that the menstrual headache is caused by a spasm or obstruction of the uterine cervix, which has the effect to prevent a ready exit of the menstrual flow. In exceptional cases, this may be true; but the reverse is certainly the rule. If it were not so, labor, either in abortus or at term, and indeed, whatever would secure the free expansion of the cervix, would cure it radically and entirely. But this woman's history disproves the theory of its being due, in her case at least, to a lesion or spasm of the neck of the womb. She has had three children, and now is worse than ever before.

Here the direct relation of the headache to the function of ovulation is shown, not only by the regularity of its return at the month, but also by a complete exemption from it during gestation and lactation. In pregnancy, and while nursing, menstruation is physiologically suspended. When this function was arrested the headache ceased, and when it was resumed the headache returned. The same was true of the period during which, for some unknown reason, she had amenorrhœa. The periodical afflux of blood to the generative organs, but more especially to the ovaries, and the nervous tension and erethism connected with the monthly crisis, appear to have been sufficient to cause the headache. As soon as the vascular and nervous energies were diverted and busy elsewhere,—in the developing uterus during gestation, and in the mammary glands while nursing her infant,—the remote cause was removed, and the effect ceased.

Proof of connection between ovulation and the cephalalgia.

This view of the etiology of "menstrual" headache is confirmed by the history of cases in which an incidental and temporary excitement of the generative system causes an attack independently of, and without reference to the monthly return. There are those who always have it after coitus. In some it follows the first indulgence of the sexual act after menstruation, or prolonged continence. In others, a sexual orgasm induced by emotional influences, especially if it is ungratified, may be followed by a severe attack of this peculiar form of headache. Incompatibility in the marriage relation is a frequent cause of it. It is sometimes due to a temporary arrest of the flow for a few hours, or rather to what has been styled "intermittent" menstruation. Or it may depend upon too scanty or too copious a discharge. In brief, in certain women, whatever mental or physical causes are sufficient greatly to derange the circulation and innervation of the internal generative organs are capable of inducing the "menstrual headache."

Headache from causes which simulate ovulation.

Exciting causes.

Suppose we interrogate this patient a little farther, and ascertain if there are not other symptoms with which we should become acquainted.

"Are you quite well, madam, with the exception of the headache?" "No, sir, not entirely; but the pain in my head, when it does come on, is so much worse than anything else, that I make no account of the other symptoms." "What other symptoms have you?" "I have a feeling, sir, as if my limbs were going to sleep. It requires a great effort for me to keep about, and I am very sensitive to the cold air." "Do you have these symptoms now, midway between the periods?" "Yes, sir." "Tell me how you feel when the flow commences, and while it continues." "I often have a kind of spasm in the bowels, which comes on just before the discharge begins, and then goes off again. Sometimes I become a little blind, and so long as I am sick there is more or less darkness before the eyes, so that I can not see distinctly." "Do these last symptoms disappear as soon as the flow stops?" "They do." "Show me where the pain is located." "It is here, sir, in the left side, right over the hip. Sometimes it is in the groin, and shoots down that leg; at other times, saving your presence, it passes into my belly. And sometimes there is a throbbing in the lower part of my back-bone." "Are you quite certain that these symptoms return every time you are sick?" "I am, sir; they are as sure to come as the flow itself."

Now, gentlemen, if there have been any doubts in your minds as to the interpretation of this case, I think they will have vanished with the close of this examination. You may sometimes find it even more difficult to locate the original lesion which has given rise to a sympathetic headache, such as that of which our patient complains; but you should always search for it. For, depend upon it, although you may fail to remedy an obscure case, if you can explain its special pathology, its cause, course, nature, and probable termination, you will have almost as strong a hold upon the confidence of the patient and her friends as if you were really able to cure it.

Search for the primary lesion.

There is no especial difficulty in diagnosticating this from other varieties of headache. The "sick" headache affects males and females indiscriminately, and sometimes affects quite young children also. It is not regularly paroxysmal. The fits have no especial relation to the menstrual cycle, but may be brought on at any time by an excess of anxiety, fatigue, or the eating of improper food. The paroxysm passes off with sleep, or is relieved by pressure, as from a handkerchief bound tightly about the head, and sometimes ends with emesis. The gastric function is chiefly deranged, and

Diagnosis—from "sick" headache.

nausea, retching, and vomiting almost always attend it. It may occur prior to puberty, and also after the climacteric. In many women the paroxysms of this headache are more frequent during the early months of pregnancy and lactation than at other times. Those who are subject to it are apt to be wretched and hypochondriacal. It is sometimes cured by change of climate.

The "neuralgic" headache is traceable to vicissitudes of weather, unusual exposure, especially to wet and cold, prolonged mental strain, insufficient nourishment, nervous exhaustion and perturbation of the mental faculties. Unless of a regular intermediate type, as in orbital neuralgia, or "sun" headache, it does not recur regularly, and has no especial relation to the menstrual function. It is often relieved by eating or drinking. The rheumatic diathesis is a strong predisponent of this variety of headache. Seamstresses and others who live upon a light and insufficient diet, who are underfed and overworked, and who drink much of tea and coffee, are very liable to it. It is sometimes caused by decayed teeth. The pain is piercing, darting, lancinating, and erratic, sometimes present in one part of the head or the face, and again in another, now superficial, then deep-seated.

From "neuralgic" headache.

The "congestive" headache, of which one sees more in the medical books and journals than in actual practice, is marked by a flushed face, redness and suffusion of the conjunctivæ, either dilated or contracted pupils, photophobia, an intolerance of noise, and a full pulse. This form of headache is usually a concomitant of some local inflammation, and subsides without any very serious consequences.

From "congestive" headache.

The "hysterical" headache differs from those of which I have spoken, in the period of its occurrence and recurrence, in the fixed limit of its location, in the fitful flow of animal spirits which accompanies it, and in the marked effect that the most trifling emotional influences have to increase the suffering. It is very likely to recur at the month, more especially if the patient has dysmenorrhœa, or spinal irritation, but is not by any means confined to that particular period. Some women always have it if the menses are delayed or suppressed. In other cases it is a sequel to menor-

From "hysterical" headache.

rhagia. The paroxysm may be caused, and may come and go, in the same manner as the true hysterical fit.

Peculiarities of the "menstrual" headache.

The proper "menstrual" headache returns with the regularity of an ague paroxysm every time the woman menstruates. If its habit has been to come on at the beginning of the monthly crisis, this habit will be persevered in. If it has been accustomed to return at the last of the month, just as the flow has almost entirely ceased, you may expect it again at the same season. If your patient menstruates once in three weeks it will not fail; if every six weeks she will not escape it. Nor does it matter if she has had an incidental attack during the inter-menstrual period. It will be all the same, whether sooner or later, whenever ovulation takes place. Pregnancy, lactation, amenorrhœa, the climacteric, or whatever interrupts the menstrual function, will arrest it. When this function is restored, it will come again. The degree of suffering in the head is not always in ratio with the quantity of blood that is lost in menstruation, neither with the intra-pelvic pain and distress that are experienced in getting rid of it. The quasi-hysterical symptoms which sometimes attend upon attacks of this headache, are incidental merely, and not at all characteristic. In the majority of cases a close and careful examination reveals either sub-acute or chronic inflammation, irritation, or neuralgia of one or both of the ovaries.

The prognosis.

The prognosis will vary with the age, temperament, and surroundings of the patient, the nature and duration of the sexual disorder, the possibility of controlling and directing her emotional states and the condition of her general health. Chronic cases are not so readily cured as those which are more recent, and therefore less complicated. The nearer the approach to the climacteric, the less promising the case. When the menses cease, however, the headache will probably stop of its own accord. Frequent child-bearing, but more especially frequent abortions, render this disease more intractable than it is under opposite circumstances. Domestic infelicity is an almost insuperable obstacle to the cure of this form of headache. The periodical engorgement of the ovaries, which is contingent upon menstruation, lights up, renews, and perpetuates the lesion of those organs, whatever it may be. If we can prevent the monthly exacerbation of the sexual disorder, and can so regulate this function that it shall become physiological and healthy, the cure is practically accomplished. Otherwise, the disease may continue and increase until the general health gives way and fatal results follow. In those who have what has been styled the "insane neurosis," or predisposition, it may finally develop into some form of insanity.

Treatment.—The first indication is to correct and control all those circumstances and habits which cause an undue afflux of blood to the internal generative organs. The eating of improper or too highly seasoned food, the drinking of wines and liquors, too much or too little of society, all those mental and moral influences that stimulate the sexual appetite, tight lacing, running the sewing machine, and constipation, are among the avoidable causes of this disease. Horseback riding has induced it, and might therefore be prejudicial. Exceptional cases are greatly benefited by the prohibition of sexual congress for the space of a week before the commencement, and a week after the cessation of the monthly flow. One of my patients insists that she is almost certain to suffer a severe attack of headache, if the act is performed in the early part of the night, when she is weary, instead of in the early morning when she has been refreshed by sleep.

Hygienic treatment.

If there is a deviation of the uterus from its normal position, it should be replaced. If there is any obstacle to the free exit of the menses, whether in the form of atresia, or flexion, or of stricture of the uterine cervix, it should be removed. The general system should be fortified against all debilitating influences whatever. In the intra-menstrual period she should be well nourished and sent to walk or drive in the fresh air and sunshine every day.

Rest at the month is an important element of cure in menstrual headache. Neither the body nor the mind should be overtaxed at this period. You should be particular in this regard, else the patient may unwittingly upset all that you have done and can do for her relief. If she is occupied as a seamstress or school-teacher, nurse, clerk, housekeeper, or what not, she should, as far as possible, avoid all excess of care, confinement and toil for a few days before, during, and immediately after the catamenia. If she belongs to the higher class, she should be advised to shun all excitement, to forego her fashionable appointments in society, parties, balls, the church, the theatre, and the opera, whenever this crisis comes, and to take the best possible care of herself until it has passed.

The extremities should be kept warm, the head cool, the skin soft and flexible, the urine free, the bowels regular, the circulation equable and uniform, more especially for some days before the flow is due. Such patients should be protected from exposure to stormy and cold weather. One of the worst possible things for them is to get the feet wet and chilled with snow-water.

When this disease is engrafted upon a neuralgic diathesis, electricity properly applied is sometimes very beneficial. In some cases relief may be obtained by having the spine and extremities thoroughly rubbed at stated intervals by one who is strong and healthy. I have known a few cases to be cured by an itinerant "magnetizer."

Electricity and magnetism.

The remedies most serviceable in this disease are those which, because of their relation to the reproductive function, are most frequently indicated in menstrual derangements. Indeed, the symptoms that pertain to the lesion upon which this headache depends are often, although not always, a better guide to the choice of the remedy than the peculiar character of the headache itself. Pulsatilla, sepia, nux vomica, belladonna, ignatia, calcarea carb., platina, baryta carb., lachesis, chamomilla, and apis mellifica are the chief representatives of this class of remedies.

Internal remedies.

If you will compare this woman's symptoms with those proper to sepia you will recognize their marked similarity, and agree with me that she should take this in preference to any other medicine. In another week she will be "unwell," and during that short interval she had better take a dose of sepia every evening. Let her report at the end of a fortnight.

PROLAPSUS UTERI WITH RIGHT LATERO-VERSION.

Case. — Mrs. — complains of a series of symptoms, from which she says she has suffered for more than a year past. She is married, but has never borne any children, neither has she ever had a miscarriage. She has dragging pain in the hips and loins, and sometimes there is strangury, with obstinate constipation. The bowels move at long intervals spontaneously, but with much effort and tenesmus, which at times are ineffectual. The stools are invariably dry, hard, and scybalous. When straining at stool, she sometimes "feels as if everything would be forced from her." All the unpleasant symptoms are increased during and for some time after the menstrual period. At times she experiences severe cramping pains in the right thigh, which come on suddenly after prolonged exercise upon her feet, or after standing for a considerable time. The only means of relief that she has found from the latter paroxysms is obtained by lying down immediately upon the left or opposite side of the body. By keeping quiet in this position for a little while the cramp-like pain subsides and soon leaves entirely. She has not been able to lie with any degree of comfort upon her right side since her ill-health began. And if she rolls upon that side while sleeping, the cramps in the right thigh will awaken her at once.. She has an almost constant headache in the region of the temples. During and after the menses, however, it is apt to be located in the occipital region. The flow is too profuse. It continues a whole week, instead of four days as heretofore. It is also too frequent, returning as often as every three weeks at the farthest.

Constipation from rectal paralysis.

You have doubtless observed the relative frequency of constipation as an attendant upon the diseases of women. One of its most common causes is a paralysis of the rectum. I have examined this patient per vaginam, and found the uterus prolapsed, and at the same time lying obliquely from right to left across the vagina. The most plausible theory of this displacement is that the descent and pressure of the womb against the bowel caused it to become paralyzed. The accumulation of fæcal matter in the rectum forced the fundus of the uterus toward the right acetabulum, and latero-version was the natural and necessary consequence. Whether the constipation really preceded or followed the prolapsus, it would be impossible to say. Latero-version of the uterus always depends upon pressure applied to the side of its body or fundus. It is incident to the history of fibroids, ovarian tumors, and to tumors within the broad ligaments. When due to either of these diseases the organ may be displaced either toward the right or the left side of the pelvis. When, however, it depends upon the pressure of a tumor caused by impacted fæces contained within the rectum, the fundus will, as in the case before us, always

Latero-version from an overloaded rectum.

be thrown toward the right acetabulum and the cervix toward the tuberosity of the left ischium. The diagnosis may be confirmed by the introduction of the uterine sound or probe.

The incidental symptoms are interesting and significant. The cramping pains of which Mrs. —— complains are referable to pressure of the corpus uteri upon the anterior branches of the sacral nerves. When she lies upon the right side, the womb falls upon those nerves, or is pressed by the distended rectum against them. When she turns upon the left side, it drops away, and the cramp ceases. When she walks too far, or is upon her feet for too long a time, the womb is more decidedly prolapsed. The nearer its approach to the perineum the more direct and positive the pressure of the rectum toward the right side of the pelvis. Straining at stool only increases the difficulty, and it is no marvel that she feels as if all the pelvic organs would be forced through the vulva.

The cramping pains.

These cramp-like pains are very similar to those which may attend upon an advanced stage of labor. In presentations of the vertex especially, when rotation occurs suddenly and the head passes rapidly through the inferior pelvic strait, direct pressure upon the sacral nerves often causes the patient to cry out that her "legs are cramping." And so also in cases in which the womb is retroverted suddenly, as from a fall or other impulse, one or both the lower extremities may be violently cramped and even paralyzed. In this poor woman's case there is no dropsy of the feet and ankles, and the veins are not varicose, because the pressure is not applied to the vessels going to the lower extremities. Those vessels emerge from the superior pelvis beneath Poupart's ligament, and are, therefore, not liable to be pressed upon by the uterus, excepting in its gravid state, after the fourth month.

One of two causes may be sufficient to account for the implication of the bladder in this case. The strangury might be caused by the displacement of the uterine cervix, or by pressure of the uterus against the neck of the bladder and the urethra. The uterine cervix is so joined with the inferior portion of the bladder that it can not be very decidedly displaced without dragging upon that organ, and giving rise to more or less of irritation, inflammation, and vesical tenesmus.

The vesical symptoms.

Hence it sometimes happens that the most prominent and persistent symptoms of uterine luxation are referred almost exclusively to the bladder. And, because they suppose that all derangements of the urinary function are due to renal disorder, patients not unfrequently consult their physician for the cure of disease of the kidneys, when they are really suffering from some form of displacement of the womb.

Such slight degrees of prolapsus, as are incident to the menstrual period and to the early weeks of pregnancy, are sometimes the cause of frequent and painful micturition. These sufferings are, however, relieved spontaneously—by the escape of the menses and the subsidence of the monthly hyperæmia in the one case, and by the final ascent of the uterus above the superior strait in the other. In chronic prolapsus all these symptoms are made to vanish, at least temporarily, by lifting the womb into its proper position.

This case illustrates the possibility of uterine displacements disconnected with abortion or with labor at term. The frequent return of menstruation, and the excess of the flow, indicate a primary disorder of this very important function.

Treatment.—There are two reasons why this woman is not well. The first is, that her rectum is paralyzed; the second, that she menstruates too freely and frequently. All the symptoms that have the least significance may be referred to one of these two causes.

Leading indications.

This is the most common form of constipation in females. If the muscular coat of the rectum has lost its tonicity through neglect of the patient to attend to the calls of nature, or to go to stool regularly every day, this bad habit should be corrected. Enemata containing olive oil, or castor oil, may be given for temporary relief, with the view of softening and removing the impacted fæces. Laxative food is of more service in constipation depending upon causes which affect the upper portion of the intestine. Some of these patients with paralysis of the rectum might eat brown bread, oat meal, figs, prunes, or baked apples until doomsday without the least benefit.

To remedy the constipation.

If the uterus is prolapsed, or so displaced as to press directly against the rectum, that pressure must be removed, or the con-

18

stipation can not be cured. And since these causes act and react, the uterine deviation may depend upon the lack of resiliency in the rectum, the presence of fæcal matter within the gut, or upon straining at stool. Pessaries are contra-indicated in case of uterine displacement with profuse and too frequent menstruation.

Empty the rectum—restore the uterus.

The most ordinary remedy for this variety of constipation, with its incidental uterine displacement, are alumina, nux vomica, natrum mur., plumbum, opium, belladonna, sulphur, zincum, and lycopodium.

Among those which are in best repute for the cure of too frequent and copious menstruation you will find calcarea carb., china, phosphoric acid, cantharis, zincum met., spongia, sulphur, creasotum, and magnesia carbonica.

This patient will take nux vomica 3d at night, and calcarea carb. 3d in the morning, one dose of each daily. She must keep off her feet as much as possible, particularly at the catamenial season.

ACUTE CERVICAL METRITIS.

Case.—Mrs. ——, aged 35, the mother of three children, the youngest of which is six years old, relates the following story: Eight days ago, at the proper time, the menses made their appearance without any unusual symptoms. On the same morning she commenced a five days' job of work upon the sewing machine. At the close of the first day's labor the flow ceased for some hours, and then, after a foot-bath and a night's rest, it returned. On the third day there was another intermission in the menstrual discharge, and on the fourth day it ceased entirely—two days sooner than usual.

She now complains of headache, with slight vertigo, the face is flushed, the pupils are somewhat dilated, noise worries her, and she can not bear the light. There are cutting, darting pains in the upper portion of the thighs and across the hips. These pains are worse on motion and while standing upon the feet. She also has a burning, bearing-down pain within the pelvis, some strangury, and great discomfort. She is very nervous and apprehensive.

The "touch" reveals the os uteri patulous, the cervix swollen, hot, dry, and exquisitely tender. She can not bear the least pressure upon it. The womb lies very low in the pelvis, so much so that when she stands upon her feet it rests upon the perineum.

Examination with the speculum shows the tumefied and tender

cervix to be congested and more than twice as large as natural, but there are no signs of abrasion, neither of ulceration. The epithelium covering its vaginal portion is intact, and there is no unnatural discharge from the external os uteri.

This is a case of acute inflammation of the neck of the womb. Writers describe two varieties of cervicitis — one in which the substance, or parenchyma of the uterine cervix is the seat of the inflammation (cervical metritis), or areolar hyperplasia (Thomas); another in which the inflammation is limited to the mucous membrane that covers the vaginal portion and lines its canal (cervical endo-metritis). These diseases are so frequent and troublesome that you will need to study their clinical history most carefully.

Varieties of.

Cervical metritis is very rare in those women who have not given birth to one or more children, either prematurely or at term. Indeed the most powerful predisponent of this disease is found in the changes which are incident to the uterine cervix during the middle and later months of gestation. The virgin cervix is firm and fibrous, almost cartilaginous in texture. Its vascularity is not at all pronounced, its dilatability is scarcely sufficient to permit the ready exit of the menses. But the modifications which it undergoes during pregnancy change the consistence of its tissues, not temporarily, but, in a sense, permanently. The contraction and involution which follow delivery do not restore the unyielding nature which is proper to the virginal cervix, and thenceforth we find it liable to diseases from which it was exempt before.

Rare in nulliparæ.

One of the most frequent of these affections is acute cervical metritis. And all of its exciting causes produce a more decided and damaging effect if they are applied at or about the time of the menstrual return. It is possible that this woman might not have experienced any ill consequences from the same kind of exercise had it been taken at another time. But, she "did not think," — a very common infirmity with patients as well as with their physicians — and therefore, she set to work the very day the flow began, intending to persevere with it during the "period."

The monthly cycle a predisponent.

Much has been said and written of the sewing-machine as a cause of uterine disease. I apprehend that it is the abuse, instead of the proper use, of the machine that works the mischief in those who run it. The trouble is that, with most housekeepers, it offers such a ready and expeditious means of doing the family sewing that they are tempted to postpone this labor until it has accumulated for weeks, and perhaps even for months. Then they go to work for days and nights consecutively, in order to despatch it, and to "get it out of the way." The instrument itself may be as innocent as the piano. It is this habit of playing upon it, or rather of working with it, continuously for hours and days together, that does the harm. If the same work were properly distributed, as our wives and daughters "practice" upon the piano — not as a business, but as a recreation and diversion, the result would doubtless be very different. In the case of those women, however, who are obliged to sit at the sewing-machine from morning until night each day in the week, in order to obtain a livelihood, it is almost impossible for them to escape certain functional and organic diseases of the womb.

Sewing machines and uterine diseases.

Whatever tends to wound, bruise, or irritate the neck of this organ may, in those who are predisposed to it, give rise to cervical metritis. Too violent exercise, as horseback riding, or riding in a rough carriage or car; misplaced, or badly-fitting pessaries; too forcible and excessive coitus; prolapsus, and the various flexions of the uterus; standing for too long a time upon the feet, as in the case of female clerks in our shops and stores, and of ladies at fashionable parties; a sudden arrest of the menstrual flow; and the extension of the inflammation in cervical endo-metritis from the lining membrane of the uterine cervix to its parenchymatous structure, are among the more common exciting causes of this disease.

Causes of acute cervical metritis.

You will readily understand how it is possible for either of these causes to develop this form of metritis by converting the physiological injection of its structures, which is necessary to their nutrition and also to the menstrual function, into a pathological congestion thereof. A local arrest of the circulation, a temporary sluggishness, or stasis of blood in its loose, connective, dilatable tissue, represents the first step in the inflammatory process. What the

Mode of operation and results.

result of this engorgement will be we can not say beforehand. If the cause is not removed and the case properly treated, the cervix may become the seat of chronic inflammation, hypertrophy, induration, and possibly of scirrhous deposit.

Differential diagnosis.

Acute cervical metritis is more likely to be confounded with cervical endo-metritis than with any other disease. In the former, the neck of the womb is swollen and tender, not only to a light touch, but also to pressure upon it from within the vagina, and through the rectum; there is no abrasion and no ulceration, no appearance of hypertrophied villi (so often mistaken for granular ulceration) and no leucorrhœal discharge. The constitutional symptoms are such as attend upon the more severe forms of local congestion and inflammation in other parts of the body. There is almost always pain in the head, photophobia, a flushed face, and such nervous symptoms as those of which this patient complains.

Prognosis.

Fortunately the organic changes in the cervix, which are the sequelæ of acute cervical metritis, develop so slowly that prompt and proper treatment may prevent the disease from becoming chronic. In most cases, however, these changes take place insidiously and in a latent manner, so that the acute stage will have passed before the physician is consulted. Doubtless the frequent return of the menses serves to perpetuate the liability of the neck of the womb, which has once been inflamed, to repeated attacks, that may finally end in establishing the chronic form of the disease in it. In those women in whom the cervix is unusually long, as well as in those who are of a relaxed fibre, cervical metritis is very apt to become chronic and intractable. The same is true if the disease occurs in women of a decidedly bilious temperament, and who may be suffering from old hepatic disorders. Chronic affections of the rectum, as prolapsus and hæmorrhoids, sometimes retard or prevent the cure of a case of cervical metritis.

Postural treatment.

Treatment. — The increased suffering which this woman experiences when she is upon her feet, suggests that she should not be allowed to walk about. The horizontal posture is the first thing you should prescribe for similar cases. You can not expect to cure them readily if the position of the patient's body facilitates and necessitates a determination of blood to the inflamed part. Especially should these patients be counseled to keep to the bed or sofa during the menstrual period, and for some days thereafter. They should also avoid all those emotional influences which might, directly or indirectly, excite the sexual system. The bladder should be emptied regularly, and the bowels not permitted to become torpid and inactive, or otherwise the intra-pelvic circulation might be so deranged as to prevent the best chosen remedies from having their desired effect.

If, in a given case, there is reason to believe that any of the causes already named has occasioned the attack, that cause must be removed. And you should act promptly. Learn the source of the mischief and remove it as soon as possible, else the most proper and appropriate time for curing the case, or at least for preventing it from developing into the chronic form of the disease, will have passed before you have accomplished anything.

Remove the cause.

As the result of an abundant experience, I am persuaded that in these cases of engorgement of the cervix uteri, with incipient inflammation of its deeper-seated tissues, "prevention is better than cure." Hygiene should go hand in hand with Therapeutics. It would not be sufficient to give this woman belladonna, or any other remedy, and dismiss her without specific instructions concerning her habits of life, of exercise, and exposure. It is just here that our knowledge of special physiology and of special pathology will render us the most important aid. It may fail to suggest the remedy for the symptoms complained of, but it will not fail to suggest what, in such a case as this, is vastly more important.

Prevention better than cure.

It might involve a species of suicide for this patient to persist in running the sewing machine. She should not ride or walk very far or frequently. A journey from Chicago to New York, before her symptoms are relieved and the next menstrual period safely passed, might render her an invalid for months or even for years. And so also of croquet, of ironing, sweeping, or prolonged standing upon the feet, whether for pleasure at a party, or for profit in a store or in school. Any menstrual irregularity should be remedied. Sexual congress should be prohibited. Pessaries and every species of artificial support,

Items.

whether within the vagina or around the body, are positively and decidedly mischievous in this class of cases. The same is true of the use of cold and astringent injections thrown into the vagina, and of most of the lotions and ointments that are applied in case of hæmorrhoids.

If you can properly attribute the attack to traumatic injury, there will be no harm in prescribing a vaginal injection, consisting of the tincture of arnica, glycerine, and tepid water. In case she has hæmorrhoids, with venous discoloration of the vagina, or a varicose condition of the veins of the lower extremities, it is best to substitute hamamelis for the arnica. Simple glycerine and water, one part of the former to five of the latter, will sometimes allay the burning heat and pain within the pelvis. I have occasionally witnessed the best effects from Dr. Sims' method of applying pure glycerine directly to and about the cervix by means of a cotton or sponge tampon which is saturated with it. In one of my cases it certainly brought away half a teacupful of serum with which the swollen and pendulous cervix had previously been engorged. It may be possible by some such simple and harmless expedient to prevent what might otherwise develop into chronic cervical metritis.

Local measures.

The internal treatment should be regulated by the obvious symptoms peculiar to the individual case for the cure of which you are consulted. This woman will take of belladonna 3d, a dose every three hours. When her symptoms are somewhat improved, it may be repeated once in six hours. Let her come again next week.

Prescription.

LECTURE XVII.

HYSTERIA.

GENTLEMEN:

Although I have already given you a clinical outline of hysteria,* the subject is by no means exhausted. Indeed, there is enough in this single topic for a whole course of lectures. For this disorder modifies and complicates almost all the diseases to which women are liable.

Case. — At 7 P. M. of yesterday, I was hurriedly summoned to the relief of Mrs. ——, aged 20 years, three months advanced in her first pregnancy, who was seized while at the tea-table with an unnatural staring and blindness, followed by a species of fit, which greatly alarmed the husband and family. I found her lying in an unconscious state upon the floor of the dining room. The eyes were staring widely and wildly, and at times the eye-balls were rolled upwards as far as possible. The pupils appeared natural, excepting at intervals of from five to ten minutes, when a general spasm of all the muscles of the extremities ensued; they would suddenly increase in size and become very large. With the approach of this symptom the face would flush, and she would roll from her left to her right side. The arms were thrown wildly about, and during the fit it was almost impossible so to hold her as to prevent her from doing herself a personal injury. Each paroxysm ended with sobbing and an attempt to articulate. The pulse was 80 and quite regular. From her manner it appeared that she was dreaming and talking, or holding intercourse with some person not present in the room, or at least not visible to the attendants. While the fit was on, the facial muscles twitched violently, but there was no frothing at the mouth, or purplish discoloration of the face. The carmine hue which came and went, however, caused her to appear very beautiful.

I ordered a plentiful supply of fresh air, the clothing to be loosened about the throat and waist, and belladonna 3rd to be given

* See pages 87 and 107 of this volume.

her (very slowly) once in twenty minutes until the fits ceased, and after that every half-hour until I called again.

9 P. M. She had only one paroxysm after taking the first dose of the medicine, but the emotional outbreaks had become more marked. She would exclaim, "Oh, so dark!" then talk incoherently, and finally cry and sob for some moments most pitifully. After a little it became evident through her speech that she was in communication with her mother, who, it was said, had died five years before. This last symptom was looked upon as supernatural, and alarmed the bystanders exceedingly. They declared it to be a premonition, and unfailing sign of the speedy departure of the patient for the land of spirits; but the husband told me that she had frequently had similar attacks, and that in all of them she had shown this same symptom.

By my advice she was carried from the sofa to her room, placed quietly in bed, the half dozen voluntary nurses discharged, and she left alone with her husband for the night. This morning he called to report that his wife had slept soundly for some hours, and now appeared quite well, although a little weak.*

Hysteria and the menstrual molimen.

Hysterical attacks usually bear some relation to the menstrual period. A woman is ill with a protracted and debilitating disease, as for example pneumonia, or typhoid fever. Perhaps she has escaped one or more "periods." But the return of the monthly cycle is shown in a peculiar aggravation of the coincident nervous symptoms. In lieu of the proper flow, she becomes unusually wakeful, restless, fitful, or disheartened. Nothing pleases or satisfies her. Her nurse is charged with neglect, she thinks that her friends have become heartless, or that her physician has lost interest in her case. In consequence her family take alarm, and unless he understands his business very thoroughly, the doctor may be led to make an unfavorable prognosis. The perturbation reacts upon the patient, who is very impressible, and the hysterical flame grows by what it feeds upon. The neighbors clamor for "counsel," or for "a change of treatment," and are permitted to have their way. The physician who is called in may or may not have tact enough to recognize the real condition of the patient. If he can separate the hysterical element, can date the exacerbation from the recurrence of the month, can proceed quietly to the cure of the origi-

* Although similar attacks occurred at the fourth, fifth and sixth months, this patient reached term without any further mishap, and was finally delivered of a healthy ten-pound child. She had no convulsions in child-bed.

nal idiopathic disease, all may yet be well. Otherwise she may continue to grow worse instead of better. The issue may depend entirely upon his skill in diagnosis. The distinctive feature of hysteria will sometimes enable you to decide whether those women who are ill with acute disease are really in so dangerous a condition as they appear to be.

Although child-bearing, if it be not too frequent or exhaustive, is a good general prophylactic of hysteria; and although pregnancy may exempt from an attack of it; the opposite effect may follow conception and the arrest of the menses. When, as in this case, the disease comes in distinct paroxysms during pregnancy, the fits are more likely to recur at or about the time the patient would have menstruated. This fact explains the liability of their developing into a form of ante-partum convulsions, of which I have already spoken; and also the increased risk from abortion, which, for physiological reasons, is more imminent at the month than at other times.

Hysteria during gestation.

Attacks of hysteria occurring as a concomitant of other diseases, or as a contingent of pregnancy and lactation, may safely be referred to some emotional excitant. The previous disease, or condition, has caused such debility and prostration, as powerfully to predispose to nervous derangement, and the patient is an easy prey to the depressing emotions. She may be borne down by influences which, under different circumstances and at other times would have had little or no effect upon her. And these circumstances include a list of avoidable causes which in themselves are so small and apparently insignificant as frequently to escape notice. We are very apt to forget — if indeed we ever knew — that it is possible for psychical causes alone to derange the blood-making process, and to poison the very fountain of life. If violent mental emotions will prevent the blood of a healthy person from coagulating when it is withdrawn from the body, they certainly are capable of destroying life, as by a slow poison, when they are brought to bear upon an organism in which the blood is already impaired and impoverished to the last degree by previous disease. I apprehend that thousands of patients have died when otherwise they would surely have recovered, because

Emotional causes of.

Possible effects of.

at a most unfortunate moment they were seized by fear and apprehension, by grief or fright, or jealousy, chagrin, disappointment, or some form of mental depression and agitation, from the fatal effects of which they could not be rallied. In illustration of this view I may mention the following

Case.—I was called from my hotel at 2 A.M., December 6, 1861, to visit a most estimable lady who was said to be dying of typhoid fever. She had been ill for five weeks under the charge of another physician, and had had a morbid fear of death from the onset of the fever. The doctor and the counsel had left her at 8 P.M., of the previous evening, after having told the family that she could not possibly survive the night. My friend, the messenger, insisted upon my visiting her and giving her something "to make her die easily," as much on his own wife's account and that of others in the house, as from motives of humanity. Her clergyman had visited her soon after the doctors left, and her friends had bidden her a final adieu. She then became apparently unconscious, and passed into a peculiar mental state, in which the nurse told me she had a vision of her mother, who had died some fifteen years before. She then began to exclaim, over and over again, "Oh, my blessed mother!" which phrase she had continued to repeat so that every one in the house could hear it. Sometimes it was spoken distinctly, and again she mumbled it, so that one could not understand what she was saying; but it was always in the same dreary monotone, which was anything but cheerful in the middle of the night, and under such painful circumstances.

I asked the nurse if the patient could see? She assured me that for several hours she had been entirely blind. Could she swallow? No. Between her exclamations, I thought I detected the woman looking at me askant and in a peculiar way. I attempted gently to part the eyelids, in order to look at the pupil of the eye, but they were so suddenly and decidedly closed as to betray a species of volition somewhat inconsistent with the alleged danger. The pulse was 115, distinct but excited. I called for some water and a spoon. When I separated the lips to put a little of the water into her mouth there was a similar resistance. The mouth was closed firmly, almost, "with an audible snap," as the surgeons say of the sudden reduction of certain dislocations. A little tact enabled me to get the water into her throat, and to compel her to swallow it. I was impressed with the idea that she was really in a semi-conscious state, and that some of her symptoms arose from a morbid desire to excite sympathy, or, briefly, that they were hysterical.

A dose of ignatia in the third decimal attenuation was given her immediately, and the nurse was directed to give another in half an hour, and a third also in case she did not become quiet and fall asleep. The room was to be cleared of all the friends who had come to witness her death; she was to be "let alone severely," and no one, excepting the nurse, permitted to remain with her. The husband and relatives were assured that the danger was more imaginary than real, and that if she could sleep and be properly nourished, she would almost certainly recover.

She soon stopped the dreary talk about her mother, became calm and fell into a quiet sleep, from which she wakened at short intervals. In the morning she was better. She took no other medicine, was well fed, and her funeral was "indefinitely postponed." Eleven years have elapsed, and she is still alive.

A practical inference.

Now, gentlemen, you shall decide whether, if some one had not recognized the real condition of things in this case, and changed it very decidedly, the circumstances which surrounded that woman in her weak condition, might not have overwhelmed her and caused her death.

Enigmatical nature of hysteria.

The well-known tendency of hysteria to imitate other diseases has in it a tinge of deceit. It may simulate almost any affection so closely, as to puzzle the best diagnostician, and to disappoint the most skillful practitioner. Or it may complicate other maladies by counfeiting single symptoms. Women of an hysterical constitution seldom pass through the different stages of an acute inflammation, or fever, without some peculiar experiences and revelations which are totally foreign to the special pathology of the disease in question. These complications may be classed as hysterical.

Suspicious symptoms.

In such cases you will observe that those symptoms which are incidental and least important, are liable to be incongruous and very much exaggerated. If, for example, such a patient has pneumonia, the physical signs will not be such as should correspond to her complaints of pain and suffering, and to the assumed character of the cough. The sputa may tell one story and her tongue another. Or, if she has dysentery, there may be a similar lack of congruity between the symptoms of which she complains, and the visible, objective phenomena. Taking the impress of this peculiar idiosyncrasy, or dyscrasia, the nervous symptoms, and especially the delirium of such a subject, in typhoid, or puerperal fever, will be very greatly modified. In each case the symptoms which are proper to the disease will be supplemented by others which are spurious, and also by a more or less decided uproar among the physical functions. And thus it may happen that your wits will sometimes be taxed to decide which is fact and which fiction. The spurious, contingent and irrelevant symptoms are the most noisy and clamorous. but not most significant and perilous. The complaint that is made is not always a reliable criterion of suffering and danger.

Hysterical exaggeration.

The hysterical subject, whether male or female, is addicted to hyperbole. The symptoms of which I have spoken resemble an over-anxious witness at court, — they testify to too much. They are actors who "mouth their part." This tendency to exaggeration is a suspicious element which will bear watching. It is so closely related to the lying propensity as almost certainly to betray its true character. You will require a large measure of tact and common sense for its detection.

Incongruous symptoms.

The gossip takes the scent of an ill-assorted marriage, and of marital and social infelicities, with the instinct of a hound and the tact of a savage. In his diagnosis the doctor is perhaps more easily deceived and decoyed. He is generally less shrewd and less skillful in his discrimination. It may not have occurred to him that symptoms, like individuals, are sometimes married without being mated. As the fruit of large experience and observation, I am persuaded that one great and essential difference between physicians consists in their varied ability to separate, to seize upon, to interpret and to remedy those symptoms which are truthful, characteristic and legitimate, to the exclusion of such as are of secondary importance, fictitious, accidental and irrelevant.

A species of malingering.

There is a species of malingering which is a curious feature in some cases of hysteria, a marked example of which came under my own observation some years ago.

Case. — A young lady of sixteen fell ill with the usual symptoms of spinal irritation. She soon complained of a loss of power to move the left arm, then the right one, and successively the lower limbs also. For eight long years the bed-ridden subject of this affliction could neither stand nor feed herself. The sympathies of the best women of the neighborhood overflowed in deeds of kindness and of charity to the poor sufferer. Finally the nurse observed that when she was left alone the patient would sometimes get possession of articles that were distant from her bed, and this without the aid of a third party. By and by a plan was arranged to discover if she really did leave her bed in the absence of others from her chamber. She was notified that for a short time she would be left alone in the house. They watched her, and ten minutes after the alleged departure of the family she was seen to rise and walk off as well as anybody. The spell was broken and she recovered immediately.

Secondary effects upon the patient.

If the consequences of this species of fraud were limited to the friends and relatives, who are usually victimized, they would be less troublesome and more easily remedied. But the worst of it is that the patient may also deceive herself. The sympathy and anxiety of her friends may cause their judgment to be too easily influenced; and the mental and physical weakness of the patient may finally lead her to believe that her symptoms are real, and not assumed, as she knew them to be at the beginning. For it is possible that a sick person may lie to himself, or herself, and not be able to detect it. In hysterics self-deception is frequently compounded with the intent to impose upon others. And you will learn from experience that it is much easier to correct the impressions of those who surround the patient, than it is to dislodge these reflex ideas from the mind of the woman herself.

Leading characteristics of hysteria.

In diagnosticating the various forms and complications of hysteria there are a few signs which almost deserve to be classed as pathognomonic. These are (1) that, as a rule, the disease is limited to females, and in them to the period usually termed "menstrual life," *id est*, between the ages of fourteen and forty-five; (2) that, while it may simulate, succeed, or complicate any other disease, its symptoms are much exaggerated, irregular, and out of proportion with those which properly belong to that disease, whatever it may be; (3) that, in general, however great the disorder among the functions, the pulse is not changed, and the appetite is more frequently excessive than deficient.

Diagnosis.—The cardiac affections with which hysterical disorders are sometimes confounded are valvular lesions, dropsy, and alleged displacement of the heart.

When they do exist, the symptoms of valvular disease of the heart in hysterical subjects are almost invariably associated with chloro-anæmia. The blood is impoverished. The rhythm of the heart's action is disturbed, and there is fluttering and præcordial oppression, palpitation and an exaggerated impulse against the thoracic parietes. In chronic cases there may be dropsy of the feet and of the face.

From valvular disease of the heart.

Physical exploration will enable you to decide between real and spurious lesions of the valves. In *bona fide* disease of the valves, either the first or the second sound of the heart is impaired in its quality, or its place is supplied by an abnormal murmur. If the first of these is implicated or superseded, we know that the auriculo-ventricular valves are diseased; if the second sound is changed, that the semilunar valves are the seat of the difficulty. In hysterical affections which counterfeit this form of endo-cardial lesion both the cardiac sounds are normal. With the first sound of the heart, however, we note the soft bellows murmur of anæmia.

This adventitious sound arises from a change in the quality of the blood, as well as from deranged innervation of the heart itself. Both sets of valves perform their function properly, and although there is palpitation and dyspnœa, yet there is little or no change in the pulse. The dropsy of the feet and of the face, when it does exist, are of hæmic origin. All the physical signs of valvular disease are lacking. There is neither patency nor constriction of the orifices, and no insufficiency of the valves that could possibly give rise either to obstruction or regurgitation.

Case.—Miss ——, aged 22, came to this city from Vermont in order to consult me for the relief of præcordial symptoms which had troubled her for three years. Her disease had been pronounced a valvular affection of the heart, and she had already been treated by three physicians. She complained of languor, lassitude, and anorexia, with disgust for meat of all kinds, of which she had eaten none for more than two years. The bowels were habitually constipated. The slightest exertion caused fatigue and a distressing dyspnœa. The recumbent posture was most agreeable; indeed, she could rest in no other. There was almost complete insomnia. When she did sleep she was not refreshed, but awakened with renewed apprehension. The complexion was pale and chlorotic, the alæ nasi and lips colorless. The pulse 82, weak and compressible, but regular. There was occasional palpitation and painful oppression of the left chest, particularly after exercise and when lying with the head low.

Auscultation revealed the bellows murmur accompanying the first sound of the heart, and I felt confident that what had been mistaken for organic disease of the valves was really chargeable to the deteriorated quality of the blood. She was treated for the chloro-anæmia, and the cardiac symptoms soon vanished. In three months she was quite well, and has continued so during an interval of six years.

From dropsy of the heart.

Women who are supposed to have dropsy of the heart sometimes complain of great difficulty of breathing after exercise, of orthopnœa, of cramping, cutting pains in the cardiac region, of stifling sensations, of a stoppage of the heart's action, or of a feeling as if it had suddenly turned topsy-turvy, of gurgling, and even as if the heart were pulsating in a collection of water. And yet all these symptoms may be found to represent a spurious affection. In diagnosticating true from false hydropericardium you should remember that, in the adult subject, the former is almost always a sequel of rheumatic pericarditis. This is not true of the hysterical disorder, which, in its objective symptoms only, resembles dropsy of the heart. In real hydropericardium the heart-sounds, the respiratory murmur, and the vocal resonance, as well as the pulse, are always implicated. The nutritive function is impaired, the blood is thin and impoverished, there is a tendency to dropsy of the joints and lower extremities, as well as to general anasarca. But in the spurious variety the very opposite is true, and no such concomitants are present.

Hydropericardium has no necessary specific or ætiological relation to menstruation and its several disorders. It is a dangerous disease, more especially if the patient is of a dropsical diathesis, or if she has had some previous difficulty with the heart, the larger blood vessels, or the lungs. Hysterical derangements are intimately connected with ovulation, both with respect to their commencement at puberty, the recurrence of the attack, the aggravation of the symptoms at the "period," the modification induced by pregnancy and lactation, and also their cessation at the climacteric. They are always more alarming than serious.

It is not an uncommon occurrence for a hysterical patient to complain that her heart is displaced! And this symptom may annoy her exceedingly. The mal-location may appear to her to be either transient or permanent. Emotional influences "bring her heart into her mouth." She suffers from violent palpitation, and sometimes from abnormal pulsations in different parts of the body. Her general appearance is healthy, her habit is plethoric, and her looks belie her sensations. The anæmic murmur is sometimes so distinctly heard by such a patient as to induce the belief that her heart is actually dislocated. As a rule you will perhaps encounter more numerous cases of this kind among healthy, bouncing Irish girls, and the fat, lazy drones of fashionable society than elsewhere. I need not tell you that the complaint has no foundation in fact.

Alleged displacement of the heart.

The hysterical cough is a species of nondescript. Its negative peculiarities are by far the more prominent. Physical exploration will not help you to judge of its cause or significance. None of the symptoms give evidence of irritating matters lodging in the respiratory passages, or of any lesion of the pulmonary organs. The cough is purely sympathetic, reflex in its origin, and serious only through its persistency.

The hysterical cough.

It is likely to be excited and aggravated by the most trivial circumstance, more especially by mental shock and emotional influences. In the case of one of my patients the slightest movement, the opening or closing of a door, however noiselessly, the footstep of an attendant, or the least current of air, no matter if she were sleeping, invariably precipitated a fit of coughing. There was some tenderness over the upper cervical vertebræ. She was cured with a few doses of silicea 6th.

Case.

Your tact will be called into exercise in order to dispel a settled conviction that such patients are consumptive. The same imitative propensity which sometimes causes a number of women to be seized with hysteria in a room where another is in a fit, leads those of an hysterical constitution to simulate a cough which does not depend upon any pectoral lesion whatever, but which may result in harmful consequences unless recognized and properly treated.

Diagnosis — from pectoral disease.

This cough is apt to be harsh, dry, barking, and paroxysmal. It alarms those who hear it more than the patient herself. In proportion to the frequency and severity of the paroxysm, the affection is sometimes complicated with spasm of the diaphragm, and the singultus annoys the patient while it amuses her. This admixture of symptoms, especially in the early stages of the disorder, causes the proper hysterical symptoms to crop out more prominently. She either laughs, sobs, chokes, or cries immoderately. If the diaphragm is very much affected, there will be more or less orthopnœa. The pulse is but slightly, if at all, accelerated, and the appetite and digestive function are intact. In case of coincident amenorrhœa, there may be vicarious menstruation in the form of hæmoptysis.

Complications and peculiarities.

You would diagnosticate the hysterical from other forms of asthma by its manifest connection with uterine and menstrual disorders. The attack generally precedes the monthly crisis and is relieved by it. The thorax feels tight and restricted. The paroxysm is aggravated by emotional causes, more especially by such as excite the passions and tend to pervert the moral nature. Even during the suffocative fit one may sometimes detect the hysterical fondness for deception. The regularity of the attack — when it returns every month — will confirm the diagnosis.

From asthma.

The hysterical aphonia is not very difficult of diagnosis. Aphonia is never an idiopathic affection. It may arise from laryngitis directly or indirectly, in which case the local and constitutional symptoms would aid you in making out its differential diagnosis from the hysterical aphonia. We may classify the prominent symptoms of the two affections thus:

Hysterical aphonia.

APHONIA FROM LARYNGITIS.	HYSTERICAL APHONIA.
1. Febrile disorder ; a quick pulse.	1. Absence of fever ; the pulse is normal.
2. The loss of voice is sudden and complete in proportion to the extent and violence of the inflammation. The aphonia disappears slowly, and is prone to become chronic.	2. The aphonia comes and goes abruptly, and without leaving any local lesion or sequel behind it. The relief is sudden and perfect.
3. There is more or less cough and expectoration, which are paroxysmal, and vary in character in different stages of the disease.	3. Cough is a rare concomitant of this form of the complaint. There is no necessary or characteristic expectoration.

APHONIA FROM LARYNGITIS.	HYSTERICAL APHONIA.
4. The inspiration is noisy, harsh and stridulous. At an early period it may be croupal, but later it is less labored and softer.	4. The inspiration is heaving, sighing, and spasmodic, the *râle* being moist and softened in its tone.
5. The dyspnœa is attended by an anxious expression of countenance. She may have fits of suffocation.	5. The features are calm and inexpressive. She is more liable to syncope than to suffocation.
6. There is complaint of angina. The fauces and uvula are congested and inflamed, with tickling, raw or burning sensations, which extend into the larynx and trachea.	6. There is a complete absence of faucial and tracheal inflammation and suffering.
7. Pain referred to the *pomum Adami*. These pains are sticking and lancinating in character.	7. There is no complaint in or about the larynx.
8. The anterior surface of the neck is sore and tender to the touch, and she will not permit one to handle it roughly.	8. Globus hystericus, with clutching at the throat. She tears away the clothing from about the neck.
9. In the acute form the aphonia usually results from taking cold.	9. Never results from this cause unless it has first given rise to some menstrual or uterine disorder upon which the aphonia is secondary.
10. Has no necessary relation to spinal irritation.	10. Is almost invariably preceded or attended by symptoms of spinal irritation, more especially by tenderness upon pressure on some of the cervical and dorsal vertebræ.
11. In the chronic form it may be due to over-fatigue and exercise of the vocal organs, or from causes which occasion a low grade of inflammation with hypertrophy or ulceration of the laryngeal mucous membrane.	11. When chronic, it invariably depends upon some uterine or cerebro-spinal lesion.

Diagnosis from apoplectic aphonia.

You should be careful not to confound the hysterical aphonia with the apoplectic. The apoplectic habit, as well as the more decided symptoms of cerebral congestion in a given case, would remove all sources of fallacy in the diagnosis of these two affections. In the hysterical aphonia, in addition to the general uproar of the functions, the result of over excitement, there is an evident hyperæsthesia of the brain and spinal cord. In the apoplectic condition the loss of voice is a tolerably certain and characteristic symptom of congestion of the medulla oblongata. The respiratory ganglia are almost certain to suffer from this engorgement, and the organs to which the pneumo-gastric nerves are distributed, first the larynx, and afterward the heart and lungs, are necessarily implicated in the resulting disorder, the cause is centric, and the consequences are apt to be disastrous. The hysterical aphonia is always more alarming than serious.

Gastro-hysterical disorders.

The gastric affections that partake of an hysterical character are almost invariably consequent upon uterine luxations or ulceration, dysmenorrhœa, leucorrhœa, pregnancy, lactation, or spinal irritation. The dyspeptic symptoms are of reflex origin, and differ essentially from those which are present in the more ordinary forms of sub-acute gastritis, gastrodynia, gastralgia, etc. In most cases of obstinate digestive derangement occurring in women during their menstrual life you will observe more or less of the hysterical complication. There is the increased suffering at the month, the fickle character of the pains, the capricious appetite, the exaggerated complaint of suffering, and the alternation of the uterine or spinal with the gastro-intestinal symptoms. I will speak of this subject more particularly at another time.

Diagnosis of hysteria from insanity.

Hysteria is frequently confounded with insanity. But the aberration of the mental faculties in the former affection is almost invariably related to disorders of menstruation, to pregnancy, or to post-partum contingencies. Moreover, as in puerperal mania, it is usually self-limited, and if not mal-treated, is neither severe in degree nor of long duration. In insanity there is evidence of real cerebro-mental disease. The reproductive function is not necessarily implicated, either as cause or effect. The delirium is more lasting. In hysteria the mind is fickle and capricious, the emotions run riot, and, as Sydenham long ago observed, the patient "observes no mean in anything, and is constant only to inconstancy."

In insanity there is a manifestation of a strong mental bias. There is usually much depression of spirits, which is the result of a fixed delusion, of which it is impossible to dispossess the mind of the patient. In hysteria a little tact will enable you to recognize a species of cunning shrewdness that is well calculated to deceive. In insanity there is an honest and grave sincerity and earnestness that will withstand any amount of analytical cross-questioning. A woman with the hysterical form of insanity almost invariably dislikes those whom she has hitherto loved the best, and towards whom she sustains the most endearing relation.

She may exhibit a decided aversion to her husband, and would perhaps even destroy her children. Removal from home, more especially if she is not permitted to see her family very frequently, will do much toward effecting a cure of her strange and temporary hallucination. In case of uncomplicated insanity the victim is as prone to suspect and to conceive a dislike for one member of the household as for another.

Hysteria is a paroxysmal disorder, with a great variety of nervous and visceral complications, none of which are, strictly speaking, pathognomonic. Insanity is not regularly paroxysmal, although it may be marked by recurring fits of greater or less duration and severity. If we except paralysis, organic nervous complications are usually lacking in insanity. Both are hereditary disorders, but the predisposition to hysteria is more marked, more easily aroused, and more easily acted upon by exciting causes than in the case of insanity. In exceptional cases they may co-exist.

LECTURE XVIII.

HYSTERIA — (CONTINUED).

GENTLEMEN :

The hysterical delirium is in many respects peculiar. It is liable to occur in typhoid, typhus, the eruptive and puerperal fevers, and also in certain menstrual and hepatic disorders. In a case either of typhoid or typhus fever, occurring in a young or middle-aged woman, if the delirium persists after the more acute symptoms have subsided, and especially if there is no particular evidence of cerebral lesion; if the paroxysms thereof return at irregular intervals, and result from trivial causes, which in one who was seriously ill would have little effect; if the mind is more than usually fitful and capricious, or if it be inclined to dwell upon a single train of ideas, which have grown out of the most ridiculous fancies; if these vagaries are *outré* and otherwise inexplicable; you will be led to suspect the hysterical complication. And your suspicion would be confirmed by any evidence of malingering on the part of the patient.

Hysterical delirium.

She will not look one directly in the face. Her eye is averted, cast down and expressionless, like that of a young man with spermatorrhœa which has been brought on by self-abuse. Or it has a roguish look, and twinkles with evident satisfaction at the alarm and discomfiture of the bystanders, upon whose sympathies she may have been playing as upon a harp. During the fit, in assumed fear of dysphagia, or from a settled determination that nothing shall pass her lips, she may peremptorily refuse to swallow either food or medicine.

The patient's manner.

She is sensitive, impressible, tearful. Her perceptive faculties are intensified. She sees and hears every motion that is made in the house. Nothing escapes her. For her to remain passive is an impossibility. She is under the dominion of an evil genius, which destroys her own peace and that of all concerned.

This form of delirium is likely to be caused or aggravated by the taking of drugs to blunt the sensibilities and to compel the patient to rest and sleep. Any of the narcotics may in exceptional cases produce an opposite effect from that which was intended. Under these circumstances they increase the perturbation and unhinge the nervous sympathies more and more. Even when the patient is easily narcotized, it is doubtless true that the habit of taking such remedies as the bromide of potassium or the hydrate of chloral, in increasing quantities, may finally work serious mischief.

Aggravated by drugs.

During the convalescence of fevers, the hysterical delirium may be suddenly developed in consequence of an incidental derangement of the menstrual process. The same is true of a tardy resumption of the ovarian and uterine functions after delivery or prolonged lactation. Until the organic processes have resumed their natural order, and the periodical discharge appears, there is danger, especially after acute disease, of the mental functions becoming temporarily impaired.

Incident to fevers.

The hysterical delirium is often present in child-bed fever, however mild its type. In this case it arises from reflex causes, and we very naturally refer the symptoms to some remote lesion of the soft parts within the pelvis. This delirium varies in its intensity with the quantity and quality of the lochia and of the lacteal secretion, being less marked and persistent if these post-partum products are freely and uninterruptedly poured out. It also varies with the gravity of the uterine lesion. Even in the most aggravated cases of delirium and puerperal mania, it is quite absurd to speak of a metastasis of uterine phlebitis, or of utero-peritoneal inflammation to the brain.

In child-bed fever.

In rare cases the hysterical delirium is complicated with a form of hypochondriasis that results from some chronic hepatic disorder. If uterine lesions are conjoined with an old organic disease of the liver, and the patient has delirium, that delirium is necessarily of serious import. Hepatic abscess may co-exist with uterine displacement, ulceration, or enlargement, and a form of delirium exist which is both hysterical and hypochondriacal. In such a case the danger is increased by the resorption into the blood of at least one of the post-organic elements of the bile, viz.: the cholesterine.

May be complicated with hypochondriasis.

It is less difficult to separate hysteria from hypochondriasis than from the more decided forms of insanity. In hysteria the mental derangement is not always, or indeed usually, of a desponding or gloomy kind. The attack comes on suddenly and without warning; is explosive in its nature. The classes of persons predisposed to the two diseases are of very different habits of thought and temperament. Those most liable to hysteria are the fitful and the frivolous, such as have not taken especial pains in the culture of the reflective faculties. Hysteria is limited almost exclusively to women. A majority of cases of hypochondriasis occur in men. Aristotle observed that "melancholy men are the men of the greatest genius." Hysteria affects the *perceptive*, hypochondriasis the *reflective* faculties of the mind. In the former it is intact and the perceptions are morbidly acute. In the latter the gloomy forebodings, the delusional insanity, impair all the mental processes; the perceptions are misinterpreted, and the judgment is perverted. When hysterical females become hypochondriacal, their thoughts almost always take a religious turn, and the delusion develops into a mild form of theomania.

Diagnosis of hysteria from hypochondriasis.

I was recently consulted in a case of this kind by my friend and former pupil, Dr. C. N. Dorion, of this city, from whom I have the following details concerning his patient:

Case.

Mrs. M——, 25 years of age, was married two years ago, but has no children. Her complexion is sallow, the menses are regular, but, for the last four or five months, rather scanty. The appetite is variable, the bowels are somewhat constipated. She suffers no pain excepting an occasional attack of headache which is not very severe. Her constitution appears to be good. Her face wears a melancholy expression. Her father is subject to fits of hypochondriasis, and one of her sisters has been insane for several months.

Last summer she made a visit to that sister, and spent some days with her in the insane asylum. Since that visit she has been very much afraid of becoming insane herself, and has a mortal dread of dying in a mad-house. She is in terror of being left alone. When her husband leaves home in the morning, she feels sure that she will never see him again. Her mind runs constantly upon religious topics, and she will sit and sing hymns for hours together. She has lost all interest in domestic affairs, and the outside world is a complete blank to her.

When lying down she fancies that it will be quite impossible for her ever to rise again, or to walk if she were upon her feet. She thinks and says that she is too weak to do anything. Occasionally there are nervous shiverings, globus hystericus, cold extremities, and, at rare intervals, an intermittent pulse. The tongue is coated white, but there is no febrile action. She broods over her certain death, her possible insanity, her sins always. When one succeeds in diverting her attention temporarily, she is apparently quite well and says that she is no longer sick. But in a short time she lapses again into the same pitiable state of mind as before. She insists that for weeks past she has not been able to sleep, even for a single hour.

The hysterical form of peritonitis.

Among the hysterical contingencies and sequelæ of labor none are more embarrassing than those which simulate puerperal peritonitis. Post-partum hysteria is sometimes very difficult of recognition. We most naturally look for it in those who in the unimpregnated state have been subject to mental unsteadiness, and who through original or acquired predisposition are considered to be "nervous." The changes incident to gestation frequently have the effect to fortify against an hysterical outbreak until "term" has arrived. But either during or subsequent to delivery the old habit is revived, and symptoms of hysteria may crop out again.

Differential diagnosis of.

In this spurious form of peritonitis the attack comes on abruptly and without any obvious cause. It may even be entirely emotional in its origin. Everything may be natural with the lying-in woman when a slight mental shock has the effect to make her alarmingly ill. There is local pain and tenderness over the abdomen. She can not bear slight pressure, the weight of the bed clothing is unsupportable, the lower extremities are sometimes but not always flexed, the abdomen is tympanitic, the urine is either scanty or suppressed. The skin is neither unnaturally hot nor cool. She has no decided chill, but may have rigors. The pulse is nearly or quite natural. If at all changed it will usually be found slower than at your last visit. The delirium is hysterical. If, for example, you attempt to administer a remedy in the form of a little powder, she will seize it and tear the paper to pieces in a twinkling. And this most deliberately and defiantly, perhaps. She clenches her teeth, closes her lips, thrusts her face into the pillow, tosses about from side to side, or persists in sitting up, even although she may be so sleepy as scarcely to be able to keep her eyes open.

Now, in genuine child-bed fever, although there is no pathognomonic lesion, any more than in surgical fever, to which it is closely allied, the symptoms differ essentially from those which I have just enumerated. If there is perimetritis, endometritis, peritonitis (ovarian or abdominal), or metro-phlebitis, the usual constitutional signs of local inflammation will be present.

Thus, in true puerperal peritonitis, we shall have a characteristic frequency of the pulse, which continues despite a copious diuresis or diaphoresis ; a decided chill at the onset of the attack, as in inflammation of serous membranes elsewhere ; severe frontal headache ; a suppression of the milk and of the lochia ; excessive abdominal distension and tenderness, which latter is greatly increased by extending the limbs or allowing the clothing to fall upon the tumor ; and a hippocratic expression of the countenance. In the worst cases the period of collapse sets in early, and the patient may die in a very few days, or she may linger for a week or more.

In private practice puerperal peritonitis is a rare affection. Probably not one-half the cases of this disease that are reported in our medical societies and journals deserve to be classed as such. The clinical history of such cases proves many of them to have been spurious, self-limited, incidental, hysterical. Any remedy capable of controlling the nervous symptoms, which are contingent upon labor, is very likely to get the credit of aborting a genuine attack of peritonitis. The same is true of the hysterical side-ache which resembles pleurisy and is so often mistaken for it ; and also of the hysterical pains which sometimes counterfeit rheumatism so closely. When you hear a physician say that he has often succeeded in curing any one of these diseases — peritonitis, pleurisy or rheumatism, in a few hours with this or that remedy, you may safely conclude that his clinical observations have not been very accurate, and that he is claiming too much for his skill.

A suggestive item.

There is a singular and significant relation between abdominal tympanites and the mental derangements, more particularly the forms of delirium, to which hysterical women are liable. It frequently happens that the degree of abdominal distension is a measure of the temporary disorder of the brain. Whether this tumefaction of the abdomen, and sometimes of the hypogastrium also, is to be regarded in the light of cause or effect, authorities are not agreed. It is incident to difficult and delayed menstruation, to the puerperal state, to abortion, to uterine displacements, and to the various forms of sexual irritation from whatever cause. It is sometimes brought on by mental shock or emotional influences of different kinds, as fear, anger, grief or disappointment. You will find in these cases that the abdomen is excessively tender to a slight touch, but not to steady and continued pressure. This distension may come on very quickly and disappear as suddenly, without being accompanied or followed by any local inflammation. I have known it to be caused by drinking a glass of ice-water, or eating a dish of ice-cream, during menstruation. In a few minutes after taking the latter the abdomen was found to be enormously swollen and the patient delirious. Similar states of the mind are incident to the tympanites intestinalis of puerperal and typhoid fevers. But, in many cases of hysterical tympanites, which are really due to derangement of function in the solar plexus and semilunar ganglion chiefly, you will observe that continued pressure upon the stomach and abdomen, when the patient's attention is diverted, will not only arrest the unnatural secretion of gas, but will cause both the swelling and the delirium to subside. This is sometimes quite diagnostic.

Abdominal tympanites and delirium.

Hysteria may counterfeit labor.

Hysteria may simulate natural labor. A marked case of this kind is reported by Dr. Hodges.*

Case.

"I was engaged to attend a married woman in her confinement for the first time, then believed by herself and friends to be about five months advanced in pregnancy. Time went on — the usual preparations were made — the nurse secured, the patient happy in the thought of becoming a mother, and pleased with the sympathy elicited from the neighbors in relation to the approaching event. In four months after the first intimation I received, I was requested, at about ten o'clock at night, to visit her, and to do so with as little delay as possible, for she had been ill all day, and was reported to be getting rapidly worse. On arriving, the pains were very severe, and of the kind attending the last stage of labor. I was pleased to hear from the nurse that the pains had been very regular all the day,

* Trans. of the Obstetrical Society of London, Vol. I, p. 339.

gradually increasing in frequency and intensity, for the hope of a night's rest was before me. They certainly were most severe and forcing, and succeeded each other so rapidly as to give the impression that the process would soon be completed, and the first casual vaginal examination conveyed to my mind the same idea, for I detected a *soft, fluctuating* tumor, filling the vagina, and which, during pain, distended and protruded it through the os externum, precisely as in natural labor when the membranes protrude. I made no observation to those around me, for the pains were so urgent and forcing that I believed the labor would be over in a minute or two; but their continued severity brought no advancement—no alteration. I then examined carefully into the cause of this apparent delay, and found that the tumor was a vaginal cystocele, or prolapse of the anterior parietes of the vagina, caused by an enormously distended bladder. The finger was with difficulty passed up behind this swelling, where the uterus was discovered with its mouth closed and of the unimpregnated size. The patient and attendants were then informed that, not only were these pains spurious, or false, or hysterical, * * * but that the patient herself was not even pregnant, which fact astonished them still more, and amused them for many a day. * * * The patient before marriage was subject to frequent attacks of hysteria, and about one year previous to this event was present at a relative's accouchement, where the pains were severe and the labor protracted."

Diagnosis of hysteria from epilepsy.

Hysteria and epilepsy are frequently confounded by those who pay too little attention to diagnosis. The points of difference between them concern the coming on of the paroxysm, the symptoms during the fit, and those which immediately follow it. In epilepsy there is usually some premonition of the spasm; the patient may fall to the floor, or the fit may come on immediately upon awaking out of sleep; the *aura epileptica* is more or less pronounced; the attack is not strictly referable to an emotional cause, but is apt to be periodical, occurring once in so many hours or days; it has no necessary relation to menstrual disorders, to the return of the month, or to enfeebled conditions of system consequent upon gestation or lactation. The hysterical fit follows some mental shock or strain; comes on gradually, usually with more or less of gastric disturbance and distress, choking, suffocation, globus hystericus, twitching and convulsive movements of the eyeballs and the eyelids; is very apt to follow in consequence of loss of sleep; and if at all periodical, it is more likely to recur at the month as a contingent of menstruation. In certain cases pregnancy and lactation may predispose to it most decidedly.

In the epileptic fit there is a sudden and total loss of consciousness. The face becomes livid and distorted; a frothy saliva flows from the mouth, and there is grinding of the teeth and biting of the tongue. The patient is entirely oblivious to all that is passing. The convulsive movements affect the muscles of the face, neck, throat, chest and extremities. The larynx is spasmodically closed, and hence the discoloration of the skin, and the temporary arrest of breathing. When the spasms reach the muscles of the extremities, those on one side of the body are apt to be more decidedly affected than those on the other. These spasms are more tonic than clonic. The movements of the patient are entirely involuntary.

In the hysterical paroxysm, if the patient becomes comatose (which is exceptional), this condition comes on very gradually and may not be complete until at the close of the fit. The face may be flushed, but it is not dusky or livid in hue; she does not foam at the mouth; as there are no convulsive movements of the lower jaw, the tongue is not apt to be bitten; and, what is quite distinctive, she displays something of volition in all her movements, and evidently "keeps the run" of what is going on around her. She sighs, or laughs, or sobs, or perhaps talks as if dreaming. The muscles of the face are seldom convulsed; the face itself is not disfigured; the larynx, which is the gateway of the respiratory system, remains open; and the movements of the extremities are always *partly* under control of the will.

The epileptic paroxysm is generally of short duration and passes off with profound sleep, from which the patient awakens without the remotest idea of what has passed since the onset of the attack. Whether sleep follows the fit or not, there is considerable dullness and hebetude of mind which may continue for hours or days, and which finally, if the fits recur very often, impair the intellect and render the patient a complete wreck.

The hysterical coma may become more profound and the patient may sleep toward the close of the paroxysm, but the rule is that the fit passes off with an ebullition of emotional feeling. She may either weep or laugh immoderately. Or she may sigh and groan and sob, and all this without any real mental anguish to correspond with these demonstrations. Her emotions run riot, and are sometimes most grotesquely jumbled together. She may know more of what has passed since the commencement of the attack than the bystanders themselves, and the only perceptible effect of a repetition of these paroxysms seems to be so to shatter her nervous system as to make her more and more susceptible to them. In many cases the fit terminates with a copious flow of pale, limpid urine.

Hysteria or "spinal irritation."

You will hardly fail to be consulted for the relief of certain hysterico-neuralgic affections of the spine. These affections are very distressing because of their chronic nature, their proneness to seize upon some of the most intelligent, gifted and amiable women in society, and because it almost always happens that before you are applied to, they will have done the very thing, and resorted to the very means best fitted to fasten the disease upon them. In these patients some portion of the spine — it may be a spot over the spinous process of a single vertebra, or perhaps the whole length of the column — becomes exquisitely sensitive to the touch. The pain may be sharp or dull, radiating, shooting, shifting, transient or permanent, and is very apt to be increased by over-fatigue of body or mind, vicissitudes of weather, as of cold and damp, strong mental emotions, sleeplessness, obstinate constipation, and the return of the menstrual crisis. It renders walking impossible in many cases, and may even interfere with riding also. The incidental symptoms vary with the seat of the local pain, but are not as serious as you would be led to infer. Indeed, the exaggerated character of the complaints that are made will prevent your confounding this with caries of the vertebræ, or with myelitis or spinal meningitis. The predisposition to this disease is the hysterical diathesis; the exciting cause may generally be found in some derangement of the menstrual function upon which the "spinal irritation" is secondary. Such patients sometimes suffer extremely from neuralgia in various parts of the body. Exercise gives them so much pain and unrest that they soon desist from taking it, and finally become bed-ridden and wretched.

Sometimes this peculiar disease locates itself in one of the larger joints, particularly in the hip or the knee. Dr. Simpson reports a case in which the pain was seated in the head of the right radius.

Hysterical affections of the joints.

The knee-joint is most frequently affected. There is the greatest dread of motion of the affected part, and the pain is said to be excruciating in degree, much more, indeed, than in case of real ulceration of the cartilages. This affection, which is comparatively frequent, was first described by Sir Benjamin Brodie, who says, concerning its diagnosis, that "There is always exceeding tenderness, connected with which, however, we may observe the remarkable circumstance, that gently touching or pinching the integuments in such a way as that the pressure can not affect the deep-seated parts, will often be productive of much more pain than the handling of the limb in a rude and careless way." A good plan is to divert the patient's attention from herself while you are manipulating the affected part, by which means you will find it possible to move the joint with little comparative complaint from her. If she insists that the limb can not be moved or straightened voluntarily, you may resort to anæsthesia by ether or chloroform as a means of making a more careful diagnosis; for it is really very important to decide in these cases whether the disease is or is not hysterical. It has frequently happened that women have been kept in bed, in the horizontal posture, for weeks and months, and even for years, when there was no actual disease of the joint itself. Indeed they have often gone through the martyrdom of blistering, cupping, leeching, salivation, and finally of amputation, for the cure of this reflex disorder.

Diagnosis of.

If you remember the distinctive characteristics of hysteria that have already been enumerated, you will be spared the commission of such blunders, and your patients saved from the prolonged suffering which, as a rule, may be easily remedied.

In the unmarried, and sometimes in women who are married but who have not borne children, vaginismus is an attendant upon hysteria. In exceptional cases the hysterical disorder appears under the form of nymphomania. Numerous instances are recorded in which ovariotomy has been attempted, when on opening the cavity of the abdomen the tumor has proved to be an hysterical phantom.

Other incidental diseases.

Nature. — But it must suffice to say that hysteria is rather a condition than a disease *per se*. This condition appears to consist in a peculiar irritability and impressibility of the nervous system, which is so modified by disorders of the sexual apparatus as to cause it to differ from every other kind of nervous derangement. This morbid irritability should be regarded in the light of a peculiar diathesis, upon which, as we have seen, almost any disease may be engrafted. Roberton says very explicitly:* "We have reason to believe that there is *as absolutely* an hysteric constitution, or congenital predisposition to hysteria, as that there is a scrofulous constitution, or congenital predisposition to scrofula; and consequently that none are liable to hysteria but only such as possess this constitution.

Hysteria not a *bona fide* disease.

"The hysteric condition is characterized by irritability, *sui generis*, of the nervous system as a whole, or sometimes more particularly as connected with certain organs; and although this condition can not propably be *originated* in the individual by modes of living, and other external circumstances, it may be aggravated by them."

In what this hysterical predisposition really consists we do not know. How it is that it reverses the finer traits and characteristics of womanhood, whether temporarily or permanently, it is impossible to comprehend. That such are among its effects is a thing of every-day observation. It is at the bottom of half the disease and the unhappiness of the sex. It may turn the wife against her husband, the sister against her brother, the daughter against her father, the mother against her child, and friend against friend the world over. Its strange characters may be traced upon every page of human history. In the affairs of church and of state, in medicine and morals, in society at large and in the sick-chamber, its influence is certain to be felt. It does not destroy life directly, but indirectly it has slain its thousands. In brief, it is the most mischievous and the most enigmatical and elusive of all those elements which enter into the formation of "poor, weak, human nature."

Its real nature is unknown.

Prognosis.—Uncomplicated hysteria is not a fatal disorder. It may, however, serve to conceal the graver symptoms of disease

* Essays and Notes on the Physiology and Diseases of Women. London, 1851. p. 237.

under cover of such as are not serious, and in this manner tends to destroy life by causing the real lesion to be overlooked. Let me illustrate: A delicate, nervous woman is seized with a sharp attack of pleuro-pneumonia. In the emergency of her sudden illness an officious neighbor is called in. This impromptu nurse has a voice and manner that serve only to excite the patient more and more, and, despite her bundle of expedients, some of which, if properly applied, might have been efficacious, the symptoms are aggravated. The reflex effect of that woman's presence and performances upon the sensibilities of such a subject is so to shock and derange them, that it may be quite impossible for the doctor when he arrives, to discriminate properly between the symptoms that are presented. He can not tell which of them are genuine and which are spurious, for the former are masked, while the latter are lashed into undue prominence. All the symptoms that are chargeable to the nurse's lack of tact, to her incompatibility and to surrounding circumstances generally, rather than to internal conditions of the patient's organism, will be likely to deceive and mislead the physician. Vesical or rectal tenesmus, globus or clavus hystericus, fugitive and excruciating local pains and spasms, a temporary diabetes insipidus, aphonia, hysterical vomiting, amenorrhœa, or a host of other irrelevant symptoms, not one of which has any characteristic relation to the original disease, are so magnified, and stand out so clearly and prominently, as to divert his mind into the wrong channel.

Illustration.

Under these circumstances, and especially if he is inexperienced, the physician may feel himself called to prognosticate a fatal issue. Taking the wrong cue, adding to the alarm instead of arresting it, and causing matters to become worse in compound ratio — for doctors are either helpful or harmful — the patient may finally die, not indeed of hysteria, but of the pneumonia which has been permitted to run its course without interruption, because it has been overlooked.

Or, if the physician in charge has had sufficient experience, and has tact enough to enable him to recognize the hysterical outgrowth in such a case, but is withal very much occupied, and weary with this class of patients especially, he may hastily conclude that she has a fit of hysteria and prescribe accordingly.

Meanwhile the real disease is making rapid progress, and before his next visit it may have become incurable.

Now it is this deceptive exaggeration that is likely to mislead, and to cause us to misjudge, to overrate, or to underrate the danger in cases of hysteria complicated with other forms of disease. Some of the verbal and objective signs are untruthful. They introduce the lying element into the record, and hence the difficulty in detecting them and in assigning their proper diagnostic and prognostic value.

General remarks.

Treatment.— Before we proceed to the special therapeutics of this affection, there are some considerations which demand our notice, and which are essential to its proper and successful treatment.

Mental remedies.

This disorder being chiefly emotional in its origin, and indeed in its very nature, it is vitally important to obtain such an influence over the mind of the patient as will serve in a measure to control the symptoms, or at least to place her in a state in which our remedies will act more promptly and efficiently. There can be no doubt that very many cases of hysteria, in some of its protean forms, have been unwittingly cured by means that were suited to occupy, divert, overwhelm, or control the emotional faculties. Such expedients are to be regarded only as auxiliaries to proper treatment, but as such they are so useful, and sometimes so necessary, that they should not be overlooked. For it has often happened that the manner and bearing of the nurse, or of some kind-hearted neighbor who has been called in, has done a thousand times more to cure these patients than the physician's prescription. The intangible, but no less potent influences of fear, faith, hope, confidence, will, reason, diversion, management, occupation of the mind, argument, concession, opposition, sympathy, indulgence of caprice, helping her to bear her burdens— whether real or imaginary— change of diet, air and scenery, are sometimes indispensable. And unless we can use them appropriately, or the patient shall happen to be accidentally brought under their influence, the best chosen remedies will utterly fail of effect.

Herein lies the difficulty in controlling and curing the various forms of hysteria. The most inexperienced among you might match a great many of the symptoms mechanically, and prescribe for them secundum artem. But, unless you are able to recognize which of them are genuine and which are not; unless you can separate the real from the spurious; unless you can refer those which are hysterical to their proper source, and succeed in reducing the emotional disturbance of the patient to order, you will fail to cure this disease.

The real problem.

Now, there are many ways of accomplishing this object. You know that hysterical patients are eccentric. For this reason it requires a large measure of tact (which can only be acquired through observation and experience) to manage them properly, and to cure them most certainly and promptly. I can no more tell you what to do in each particular case of hysteria than I could define the odor of small-pox or of measles. But it is possible to give you some general directions that shall be useful.

In the first place, if you desire to be most successful in treating this class of diseases, you should maintain your distinctive character as physicians. For there is a species of mutual reserve and respect which should separate the physician from his patients, and which invest him with a peculiar influence over them. If this is properly maintained, it need not subtract from the social character and position upon which so much of his general reputation depends. But it will give him an immense advantage in the management of every kind of hysterical disorder, to which so many of his lady patients are subject.

Something depends upon the doctor's habits.

Nor is a highly-wrought, delicate, impressible, nervous woman likely to be benefited by the advice of a physician whose personal habits and manners are repulsive to her, and whom she is compelled to tolerate rather than esteem. In this, as in other matters, trifles have great weight. I have known a brother practitioner, who was skillful and competent, to be discharged by such a patient for the reason that "he never wore a decent cravat." His slovenly habit more than counterbalanced the effect of his remedies, and, while he continued to visit her, his patient grew worse instead of better. The good influence of one physician may be crippled by his loquacity, another is too taciturn; a third asks too many, and a fourth too few questions of the patient; one brings too full a budget of news from a neighbor; another is eternally canvassing

Also his personal address, etc.

for his school of medical practice, his church, his club, or his political party; one is too cross, while it is alleged that another is "altogether too kind."

This is but a scanty list of personalities, any one of which may serve, in this class of diseases especially, to neutralize the curative effect of his remedies. You are not to suppose that they are insignificant merely because they are not alluded to in your text-books. Whatever can by any possibility constitute an obstacle to recovery is important and worthy of your attention. Fortunately most of these vexations are avoidable. You will not all excel in obtaining the confidence of your patients, and in bringing them into that passive state in which they can be most readily cured. But each of you can by education acquire such a measure of tact and of adaptation to caprice and circumstance as will multiply your resources and render you many times more useful to them.

The smallest items not always trivial.

I am so confident that a lack of sympathy, a dearth of feeling, a real incompatibility of temper and taste between the physician and his hysterical patient may cause his treatment to result in more of harm than of good, that, in case this obstacle can not be otherwise removed, I think it better to withdraw and to let another physician be called. Indeed, I have sometimes voluntarily discharged myself, after having frankly told the patient and her family that, for some unknown reason, my remedies had failed to cure her; and that, in my judgment, such a change was what she most needed. Under similar circumstances we would not hesitate to discharge the nurse whose every movement was annoying to the patient and antagonistic to her comfort and welfare. And I do not know why the same rule should not also apply to the doctor. If a new face and a new method of prescription will work the desired change in her feelings and her symptoms, by all means let them be tried. For these things can operate through the emotions, and may entirely supersede the necessity for remedies of whatever kind. And by following this rule, although you lose the credit of curing one such patient, you will gain the reputation of saving another; for, when the wheel turns around, your face and your manner may be the

Incompatibility between physician and patient.

How to remedy it.

one thing needful in a similar case which your professional neighbor has failed to relieve.

In lieu of controlling the emotional outbreaks and suffering in hysteria, by the personal tact, character and magnetism of which I have spoken, these subjects are often brought under the quieting influence of narcotics and anti-spasmodics of various kinds. But such medicines are mischievous, and should be given under protest and exceptionally, or rather not at all. One reason why there are so many nervous women in our day is, that the habit of taking such drugs is almost universal. And every few months a new one is added to the list. Thousands of women, who should be well and healthy, are just now under the slavish dominion of the hydrate of chloral and the bromide of potassium. The taking of these substances habitually begets a predisposition to nervous disorders which grows apace. So that if there were no other reason for withholding them from our prescriptions, we should not give them freely and indiscriminately, lest the habit be formed in consequence.

Narcotics and Anti-spasmodics.

Objections to.

There are, however, exceptional cases in which this means of temporary relief can not be rationally excluded. When from excess of pain, fatigue, or excitement, it is absolutely impossible otherwise to procure the needful rest, they are perhaps permissible. But these are exceptional cases in which we must choose between two evils. It may be better to compel sleep, to overwhelm the nervous centers, and to run the risk of the secondary consequences of such an expedient, rather than let the patient wear herself out with unrest, extreme pain, or protracted insomnia.

Sometimes permissible.

Concerning the propriety and advisability of alcoholic stimulation in the weakened conditions of the nervous system, which predispose to, and attend upon hysterical disorders, physicians are not agreed. One class, of which Dr. Skey is the modern representative,* considers them indispensable, and insists that they should be given freely and promiscuously. On the contrary, what might be called the denunciatory school is equally positive that in all forms alcohol is always injurious.

Alcoholic stimulation.

* Skey on Hysteria. A. Simpson & Co., N. Y., 1867.

This involves a question which can not be settled for you in the lecture-room. If you are satisfied that these agents can be utilized in correcting the mal-nutrition and depraved vitality from which this class of patients often suffers preëminently, it will be your duty to prescribe their sparing and transient use. If you need to husband the vital resources of one who is exceedingly weak, and almost bankrupt in strength, and are satisfied that alcohol, or tea, or coffee will diminish disassimilation, and prove a veritable "savings bank to the tissues," as Moleschott so quaintly terms it, you should not withhold them.

Under certain circumstances it may be quite as necessary to furnish a rapidly oxydizable material to the organism, as in other conditions it is to supply oxygen itself. I might insist that wine, brandy or whiskey have never been of the least service in any case of hysteria. But that would not alter the facts. Individual observation is too limited to justify such assertions. Indeed, these arbitrary rules have very little to recommend them. I have known weak, nervous, delicate women to be disabled and bed-ridden for months and years because their physician obstinately denied them the little stimulus which they craved, and the temporary use of which would have set them upon their feet again, without doing any possible harm.

Folly of dogmatizing.

So far as my own experience extends, I have found it best to discriminate carefully, and to prescribe one or another of the different preparations of alcohol only when I could not do better, and when there was no especial danger of reviving an old habit, or of forming a new one which would result in intemperance. There is an essential difference between giving wine or brandy to the extent of complete narcotism, or endorsing its persistent use until one's patient is in a state of chronic alcholism, and the judicious and temporary employment of it as an available stimulus in an emergency. And let me tell you that there is not one-hundreth part the danger of our making drunkards of women that there is of making topers of men.

Qualified use of stimulants.

The exercise should be regulated most carefully. Many women become fatigued almost beyond measure who, strictly speaking, take little or no exercise. With the majority of these persons the fault is not that their time is not occupied, but that they lack the stimulus and benefit of

Proper exercise.

variety of occupation. Their house-life is a species of tread-mill round of work and worry, with little or no change whatever. What this class needs is diversion, a combination of mental and physical exercise that shall keep all their faculties in healthful play. If a woman wears out her nervous energies in household drudgery, you must prescribe a change of habit, and season her cares with a little of the spice of the outside world. Fresh air and sunlight, society, travel, music, literature, or an additional servant may be useful ingredients in your prescription.

Among what are called the "better classes," with whom life is a listless, perpetual holiday, a predisposition to hysteria is frequently nurtured or acquired. With many women the seeds of this disorder have been sown in boarding-school. Boarding-house life and hotel life, in America, are nurseries of hysteria. This kind of life subjects its victims, who are without proper and constant employment of their time, to vicissitudes of excitement, and of personal experience that are inimical to health. The nervous systems of these women suffer most severely. Their life is an aimless, artificial one, with a large margin of leisure which is apt to be wrongly appropriated. It is almost impossible for a gifted and attractive young or middle-aged lady to escape the perils of such a home, if indeed it deserves the name.

Hysteria among the "better classes."

And, since it will not always be possible for you to locate these patients just as you could wish, any more than to mate them properly, you will be forced to counteract such influences in the most practicable manner. If they have the means and the disposition, persuade them, if possible, to settle in homes of their own, where proper domestic cares may occupy a share of their time and attention. Thousands of women would be cured of the hysterical tendency if they were blessed with comfortable homes, and removed permanently from the corrupting influences to which they are otherwise subjected. It is sometimes absolutely essential to remove them from a house in which everybody knows everybody's business, and in which no woman has any business. You can also accomplish a great deal by the exercise of a little tact in keeping these patients busy with something useful, instructive and profitable. One may perhaps become interested in a course of reading which you

Domestic occupation.

shall map out for her. Another might be made to forget her complaints if she were to resume her music, her French, or her German; or to participate in one or another of the charitable objects and missions, in which some of the best women of our day are so much engrossed. One should see more of society, and another less. All need some kind of diversion, some mental occupation, some change which shall divert their thoughts from themselves, and especially from a morbid stimulation and gratification of the sexual appetite.

Cultivation of proper mental habits.

You will sometimes have to counteract such domestic infelicities as, by the constant fret and friction which they induce, serve to keep those who are predisposed to hysteria, always on the sick list. This woman may be cured by getting her out of sight of her own servants; and that one, if she can escape the neighborhood in which she is certain to see or hear something of others, men or women, against whom she has conceived an inveterate dislike.

Remove domestic infelicities.

The hysterical irritability is very apt to accompany, or to be engrafted upon a jealous and unhappy disposition. It certainly is much easier to prescribe than to furnish contentment to such persons, but example and precept will accomplish wonders, even although, like the third party who attempts to make peace between man and wife, we sometimes incur considerable risk in giving our advice. In all this you will be compelled to take a leading character in the old play of Tact *versus* Talent. And I am anxious that you shall not appear upon the stage of practical life as physicians without ever having had a rehearsal. For, in the cure of hysteria especially, the largest share of the work to be done may depend upon these common-place matters.

Contentment.

LECTURE XIX.

TREATMENT OF HYSTERIA (CONCLUDED).

GENTLEMEN:

From the time of the Greek midwives, who, according to Galen, were the first to employ the word Hysteria, its treatment has been divided into that proper for the paroxysm and that for the interval.

Treatment during the fit.

When you are called to relieve a woman who is in "a fit of hysterics," you must know what to do. First, you should be self-possessed, and not in a flutter. Allow nothing to surprise you. Be cool and collected. Look upon the most startling developments as matters of course. Do not give a hasty opinion as to the result. Qualify your prognosis, and above all things do not be in a gloomy, despondent state of mind yourself. Have the patient placed in a comfortable position upon the bed or sofa. Let the head be slightly raised, and if need be, held by an assistant. Have the forehead and face bathed with cool or cold water, or cold compresses laid across the forehead and temples. Let her have a plentiful supply of fresh air. If it blows from the window directly into her face, so much the better; or she may be fanned by the nurse. All ligatures in the form of corsets and garters, etc., should be removed. The dress should be thrown open at the throat especially, and only enough force applied to keep her from inflicting bodily injury upon herself and others.

Available expedients.

The usual restoratives consist in allowing her to smell of ordinary spirits of camphor, ammonia, musk, cologne water, chloroform, ether, alcohol, vinegar, the fumes of a burning feather, or of a lighted match. Sinapisms and the warm foot or sitz-bath, vigorous rubbing by a strong, healthy person, dashing cold water upon the head or spine, the application of heat, electricity, and the use of brandy, coffee, camphor, sulphuric ether, ice water, or a solution of some salt of valerian by injection into the rectum, are among the available expedients, which may be tried before the patient is able to swallow. Sometimes the paroxysm will be relieved almost immediately by firm pressure upon the hypogastrium. More frequently it will pass away insensibly under the influence of delicate attention and quiet, and proper sympathy which tend to soothe and calm the excited feelings. Or it may terminate by your sending out of the room some person who is well enough disposed, but who is especially obnoxious to the patient.

Precaution—Tact.

If the fit has been induced by anger, or some fancied slight, or disappointment, or by mental anxiety or grief, no allusion to the cause or to the possible consequences of the attack should be permitted within hearing of the patient. Indeed, the greatest care should be taken to turn the current of conversation, if there is any in the room, into quite another channel, else it may prolong the disorder. Whatever is said should be calculated to divert her attention from herself, and thus indirectly to restore the will to its supremacy over the emotions, for when the will of the patient is in league with the emotions it adds fuel to the flame to persist in telling her how very ill she is. The better plan is to speak of something quite foreign to her present condition and surroundings, and to try to interest those who are present in the subject matter of conversation. This will be a mild means of counter-irritation, or diversion, which will serve to benefit the patient, who is unwittingly being toned down by your tact.

Don't scold.

It is the habit of some physicians to scold such a patient, or to declare contemptuously that she has "nothing but hysterics," and to refuse to do anything for her. This is positively and unprofessionally cruel, for, while it lasts, the suffering is as real as in any other disease, and the patient as deserving of sympathy and relief. Doctors are servants. And whether you are sent for in the middle of the night, or while at church, or at a social party, to visit an hysterical patient, you should carry with you as large a measure of good-nature as if you were going to a case of puerperal peritonitis, or of some other serious disease.

Most frequently, however, the paroxysm will have ended before your arrival. If she remains obstinately silent and refuses to answer your questions, give her the medicine, and wait until she gets ready to speak. This let-alone species of indifference on your part will hasten the crisis, and after a fit of weeping, she will be communicative enough.

For her taciturnity.

Concerning the treatment between the paroxysms, I wish in the first place to insist that you shall not be misled by the incidental and irrelevant symptoms which are so common in all forms of hysteria. I have often thought that if it were possible to treat our hysterical patients just as we are compelled to treat infants when they are ill, that is, without regard to their subjective sensations, the special treatment of this disease would be greatly simplified and much more successful. For it is the peculiar rendering, the exaggerated estimate, the misinterpretation of the sufferings experienced, that will sometimes lead you to wish that such a patient was as mute as a child that is only a month old.

Treatment in the interval.

I know that it is very difficult to discard worthless symptoms without at the same time eliminating some which are really valuable and important, and yet, I tell you frankly that, in my judgment, a majority of the symptoms, more especially those derived from the tongue of an hysterical patient, are of no practical significance whatever. You cannot depend upon them. They are compounded of shrewdness, cunning, trickery, deceit, a morbid imagination, real suffering, and reflex irritations of all kinds, which confuse and confound us at every turn. One of my medical friends says that a hysterical patient is "a pathological kaleidoscope." It is so absolutely impossible to prescribe for the totality of the symptoms that, in many cases of hysteria, you will be compelled to abandon the idea; for when they change like the hues of the chameleon, and are as irreconcilable, incompatible, and contradictory, as they often are, you would need as many remedies as there are single, individual symptoms, and these might have to be changed several times daily.

Necessity for caution in the exclusion of symptoms.

May be too kaleidoscopic to be covered by any single remedy.

As a prospective improvement upon the ordinary unsatisfactory and unsuccessful method of combating hysterical symptoms, let me counsel you to direct your treatment, 1st, *Against the hysteri-*

cal diathesis, and 2d, *Against the symptoms which properly belong to the lesion, of which the hysterical attack is either the consequence or the concomitant.* Physicians recognize the practical significance of the rheumatic, the gouty, the tuberculous, and the syphilitic diatheses. In the treatment of almost every variety of disease of which their existence can possibly complicate or modify the symptoms, they receive due consideration when we make our prescriptions. The hysterical predisposition is equally pronounced and equally deserving of attention. Its treatment is more decidedly hygienic and prophylactic, than medicinal. It prescribes the removal, if possible, of all the causes which might originate or perpetuate this disorder. It regulates the mental and physical exercise of the patient, her habits of eating and sleeping, her social and domestic life, and everything, in short, which can influence the functional operations of her nervous system. It places particular stress upon these matters in her case because of her constitutional bias towards hysteria. It recognizes that health cannot be restored unless the proper physiological conditions for its restoration and maintenance are supplied.

General rules.

For the *hysterical diathesis.*

A knowledge of this diathesis will sometimes aid in the selection of our remedies. The relations of belladonna, ignatia, caulophyllin, agaricus, hyoscyamus, lilium tig., gelseminum, ether, moschus and valerian to this peculiar predisposition are well known to the profession. They are sometimes given with excellent effect as hysterical prophylactics, and may finally eradicate the disease altogether. As intercurrent remedies they may be equally useful. The choice between them will depend upon a few "characteristic," objective, cardinal symptoms.

Remedies to counteract it.

The diseases of the generative system are the most usual concomitants of hysteria. Disorders of menstruation underlie a large proportion of the cases of this disease. Dysmenorrhœa, amenorrhœa, too scanty, too copious, irregular and too frequent menstruation may need to be cured before the symptoms of hysteria will disappear. For each of these affections you should therefore prescribe as carefully as possible, taking only such note of the hysterical outgrowth as will enable you to counteract the predisposition of which I have

Coincident menstrual disorders.

spoken. The chief thing is to cure the menstrual irregularity, after which the contingent symptoms will disappear of themselves. Remove the cause and the effect will cease. Cure the idiopathic lesion, and the sympathetic, nervous, accidental symptoms will vanish.

The careful study of the legitimate symptoms.

This method of procedure will enable you to discriminate between the legitimate symptoms, which are reliable, and those which are not. It will not, however, do away with the necessity for close and careful study of those symptoms, and a proper adaptation of the remedy to the cure of the menstrual difficulty. You will proceed to remedy that disorder, whatever it may be, with little or no regard to the hysterical phenomena, however noisy and clamorous they are.

Coincident lesions of the uterus, ovaries, etc.

The same rule applies to organic disease of the ovaries, and of the uterus, to uterine displacements and ulceration, to hypertrophy and neoplasms of the womb, to leucorrhœa, abortion and its consequences, to vesical and rectal irritation, inflammation and ulceration, which so frequently exist in connection with hysteria. The symptoms that properly belong to these several affections are those which are most significant, and which will afford the real indications for the cure of the case. There is no objection to an intercurrent remedy for the relief and removal of a contingent delirium, globus or clavus hystericus, the hysterical stitch in the side, or the infra-mammary pain; but your chief concern will be to recognize and cure the lesion from which so many of the symptoms are proliferated, but upon which they are in a sense supernumerary.

Also of other organs, which are themselves secondary.

So, also, with the gastro-alimentary, hepatic, cardiac, cerebral, spinal and renal difficulties which sometimes attend upon hysteria. These complications render it still more difficult to cure. For they may be, and often are, themselves secondary upon some inter-pelvic disorder. Under these circumstances you will be compelled to analyze the symptoms, to go back to their first cause, and in selecting the remedy, to recognize the relative importance of the uterine and the ovarian symptoms.

For example, in a case of utero-gastric or utero-cardiac disorder, the symptoms that are referable to the pelvic viscera may afford a more reliable guide in the treatment than the gastric or the cardiac symptoms, separately considered. One of my patients had an intractable emesis which the best chosen internal remedies failed to relieve. In addition to the vomiting, she had a great variety of hysterical symptoms, which alarmed her family exceedingly. Feeling confident, at last, that in her case the remote cause was located within the pelvis, I proposed a vaginal examination. The touch revealed the uterus badly prolapsed. It was replaced and kept in position, and not only did the vomiting cease, but the hysterical symptoms also were cured from that moment.

Utero-gastric and utero-cardiac derangements.

Case.

Another lady suffered from violent attacks of palpitation of the heart. Her physician had decided that she really had organic disease of the heart. These attacks of palpitation followed riding, walking, defecation and coitus. They had occurred repeatedly at intervals for more than three months, when I was called to see her. The nervous system had become so much involved that these paroxysms finally merged into a species of hysterical fit. Vaginal examination with the speculum disclosed an abrasion of almost the whole of the anterior lip of the os uteri. I applied the oleaginous collodion a few times, ordered her to keep off her feet, and in a fortnight the heart disease and its hysterical outgrowth had entirely disappeared. She has had no return of either affection within the last three years.

Case.

These cases are exceptional, but they will serve to illustrate the importance of striking at the root of the real difficulty, when it is possible, instead of contenting yourselves with lopping off a branch here and there in the shape of an impertinent symptom, or class of symptoms.

Hysteria occurring at the climacteric period, or during pregnancy, labor, the parturient state, or lactation, will need to be treated with especial reference to these states or conditions, which are prime factors in the production and modification of its symptoms.

Other complicating conditions.

During the winter I shall have frequent occasion to elaborate and apply these general rules for the treatment of Hysteria. I will therefore spare you the infliction of a lecture upon its special therapeutics this morning. In the present connection it must suffice to remind you that it is one thing to put an end to the hysterical fit, by the use of such expedients as any old nurse could suggest and apply, and quite another thing to treat the various forms of this disease intelligently, thoroughly and successfully. For no other affection is so complicated, so enigmatical, so persistent, and so trying in every respect. And yet there is no other more amenable to rational, persevering and appropriate treatment.

IRRITABLE ULCER OF THE UTERINE CERVIX.

Case.— Mrs. B——, aged 40, has been ill for two months past. All her sufferings are referred to the epigastric region. She is subject to cramp-like pains in the pit of the stomach, which are sometimes so severe as to threaten her life. These paroxysms bear no relation to her meals, are not influenced by the variety or quality of her food, nor are they assuaged or aggravated in any manner by eating. They are quite as apt to return during the night as in the day. She has slight nausea, but no vomiting; is very thirsty, and the bowels are costive. The tongue is pale but not coated, the lips are blanched, the oral mucous membrane looks as if it would readily become ulcerated, as in stomatitis materna. She is the mother of four children, the youngest of which is three years old. Has never had stomatitis. Has always menstruated regularly, but, for some months past, has observed that the flow is less free than formerly. She has no pelvic pain or distress of any kind, but is at times annoyed with a copious leucorrhœa, which she describes as purulent and very weakening. The discharge is increased by prolonged exercise, as by washing, or by walking a considerable distance. She has been treated for the gastric difficulty for some weeks past, but without the slightest relief.

Reflex relations of uterus and stomach.

No physiological fact is more certain and more significant than the reflex relation which connects the uterus and the stomach. This relation is especially marked between the uterine cervix and the stomach. This poor woman is the victim of utero-gastric irritation which is so decided as to make her wretched and to cause her a great deal of pain. But the pain and suffering are located exclusively in the epigastrium. From the mere symptoms which she has given us one would not be led to suspect any uterine complication. Even the leucorrhœa would not necessarily be due to ulceration. It might be catarrhal, and, at her age, critical in character, more especially as the quantity of the menstrual flow is gradually diminishing.

The speculum not always necessary.

In treating this class of cases in private practice it is not always advisable or necessary to subject the patient to an examination with the speculum. The better plan is to remember these reflex relations, and to try if possible to cure the patient without placing a premium on the indiscriminate use of this means of diagnosis. But where the disease of the stomach, the heart, or any of the more important viscera does not yield to well-chosen remedies, you will be justified in proposing to search for the remote cause within the pelvis. And not unfrequently you will discover a latent and unsuspected lesion of some kind which will be quite sufficient to account, not alone for the peculiar nature of the individual symptoms, but also for their persistency in not yielding to treatment.

The uterine lesion may be latent.

That there may be very extensive and serious disease of the pelvic organs, without a corresponding degree of suffering, indeed without the patient or her physician having suspected anything of the kind, is a fact beyond question. It is altogether probable that the ulcer which some members of the class saw in this case, in the ante-room just now, has existed from the commencement of this woman's illness. I have seen examples of the kind in which a similar lesion must have continued for months, and even for years, without being recognized. Such an oversight is quite as inexcusable as it would be to treat a patient's throat or lungs for months together without ever having made a physical examination of the parts affected.

Removal of the protective mucus.

The surface of these uterine ulcers, in all such as are benign and not malignant, or specific in character, is usually covered either with pus, or with a bland, somewhat gelatinous mucus, resembling the white of an egg. These coatings are protective, and should be removed very cautiously, else the free surface of the ulcer may be wounded, and its appearance very much changed. If you will take a bit of cotton wool, or of soft sponge in the grasp of the forceps, pass the instrument carefully through the speculum, and when it approaches the cervix uteri, give it one or two turns upon its own axis, very gently and cautiously, you can wind the mucus about it in such a manner as to remove it from the surface of the ulcer without injuring it in the least. But if you mop it off roughly, your examination may be of little practical advantage, at least in so far as the differential diagnosis of uterine ulceration is concerned.

Appearance of the ulcer.

The irritable ulcer is irregular in outline, and varies in its depth. It looks as if it had been cut out with a "punch," the base thereof being considerably depressed below the level of the mucous membrane covering the uterine cervix. This mucous membrane is sometimes red, inflamed, and even œdematous, but again, as in this case, it is almost as colorless as cartilage. The bottom of the ulcer is of a dark red cranberry hue. Sometimes its vessels are so surcharged with venous blood as to cause it to be almost black in color. The granulations are very vascular, and bleed upon the slightest touch. Such patients sometimes complain of a slight flow of blood after exercise and after coitus.

A sign of depraved vitality.

This ulcer implies a low grade of vitality. As in the case of irritable ulcers located on the shin, examples of which you have seen in the surgical clinic, it depends upon a morbid state of the general constitution, and a depraved habit of the patient. The digestive system is almost always deranged. The patient is badly nourished. The mucous membranes elsewhere are not healthy, but pale, easily inflamed, and readily become ulcerated. This poor woman's lips and alæ nasi confirm this view. They have a pearly, exsanguine look, and her tongue has the ragged appearance of one which has been badly ulcerated. The gums are not healthy, and there is every reason to suppose that the lining membrane of her stomach has participated to some extent in this tendency to inflammation and ulceration. Hence her indigestion, inanition, general ill-health, and uterine ulceration, which, with its consequent leucorrhœa, are increased sources of weakness and disease.

Not limited to the poor.

But you must not suppose that this variety of ulceration is limited to the poorer classes of society. Indeed, the most marked examples of this disease are sometimes met with among those who have "lived too well," as the phrase is. These persons have brought on indigestion, and a depraved state of the nutritive function by eating irregularly and immoderately, by drinking too much wine and spirits, and developing an irritable, nervous temperament that has predisposed to this species of cachexia. It sometimes follows excessive loss of blood, as in hæmorrhage from abortion, and may be due to too prolonged lactation.

Treatment.—When there is reason to believe that uterine ulceration proceeds from, or is perpetuated by some digestive derangement, it is of the first importance to correct that disorder, whatever it may be. For this purpose the diet should be carefully prescribed, such aliment being chosen as can be most readily digested and assimilated. Albuminous articles are preferable. Lean meats, milk, the white of eggs, oysters and fish in their season, good bread, rice and farinaceous food, afford a sufficient variety. Fruits will furnish the vegetable acid, which is sometimes an excellent antidote to this cachexia. In case of indigestion, peaches, apples, pears and cherries should be cooked before eating them. This is especially true if they must be procured from the market.

Cure the indigestion—Diet, etc.

It is also desirable in this class of cases to husband the resources of the patient's system as much as possible, by closing any drain which may be exhausting her little stock of strength. Hæmorrhage, too excessive or prolonged lactation, diarrhœa, leucorrhœa, night sweats, copious expectoration, or diuresis, may need to be remedied before you prescribe for the ulceration itself. Fresh air, sunlight, diversion of the mind, and the cultivation of a good morale, are as requisite here as elsewhere.

Stop any drain.

The class of remedies most frequently indicated are arsenicum alb., nitric, muriatic or sulphuric acids, sulphur, rhus toxicodendron, baptisia tinctoria, hydrastin, and arsenicum jod. Incidental remedies may be given for incidental symptoms, but we can not be very far wrong in prescribing the first of these for Mrs. B. She will take a dose of arsenicum alb. 6th, morning and evening, and report on our next clinic day.

Internal remedies.

But it is not sufficient merely to regulate the diet, the exercise, and the hygienic condition and surroundings of this class of patients. Some kind of local treatment is called for, and may, if properly selected and applied, assist in the cure. Although, as I have already said, Nature extemporizes a coating for the ulcerated cervix uteri, still that coating is not always sufficiently protective to prevent the contact of the atmosphere and of acrid discharges, which may serve to interrupt the healing process. And although it is in a measure protective, that mucus is not properly, or in any sense curative. Therefore we find it advisable and necessary to substitute this natural covering by a better one, one that shall serve to keep the part protected against harmful influences, and which is, at the same time, possessed of healing properties. You may sometimes apply the baptisia, calendula, hydrastin, or, if you prefer, the same remedy which you have ordered to be taken internally. Simple glycerine will sometimes be sufficient. When either of these substances are given by injection, the vagina should first be syringed out thoroughly, in order to remove foreign matters, mucus, etc. After taking such an injection, the patient should lie upon the back, with the hips elevated, and without moving the body or shoulders for a considerable time. These injections may be repeated twice or thrice daily, according to circumstances. Where the leucorrhœal discharge is purulent and copious, as in this case, I prefer the calendula with glycerine.

Local treatment.

In this case the near approach of the climacteric may interfere somewhat with a prompt and radical cure of the ulceration. For, although all forms of uterine ulceration heal more slowly and less certainly at the change of life, you will find the irritable ulcer especially liable to become chronic, or, if healed up, to break out again.

THE DIFFERENTIAL DIAGNOSIS OF PREGNANCY.

Case.—Mrs. ——, aged 39, has not menstruated within the last fourteen months. About the time the menses ceased she had a severe attack of dysentery, which continued four weeks. This was accompanied and followed by evident inflammation of the bladder, the vagina, and possibly, also, of the womb, from which she convalesced very slowly. Five months and a half later, she married. Her husband remained with her only two days, and then left on plea of business in a distant State. In that period only two attempts were made at coitus, in neither of which did the male organ penetrate the vagina. She suffered extreme agony in these ineffectual attempts at intercourse.

During the interval, which is now eight and a half months, the husband has never returned. Four months ago she observed that the form of her abdomen began to change, becoming more and more prominent in the left inguinal and hypogastric regions. Sometimes the tumor subsides considerably, and afterwards becomes as large as before. The only unusual sensation she has experienced was that resembling the gurgling of a liquid, which seemed to pass upward from the left hypochondrium toward the umbilicus. The abdomen is now as large as that of one who is eight and a half months advanced in pregnancy, but the chief enlargement is upon the left side. She has had no morning sickness, no caprice of appetite, no urinary trouble, and no headache since she incurred the risk of becoming pregnant. The breasts are somewhat enlarged and tender, and the areola about the nipple is quite distinct. Physical examination of the abdomen by auscultation reveals a sound resembling the placental souffle, but it is not very decided. We have failed, after several examinations, to detect the fœtal heart-sounds.

Its great importance.

Although the whole generative function is physiological, and does not necessarily include any morbid process whatever, still its contingencies are so numerous, and the changes which it develops within the pelvic and abdominal organs are so pronounced, and withal so similar to those which attend upon certain diseases, as to render the diagnosis of pregnancy a very delicate and difficult matter. It may involve the position of your patient, and others also, in society and in the church, loyalty to the marriage relation, and legitimacy of offspring, as well as questions which are purely professional in their character, and which concern the proper treatment of the case in hand. How to decide whether a woman is or is not pregnant, is one of the lessons which you should learn most thoroughly. For nothing would so damage your reputation, as skillful practitioners, as to decide it wrongly.

Suppression of the menses.

In many respects the case before you is a very interesting one. The menses have been suppressed for a long period. And, although women sometimes reach the climacteric before their fortieth year, there is reason to believe that we should not attribute the arrest of function in her case to this cause. If there was no uterine tumor, no development of the abdomen, and none of the other signs of pregnancy were present, we might, perhaps, charge the suppression of the accustomed flow to "change of life." If she had not suffered from disease of the pelvic organs, and the suppression had not already existed before her marriage, the case would be different. As it is, we must remember that many other causes beside conception may interrupt the regularity of the menstrual function. Inflammation of any portion of the generative intestine, the vagina, the uterus, the Fallopian tubes, or of the ovaries, may cause an amenorrhœa which shall lead us to suppose a woman to be pregnant. So also inflammation of the bladder, the rectum, the intestines, and even of the lungs, may have the same effect, directly or indirectly. Displacements and deviations of the womb sometimes arrest the flow by obliterating the canal of the uterine cervix. The presence of polypi, fibroids, hydatids, and other tumors within that organ, may have the same mechanical effect. Atresia of the cervix, in consequence of the use of harsh astringent injections, or of the application of caustics, or of inflammation caused by an improper or ill-adjusted pessary, or of the bungling and harmful use of instruments in abortus or in labor at term, may also cause a suppression of the menses.

Therefore, while this symptom is regarded by women themselves as an almost certain sign of pregnancy, physicians look upon it as equivocal, and not by any means positive. We can not rely upon it in a given case. This woman has not menstruated for fourteen months. The period during which the arrest has continued is longer than that proper to gestation. Shall we therefore conclude that she is not pregnant, because she has passed the ninth month without being delivered of a child? That would not be a safe or satisfactory conclusion. For, in some cases, the catamenia are arrested for weeks and even for months, and conception takes place before they have been restored. This often happens with women who become pregnant again while they are nursing their children, and before they have begun to menstruate after delivery. So our patient might have had a suppression of this flow for six months or more, and then have become pregnant after her marriage, and before the menses had re-appeared.

An uncertain sign.

With respect to this symptom, therefore, there are so many irregularities, complications and exceptions that it is not to be regarded as a positive sign of pregnancy. At best, it is only corroborative. Taken in connection with other symptoms, it may help to settle the diagnosis, but singly and alone it is of very little consequence. An additional reason why we should not place an exclusive dependence upon it is that we are always compelled to take the patient's version of the facts in the case. If she is anxious to have children, or, for any ulterior reason, desires to have it decided that she is pregnant, she may claim that for a given time she has not menstruated at all, when this is not so. Or if, on the other hand, she is disposed to mislead the doctor, she may insist that her courses are regular, and normal in every respect, when, in truth, they have not appeared for months.

Marriage as a remedy for suppression.

It is the habit of some physicians to prescribe marriage as a remedy for suppression of the menses, with almost a total disregard of its cause, and of the consequences of taking such advice. It is my duty to warn you against this practice. For it is altogether wrong. Thousands of persons have been made wretched, while few, very few, have been cured by it.

Uterine obliquities.

In pregnancy it is not at all uncommon for the abdomen to be developed upon one side more than upon the other. Usually, however, the uterine tumor inclines to the right hypochondrium, for the alleged reason that the rectum pushes it in that direction as the womb passes above the superior strait at or about the fourth month. In this case, however, the tumor is at the left side, and has been from the first (left lateral obliquity). Its size and prominence, according to the patient's story, appear to vary somewhat, a fact which is easily enough explained upon the theory that there is an accompanying meteorism of the abdomen, which subsides of itself and recurs again. This would also account for the gurgling sensation, which is incidental, and not, in any sense, distinctive of pregnancy.

We need not discuss the negative value of the absence of morning sickness, nausea, caprice of appetite, quickening, headache, toothache, vesical tenesmus, and other occasional symptoms of pregnancy. In many examples of gestation, they are wanting altogether from first to last. If she has really passed the eighth month, ballottement would not be available.

But the changes in the areolæ about the nipples, and in the breasts themselves, are more significant. In pregnancy, whatever changes take place in these glands affect both breasts alike. This is not true of any disease to which they are subject. Consequently, when you find that both these organs are becoming larger, warmer, and softer, especially in those who have not already borne children, or been pregnant before, or if there is a slight secretion of milk, it is a suspicious sign of pregnancy. More especially is this true if the nipple is more erectile, vascular and granular on its exterior and tip than it has been, and if the circle of discoloration about it is more pronounced and decided. Here you have a good illustration of this subject. You observe the glandular follicles about the nipples are considerably enlarged, and that they pour out a quantity of fluid which gives the areola the appearance of having been oiled. The cellular tissue beneath and within the nipple is in a state of turgescence. The discoloration about the nipple is so marked that you can see it across the lecture-room. This looks as if our patient were really pregnant, and some authorities would decide the question upon the evidence afforded by this single symptom. But we must look a little farther.

Changes in the breasts.

If we could detect the fœtal heart-sound, resembling the ticking of a watch beneath the pillow, we should have a positive and unmistakable sign of pregnancy. But this we have failed to elicit. And yet it may be present. The mere fact that we fail to detect it, is no sign that a woman is not pregnant; while, if it can be heard, we *know* that she is *enceinte*. It is not safe, however, to depend upon a single examination in a case of this kind. For you may imagine that you hear it when you do not, or it may be impossible to hear it today, and the easiest thing in the world to note it to-morrow.

The fœtal heart-sound.

The uterine souffle is so frequent an accompaniment of abdominal and uterine tumors, aneurism, etc., as not to afford any reliable criterion of the pregnant state. At best it is only a confirmatory sign, which may be classed as a probable, but not as a positive symptom of pregnancy.

The uterine souffle.

There is still another means of exploration that, in a case so advanced as the one before us, may help to settle the diagnosis of pregnancy. If this woman really conceived eight and a-half months ago, the changes which have taken place in the uterine cervix should be quite marked and decisive. And so I find them to be. The neck of the womb is shortened and almost obliterated, soft, somewhat patulous—although she is a primipara—and in such a condition as can only attend upon gestation.

Changes in the cervix.

This, therefore, enables us to decide that Mrs. —— is undoubtedly pregnant. In reaching this conclusion, we rely upon the changes in the breasts, the discoloration of the areolæ, the characteristic softening and shortening of the cervix uteri, the abdominal development, and the placental souffle. All of these symptoms are taken collectively, and within the space of a month, at least, I have no doubt but that our diagnosis will be confirmed, (*Exit the patient.*)

Some of you may have doubted the possibility of conception without penetration of the male organ during coitus. Numerous cases are recorded in which this result has followed imperfect intercourse on account of some mechanical obstacle, as an imperforate hymen, or an inveterate vaginismus, and the like. In resolving such doubts you have only to remember that the essential condition of impregnation, is that the vitalizing part of the male semen shall be brought into contact with the ovum of the female somewhere within the generative tract. The discharge of that semen within the vulva may, under certain circumstances and exceptionally, produce the same result that would follow the complete act. But such cases are by no means so frequent as some have imagined.

LECTURE XX.

THE SPONGE-TENT AS A MEANS OF DIAGNOSIS IN DISEASES OF THE BLADDER AND URETHRA IN WOMEN.

GENTLEMEN:

Some of you are already familiar with the fact that the female urethra may be so dilated as to admit of the introduction of the index finger. You have seen me perform this operation by means of the dressing forceps, Atlee's uterine dilator, and the sponge-tent. Of late this expedient has been quite frequently resorted to for the removal of stone from the bladder without cutting.

A new use of the sponge-tent.

Here is a sponge-tent that I wish you to examine carefully. Ten minutes ago it was removed from the urethra of one of my lady patients, and it presents some appearances which it is quite probable you have never before observed. Its base is as large as a silver dollar. It is of unusual length, and is composed of the best sponge. Excepting only at its smaller extremity, it is as clean as if it had just been washed. There is not a shred of mucus or a drop of blood upon it anywhere else. At its tip, however, you will see a quantity of pus which is slightly streaked with blood.

Case.

My patient has been ill for some weeks with a violent, non-specific urethritis, Under the appropriate treatment, which I have already detailed to you,* the inflammation of the urethra was entirely cured. But there remained a frequent desire to urinate, inability to retain the urine for more than an hour at a time (unless she was riding in her carriage), an occasional deposit of a creamy-looking matter in the bottom of the vessel, and more or less of vesical tenesmus. Some of the symptoms resembling those of stone in the bladder, and all of them failing to respond to the usual remedies, I determined to

* See page 181.

dilate the urethra for the purpose of further exploration. This was first done by means of the instruments named, and afterwards by the introduction of a series of long sponge-tents at intervals of three days. Each time that I have removed the tent it has presented the appearance so well shown in this specimen.

The use of the tent in this case enables me to locate the seat of the ulceration very definitely. I know by the appearance of the sponge that the urethra is in a healthy state, and that the pus which has been discharged with the urine came from some portion of the bladder. Having stretched the vesical sphincter with the dilator, so that the urine escaped freely, and afterwards introduced the tent to the same distance, by actual measurement, I am confident that its tip was applied to and within the neck of the bladder. The thick, creamy pus, which has been brought away by the sponge, was not sufficiently fluid to have run down from the cavity of the bladder, but was evidently taken up by it directly from the diseased surface at its neck. The distal extremity of this sponge looks exactly as if it had been applied to a suppurating ulcer on the integument.

I am, therefore, justified in feeling as confident in the diagnosis of ulceration of the neck of the bladder in this case, as if I had seen the ulcer. Indeed this means of exploration has certain advantages over the endoscope as applied to diseases of the urinary passages in the female subject. It is more simple and available. It does not require an especial and expensive instrument. It furnishes a sample of the discharge, and dilates the urethra so as greatly to facilitate the local application of remedies, if it shall be deemed desirable.

There is no harm in dilating the female urethra quite rapidly. For this reason, and because it lessens the duration of suffering, we choose a freshly-made tent, one that will soften and expand very readily. The patient should be placed upon the back, with the hips brought to the edge of the bed. The feet may be put each in a chair at the side of the bed, as if you were intending to apply the obstetric forceps. Then take Atlee's uterine dilator, or the long dressing forceps, have them well oiled, or anointed with glycerine, or with soap from the dressing-table, introduce them carefully into the urethra, and separate the blades so as to

Mode of applying.

stretch the passage from right to left, and from above downwards. Upon the removal of the instrument the tent can be pushed in carefully and steadily, until it has reached the neck of the bladder. Hold it there for a few moments until it begins to soften, else, being pointed and somewhat conoidal, it may be forced out by a sort of peristaltic spasm of the adjacent muscles. You may leave it within the urethra for from half an hour to one or two hours, but not longer. For it will soften and dilate much more rapidly than if it were in the canal of the uterine cervix; and besides, an early removal will give you a better idea of the condition of the neck of the bladder than if it were allowed to remain for any considerable time. It need not be carbolized.

If the passage is very narrow, or has been inflamed, it is better to begin with a small-sized tent, and afterwards to use larger ones. The sponge is certainly preferable to the sea-tangle, or slippery elm and other material, because it is less hard and irritating when first introduced, and because it does not need to be retained so long in the urethra. The bladder should be emptied before beginning the operation.

The tent in urethritis.

I have used the tent also in very obstinate inflammation of the urethra, and have thus been enabled to recognize, locate and treat an ulceration of its mucous membrane much more directly and successfully than I could otherwise have done. The topical employment of remedies to the inflamed urethra might easily be secured by means of medicated tents and bougies.

A practical hint.

In dilating the urethra for the purpose of bringing medicated substances and injections in contact with the neck of the bladder, and with the upper portion of that canal, it is best to stretch it only at its inner extremity, by means of one of the instruments named. This leaves it funnel-shaped, and, while the patient lies upon her back with the hips raised, secures the retention and contact of the substances injected. An ordinary hard-rubber intra-uterine syringe will answer a better purpose than a more complicated one for throwing these injections into the female urethra, and even into the bladder, when it is necessary.

SIMPLE ULCER OF THE UTERINE CERVIX.

Case.—Mrs. T——, aged 28, mother of one child, has been ill for six months. She complains of weakness and debility, which incapacitate her for her daily duties. There is a great deal of pain in the sacral region, dragging in the loins, and bearing-down sensations when she is upon her feet for any considerable time. Internally she feels a sense of swelling and fullness within the vagina, and of burning at its upper portion. At times there is quite a free leucorrhœal flow, which is of a bland unirritating character. Examination with the speculum reveals a simple ulcer of the size of my thumb nail, situated chiefly on the posterior lip of the os uteri, and extending within the orifice.

The subjective symptoms of this, as of most other varieties of uterine ulceration, are not peculiar. The patient may complain of pain in the sacrum, the hips, the thighs, the coccyx, the symphysis pubis, the hypogastric, or the ovarian regions. There is a sense of weight and fullness, of weakness and bearing-down in the region of the womb. She has, perhaps, great lassitude, with an almost insuperable dislike of mental and physical exertion. Leucorrhœa and painful menstruation are frequent and troublesome concomitants. In some cases, as in this one, there is a sense of tumefaction, and of local heat in the parts affected. This symptom is especially tormenting after the menstrual discharge has ceased, and also after coitus. Not unfrequently there is an aversion to sexual congress, and when complicated with vaginitis, the act is likely to be followed by a bloody discharge. The reflex hysterical symptoms are numerous and varied. Such patients are prone to be hypochondriacal, and sometimes exhibit strong tendencies towards insanity.

Subjective symptoms.

The objective local symptoms revealed by the "touch" and the uterine speculum are peculiar, and we must rely upon them as diagnostic. The ulcer, the shape of which is irregularly circular, may occupy one or both lips of the cervix, although the posterior lip is its most frequent seat. For this latter reason the slightly curved speculum is sometimes preferable in making an examination. The lesion sometimes extends within the os and along the cervical canal. On removing the accumulated secretion from the

Objective local symptoms.

orifice with a pair of long dressing-forceps and a bit of charpie or cotton, and expanding the bi-valve speculum, if you use it, the ulcer is freely exposed. There is necessity for care in all these manipulations of the cervix, on account of the extreme delicacy of the structure implicated. This ulcer within the os and the canal of the cervix is sometimes the last and most difficult part to heal. Indeed it often happens that such cases are dismissed as cured, when only the mucous membrane exterior to the orifice has been healed.

Appearance of.

The simple ulcer is superficial, not excavated, and its margins may be irregular, wavy or stellated. In some cases its borders are slightly raised and cord-like to the "touch." The color is usually scarlet, evincing a remarkable degree of vascularity. Sometimes however, it is of a dark or dusky-red hue, resembling erysipelas. This blush may extend beyond the border of the ulcer itself. The more protracted the case, the darker and more livid the complexion of the ulcer. The surface is almost always covered with a muco-purulent secretion, which must be wiped off carefully.

In an acute case the part looks as if a corresponding extent of its investing epithelium had been stripped off. Sometimes there is a simple erosion, which Kennedy has compared to excoriations of the glans penis, and to aphthous ulcers in stomatitis. The cervix is swollen, congested and sensitive. When the lesion has existed for a considerable time, it has a suppurating surface, and it becomes the source of an intractable and exhausting leucorrhœa. At this stage the simple ulcer may degenerate into the fungous, or granular variety, of which we shall have more to say hereafter.

Causes.

The most common causes are painful, forcible and too frequent intercourse; coitus during or directly after menstruation, while the utero-vaginal mucous membrane is very vascular and sensitive to mechanical injury; disproportion in length between the male organ and the vagina; the injudicious use of astringent and harmful injections per vaginam; cold; insufficient clothing of the inferior extremities; vaginitis; and friction of the parts from walking when the uterus is prolapsed upon the perineum, are among the more frequent causes of simple ulceration of the os and cervix uteri. Tyler

Smith is of opinion that the corrosive properties of the leucorrhœal discharge may occasion this form of ulceration, when brought into contact with the surface.

This form of uterine ulceration is especially apt to occur soon after marriage; or it may be caused by too prolonged nursing. According to eminent authorities, among whom are Churchill, Bennett and Whitehead, it may result in abortion and sterility.

The treatment proper for this variety of ulceration is constistitutional and local. The internal remedies most frequently indicated are, arsenicum alb., arsenicum jod., nitric acid, belladonna, arnica, ignatia, aurum mur., nux vomica, sepia, and sulphur. Incidental complications, of course, require intercurrent and appropriate remedies.

Treatment.

The local treatment should be as soothing as possible. The principal indication in most cases is to prevent the contact of the vaginal mucus and of the leucorrhœal discharge, and so to protect the denuded surface from the influence of atmospheric air as to facilitate the reproduction of the proper epithelial tissue. If the ulceration is of traumatic origin, you may prescribe vaginal injections of dilute arnica with glycerine. If the leucorrhœa is purulent, or muco-purulent, it may be better to substitute calendula for the arnica. Other topical expedients are injections of an infusion of flax-seed, or of dilute glycerine, which does not become rancid; the direct application to the ulcer of a watery solution of gum tragacanth, or of a solution of loaf-sugar; painting the ulcer with collodion, or with glyceroles of iodine, hydrastin or aloes. Latour's oleaginous collodion is preferable to the ordinary collodion, because it does not cause pain by its shrinking.*

Topical treatment.

THE SEQUELÆ OF ABORTION.

This patient was brought to the Clinic by my friend, Dr. W. W. Wilson, whose notes of the case I will read you:

Case.—Mrs. ——, aged 39, English, the mother of two children, has always enjoyed good health until now. She has never been

*℞. Ether sulph., grammes 400.
Alcohol, " 100.
Gun cotton, " 35.
Ol. ricini, " 35.
Mix the three first ingredients thoroughly, and when dissolved, add the castor oil. Apply with a camel's hair brush.

troubled with female weaknesses of any kind, and never aborted before. She became pregnant during the latter part of April, and by the advice of an old midwife, took vaginal injections of warm water twice daily, for the purpose of promoting an easy labor at term! On the tenth of June (at the sixth week), she came by railway from Indianapolis to Chicago. The next morning after her arrival, not having any warm water convenient, she took an injection of cold water instead, and this was applied with a common rectal syringe. The shock was such that she fainted, and in a few minutes aborted, everything coming away with a gush.

A physician was called in, who arrested the flow entirely, and the next day she felt so well that she did the washing for the family. That night she was seized with cramps and great pains through her body and limbs. Another doctor came, who said that she had inflammation of the bowels, and treated her accordingly. Since that time she has had four other physicians in turn, one of whom treated her for neuralgia of the liver (!), another for dropsy, a third for enlargement of the womb, and the last for dyspepsia.

I was called Aug. 31, and found her in great pain and distress, respiration labored, pulse 125, feverish and talking incoherently. The pains were paroxysmal, like those of labor, but were confined to the left ovarian region. On examination, I found the uterus and vagina normal, except that there was a slight, whitish discharge from the os uteri. Ordered pulsatilla^{200} every two hours, and the local use of the extract of hamamelis.

Sept. 1. Much easier. The pains have almost entirely ceased. Bell.^{200}.

Sept. 2. Still improving, but restless and cannot sleep. Continue the belladonna, but in addition to take three doses of coffea^{30} between 4 and 10 p.m.

Sept. 3. Husband reports his wife better. Slept well all night. Continue the same remedies.

Sept. 5. Found my patient sitting up and relatively comfortable. Bryonia^{200} every three hours, and zincum valerianicum 3 dec. a powder at night.

Sept. 8. The menses came at 10 A. M. Says she is well, but very weak. China^{200} every three hours.

Causes of abortion.

There is no single respect in which women differ more decidedly than in the readiness with which they abort. With some the slightest causes will induce a "mishap." A misstep, a rough ride in a carriage, climbing stairs, a long walk, a severe cold, coughing, sneezing, an attack of dysentery or diarrhœa, nausea, dysuria, a severe toothache, mental anxiety, or even jumping out of bed suddenly, have been known to cause it in those who were very susceptible. On the other hand, there are some women, who, no matter what they do, or suffer, are in no possible danger of miscarrying. They incur every risk without the least concern, or if so wickedly disposed, may try every means to induce an abortion, but without effecting it. The former are often disappointed in being unable to carry their offspring to term; but sometimes take advantage of their idiosyncrasy to put an end to intra-uterine development. The latter are often victims of their own or others' temerity in trying to interrupt the wonderful process of gestation, and thousands of them suffer the remote consequences of such conduct in the form of uterine diseases which are sometimes entailed upon them for life.

Toleration of injuries during pregnancy.

But nature has thrown certain safeguards around pregnant women which generally exempt them from harmful contingencies, and help them to pass through the ordeal of maternity with less of danger and risk than you would at first suppose. As pregnancy advances she develops a species of toleration to processes that are new and peculiar. She even counteracts and antidotes the mischievous interference of doctors of every grade, and nurses of all sorts, with her prerogatives. In this woman's case, the warm water injections happily did no harm. She could bear them with impunity. But the shock of the cold water, and especially when taken so soon after the journey, caused an almost instantaneous abortion. Perhaps she might have taken this injection at another time without any ill effect; but, the probabilities are that while the habitual use of the warm water developed a toleration for it, the cold application could not be borne at all without mischievous results.

Sophistries of the Abortionist.

I regret to say that there are physicians who do not regard an abortion at the early period of six weeks as an affair of the least consequence. They will tell you that prior to quickening the embryo is not alive, and that there is no particular necessity for ministering to its welfare or for shielding it from harm. But let me say, that the moment the ovum escapes from the Graäfian follicle, that moment it ceases to be a part of the maternal organism. This is as true in case of fecundation as it is in menstruation. Arrived in the uterine cavity, the egg is no more a part of the mother than is the egg of the bird when laid in its nest to await future development, or that of the snake when dropped into the grass before being fertilized. It represents a separate organization, which, although incapable of maintaining a separate existence, is as really independent as the infant at birth, or its father at forty.

Once the conditions for conception are supplied, and the vitalizing portion of the semen masculinum has impressed itself upon the ovum somewhere along the course of the generative intestine, the first step in the reproductive series has been taken. From this time forth, whatever imperils the integrity of that germ, implicates life; and whoever intentionally intercepts the wonderful changes incident thereto, *unless to save life*, is a veritable murderer—no more and no less!

The embryo is alive.

Whether prior or subsequent to the formation of the placenta, the dependence upon the mother for subsistence is substantially the same. No one familiar with the organization and function of the chorion can doubt this. The physical laws that regulate the supply and waste, the nutrition and detritus of germ-life, embryonic life, and fœtal life, are identical, and there is nothing in the mode of their operation which could lead us to infer that from the moment of fecundation, the whole process of intra-uterine development is not of the greatest importance.

It is no argument against the vitality of the smallest embryo, that direct vascular and nervous attachments between it and the endometrium have never been demonstrated. Blood-vessels have never been found in cartilages, ligaments, the epithelial tissues, and the epidermis. We may as well declare them inanimate for similar reasons. Moreover, the fact that direct means of communication between the mother's organism and the fecundated ovum, prior to the formation of the placenta, have not been discovered, is not to be received as proof of their non-existence. Reasoning by analogy, we know that the means of preserving life therein are not lacking.

The fertilized human ovum is not like the seed that has been wrapped in an old mummy, and left for centuries to await the conditions for its development. Its growth is steady and constant, progressive, physiological and positive. The qualities it has derived from either parent are preserved. The predominant traits of temperament and predisposition, the idiosyncrasies and individualities that go to make up the separate being in subsequent life, are there *in esse*. The hereditary features, and physical bias, the mental capacity and character, which are latent and undiscoverable to us, are nevertheless epitomized in the developing germ. If, prior to quickening, the mass were inanimate or dead, this could not be true ; nor would it be possible, when two or three months had elapsed, for the mother, however imaginative, to imprint such *paternal* characteristics as are frequently inherited upon her offspring. The very fact that these peculiarities are perpetuated is proof positive of constant development and physiological change.

Quickening not the first sign of life.

Quickening is not a reliable criterion of the vitality of the embryo, for the obvious reasons that it does not begin at a fixed and determinate period of pregnancy ; that it is frequently lacking throughout gestation ; that it may be confounded with abnormal sensations of various kinds ; and that the force of the impulse felt by the mother may be very strong in case of a weakly infant, or *vice versa*. It is more than possible that fœtal movements may occur for some weeks before they are recognized by the mother. Auscultation of the abdomen discloses the existence of these movements before the pulsations of the fœtal heart, or even the placental souffle can be heard. Not long since, a mother told me that, after its birth, a fœtus of a little more than two months kicked quite violently ; and at a very early period of gestation they have been known to breathe and cry when suddenly expelled the uterus.

Abortion as a cause of disease.

From my frequent allusion to abortion as an indirect cause of many of the diseases of women, you already have an idea of the importance of this subject. For the whole question of its prophylaxis, the right, and wrong, and responsibility of it, must be settled by medical men. Nothing could be more natural than for a sudden and forcible interruption of the textural changes and sympathetic relations, peculiar to pregnancy, to result in more or less of disease and disorder. The ovaries, the mammary glands, the uterine walls, vessels and lining membrane, and the nutritive and nervous systems are especially apt to suffer; and, strange to say, with certain exceptions, the earlier the period of the abortion, the greater the liability to these unfortunate sequelæ.

Sequelæ of abortion.

The list of these contingent and consecutive ailments is a long one. It includes the different forms of ovarian inflammation, ovarian dropsy, every species of menstrual disorder, peri- and para-metritis, metro-peritonitis, hæmatocele, the formation of moles, hydatids, fibroids, and uterine polypi, uterine displacements, uterine and vaginal fistulæ, subsequent abortion, atresia of the cervix uteri, sterility, hysteria, dyspepsia, neuralgia, leucorrhœa; malignant diseases, as cancer, at the climacteric, and mania.

Such an array of the possible consequences of abortion, whether accidental or induced, should lead you to make an especial effort to prevent it, whenever it is possible. I have placed upon the black-board a table of the causes of abortion, which you would do well to copy into your note-books, and study at your leisure:

I.—CONSTITUTIONAL OR PREDISPOSING.

1.—Plethora,
2.—Anæmia and Chlorosis,
3.—The Scrofulous Diathesis,
4.—The Menstrual Molimen,
5.—Zymotic Diseases:
  Syphilis,
  Mercurialization,
  Variola,
  Scarlatina,
  Diphtheria,
  Cholera.

II.—LOCAL, OR ORGANIC.

1.—Malformation of the Ovum.
2.— " of the Membrane (moles, hydatids).
3.—Placental Abnormalities:
  Mal-location of, (placenta prævia.)
  Organic disease of,
  Detachment of,
  Fatty degeneration of,
  Calcareous ditto.

III.—REFLEX, OR EXCITING.

1.—Centric:
  Emotional, as Fright, Anger, Grief, etc.,
  Direct blows upon the head or back,
  Cerebro-spinal meningitis,
  Cerebro-spinal effusion,
  Hysteria and Epilepsy.
2.—Ecentric:
  Parotidean Irritation,
  Thoracic do.
  Mammary do.
  Dental do.
  Gastric do.
  Rectal do.
  Vesical and Renal Irritation,
  Vaginal Irritation,
  Falls, jumping, blows, etc.,
  Functional and Organic Disease of the Womb,
  Ditto of the Ovaries,
  Death of the Embryo,
  Shock from cold injections, cold bath, etc.,
  Genital irritation (coitus),
  Do. do. (instrumental).

IV.—MEDICINAL.

This class includes the various emmenagogues, or oxytoxics, which have been known to cause the uterus to empty itself of its contents, among which are tansy, (tanacetum vulgare), ergot, (secale cornutum), cotton plant (gossypium herb.), quinine, cantharis, electricity, and some others.

You could not have a better illustration of the importance of this subject than the history of this case affords. It is more than possible that, until my young friend here was called to the rescue, no one had an intelligent idea of this poor woman's condition. The first doctor who came to her, and who sealed up the flow so promptly, should have impressed upon her the absolute necessity for rest and quiet. He should have insisted upon her remaining in bed, with as much care, and for as long a time as if she had just passed through labor at term. If he had taken this precaution, and given her no medicine whatever, she would probably have recovered without any untoward symptoms.

But he did nothing of the kind, and the consequence was that she became very ill, and, worst of all, was subjected in turn to the tender mercies of several other incompetent doctors. One said that she had enteritis, another neuralgia of the liver (!), a third hypertrophy of the womb, and a fourth dyspepsia. Their diagnosis was wrong, and hence their treatment could not be right. She grew worse instead of better.

Ill effects of wrong diagnosis.

This brings us to the practical lesson that I wish to draw from the case before you. It concerns the difficulty of diagnosticating the diseases that may accompany or follow abortion. For I am confident that this patient's experience at the hands of her physicians is by no means an uncommon one. In truth it is very difficult, and sometimes quite impossible, to decide whether this or that class of symptoms of which women complain is or is not referable to abortion as a cause. The perplexity is increased by our liability to confound it with delayed or painful menstruation, menorrhagia, membranous dysmenorrhœa, and by the possibility that the patient, if so disposed, may deceive us, by leading us to believe that she has miscarried when she has not, or *vice versa.* Add to this that in many cases the diseases of the womb and of the ovaries which follow abortion run a latent course; or they may partake of just enough of the hysterical "mimicry" to counterfeit other diseases, as for example peritonitis, enteritis, cystitis, etc.

Difficulty of recognizing the sequelæ of abortion.

A recent writer* has published the following table upon the

* Dr. Van de Warker, in the Journal of the Gynæcological Society of Boston, vol. IV, pp. 297-8.

differential diagnosis between spontaneous and induced abortion :—

Accidental and Spontaneous Abortion, to the Third Month.	Instrumental Abortion, to the Third Month.
1. Ovular abortion may occur and simulate dysmenorrhœa. Later; a gradual climax of symptoms, thus: loss of appetite, depression of spirits, pain in the loins, weight at anus or vulva, pain in breasts, followed by hæmorrhage and expulsive pains in the uterus.	1. Marked constitutional disturbance from the first. Rigors, fainting or collapse, severe pain in the hypogastrium, often extending over the entire abdomen, and marked tenderness on pressure.
2. From accident; sharp pain in the back, loins, or abdomen; often an interval of a day or two, or more, and then pains renewed violently and bleeding.	2. Expulsive pains before the hæmorrhage Pain severe in the back, and in a line from the umbilicus to the sacrum, pain and hæmorrhage occurring together. Large clots.
3 Evidence of history; habitual abortion, previous ill-health, or plethoric state.	3. Evidence of history. Previous good health. Evidence of habitual abortion absent, or doubtful.
4. Often a history of uterine displacement.	4.
5 As a rule the pulse rarely reaches 100.	5. As a rule pulse from 100 to 120.
6. As a rule, there are no symptoms of inflammatory complications of the uterus or the abdominal viscera.	6. As a rule there are always symptoms of inflammatory complications, and tenderness on pressure over the uterus. Os and cervix enlarged and extremely tender to the touch.

Treatment.—In case of threatened abortion, it will become your duty, whenever possible, to prevent it. If, however, delivery is inevitable, you must conduct it to a safe termination for the mother. But your interest in the case will not end with the expulsion of the embryo, or the birth of the fœtus, as the case may be, any more than the surgeon's interest in his patient should end with the operation of cutting off a leg, or stitching up a wound. Success may depend wholly upon the after-treatment.

First, then, as in surgical fever following bodily injuries and surgical operations, *rest* is the great remedy. A woman, the lining membrane of whose womb has been forcibly torn off in an early abortion, perhaps, by the use and abuse of instruments, or whose placenta has been prematurely detached in miscarriage, is as unfit for exercise as the man who has but just undergone an amputation of the thigh. Under these circumstances it is as necessary and proper that the uterus should repose quietly as that the stump should not be injured by the patient's hobbling around.

Rest.

I know there are women who ignore and disregard these precautions, and who do really escape any very serious consequences. But, depend upon it, these cases are exceptional. Thousands of them suffer and die of obscure, or more obvious, uterine disease as the result of a lack of care after a miscarriage. It is no uncommon thing for women to leave home on a long journey directly after "getting through," or even while they are in danger of aborting on the way. And some of you know from experience what it is to have such patients come to you from a neighboring town or city directly after an "operation," looking to the murder of the little innocent, has been performed. In this case the unknown city doctor kills the offspring, while, despite your best efforts, the ride and the excitement may cost the mother her life.

Arnica.

The analogy between the post-partum effects of abortion and the sequelæ of a severe injury, or surgical operation, suggests the use of arnica both locally and internally in these cases. The strong tincture may be diluted in the proportion of one part of the arnica to six of water, and applied by means of compresses over the hypogastrium and pudenda. If the patient flows freely, or is particularly addicted to hæmorrhage, the water should be cold; otherwise, if she prefers, it may be tepid or even warm. You can advise whatever attenuation of arnica you choose to be taken internally at the same time.

Arnica with aconite.

A very common, and a very useful prescription, of the stereotype sort, is to give aconite and arnica in hourly or less frequent alternation. These remedies are wonderfully efficacious in warding off the incidental fever and traumatic inflammation. This prescription may serve you a good turn in case you find it impossible to visit such patients very often or regularly. It should be given as soon as the delivery and its immediate dangers are passed. Aconite is particularly indicated if the miscarriage was caused by fright, and has been followed by fear and dread of fatal consequences.

Belladonna.

In case of the development of quasi-inflammatory symptoms, as in the spurious peritonitis, of which I have already spoken,* ovarian irritation or neuralgia, undue determination of blood to the pelvic viscera without hæmorrhage, excessive perturbation, unrest, and nervous irritabil-

* See page 297.

ity, with more or less acute pain, local or general, I know of no remedy so useful as belladonna. Atropine in the third decimal trituration will somtimes remove these symptoms like a charm.

Chamomilla, colocynth, ignatia, hyoscyamus, and other polychrests will be useful under appropriate indications. If the pains assume the character of genuine after-pains, camphora, caulophyllin, belladonna, or nux vomica, may be required. If real metritis, phlebitis, or cellulitis shall result, the case will become more serious, and you will need to study very closely in order to find the appropriate remedy or remedies. Do not forget to give due weight to the accidental, as well as to the emotional causes of these secondary disorders. But I need not repeat what I have already said concerning their treatment.

Local treatment.

If the abdomen is tympanitic, and exceedingly tender to the touch, order the dry, hot, bran poultice, or the application of dry heat by means of plates wrapped in flannels, or have the abdomen covered with cotton batting, or hot flannel. If the pain is circumscribed, and limited to one or the other ovarian region, it is possible that relief may follow a change of posture. Have the patient "change sides," and learn if she cannot lie with more ease upon one than upon the other. Forbid cold drinks while she is suffering, and let all her clothing, and that of the bed, be warm and dry. The chamber should be well ventilated, but do not allow a draft of air to pass near or over the bed. Place the patient in the most favorable position for regaining her health. And, what is sometimes as important as anything beside, see to it that officious neighbors and nurses, (and doctors too,) do not swarm about your patient in your absence.

This woman is practically cured, and I will not change the prescription; for it is a good rule in medicine as well as in morals to "let well enough alone."

LECTURE XXI.

CHRONIC CERVICAL ENDO-METRITIS, OR ENDO-CERVICITIS.—UTERINE LEUCORRHŒA.

GENTLEMEN:

Inflammation of the mucous membrane lining the uterine cervix is especially interesting because of its clinical relation to what is commonly known as uterine leucorrhœa. This patient came under our care six weeks ago. She is now almost well, and I present her as an illustration of the importance, nay, the absolute necessity, of a correct diagnosis as a condition of cure in some of these cases, and for the purpose of showing you that the simplest remedies are sometimes the most efficacious. Her clinical history, as recorded on her admission, is as follows:—

Case.— Mrs. ——, 28 years of age, the mother of two children, has been an invalid for two years past. Her ill health dates from her last accouchement, which was normal in all respects. She, however, "got up" very slowly, and was weakly during lactation. She still nurses her child, which is a big, hearty boy; and being obliged to take the entire care of him, she holds and carries him most of the time. She has not menstruated since her confinement.

She complains of aching in the loins, a dragging sensation about the hips, which extends to the thighs, and bearing down pains and pressure within the pelvis, "as if everything would be forced from her." This latter symptom is worse when she rises to her feet from the chair or couch. She also has a leucorrhœal discharge, which is thick, creamy, and sometimes more watery and copious. The freer this flow the greater her debility and prostration, and the more severe and distressing the pain in the back. Upon arising in the morning this discharge is often so profuse as to cause her to be faint, to destroy her appetite, and to incapacitate her for her household duties. She finds it impossible to stand more than a few minutes at a time, and can not walk but a short distance without being very much fatigued. She enjoys a short ride, providing the carriage is easy and the road is not rough.

At times she has a burning pain which, she thinks, is in the mouth of the womb. Intercourse is almost intolerable. The bowels are badly constipated; the appetite poor and capricious, with more or less of nausea and loathing of food, especially in the morning. Her eyes are so weak that she can not read or sew more than five or ten minutes at a time without pain, indistinct vision, and lachrymation.

The touch reveals a tumefaction and tenderness of the cervix uteri. The womb lies very low in the pelvis. The external os uteri is patulous, and its lining membrane everted. A thick, albuminous mucus was taken directly from the canal of the cervix and subjected to microscopical examination. There is no visible ulceration, although she has been treated by three physicians for that disease. The neighboring organs appear to be healthy.

I have already spoken of cervical metritis, or inflammation of the parenchyma of the uterine cervix.* The case before us is one in which the lesion is limited to the mucous membrane that lines its canal. It is styled cervical endo-metritis, or endo-cervicitis, to distinguish it from corporeal endo-metritis, internal metritis, or inflammation of the proper uterine mucous membrane, which is found within the cavity of the womb. For while you would naturally suppose that these two affections would often coexist, the fact is that they are almost as distinct and as little related to each other as are bronchitis and *bona fide* pneumonia.

Extent of the cervical mucous membrane.

Those of you who are not practically familiar with this disease may be disposed to question whether such a limited extent of inflammation could really induce very serious or persistent symptoms and ill health. The uterine cervix is only one and a quarter to one and a half inches in length. But the mucous membrane that lines its cavity presents a very considerable surface. Its rugæ, or plicated folds, are numerous; it is reflected over the arbor vitæ uterinus, and dips down into each of the little glands within the cervix, of which, according to Dr. Tyler Smith, there are as many as from two to three thousand. In an ordinary case of endo-cervicitis, therefore, a larger extent of mucous membrane is inflamed than you would at first have supposed possible.

A glandular lesion.

And not only is this lesion an extensive one. The necessary implication of the glandular apparatus develops a disorder of secretion which depletes from the patient's general strength, complicates the case, adds to the suf-

* See page 274.

fering and retards the cure. Every well-marked example of endo-cervicitis is accompanied by a more or less copious and intractable leucorrhœa. And, although it does not come from the cavity of the womb, this discharge is commonly regarded as uterine. Hence, a majority of writers treat of this cervical leucorrhœa, which is a contingent and consequence of inflammation within the cavity of the cervix, and exterior to the os internum, as *uterine catarrh*. As applied to this disorder the term is a misnomer, and calculated to mislead. For there is as great a difference between the character of the flow in true uterine catarrh, and in proper cervical leucorrhœa, as there is between the rusty sputa of pneumonia and the mucoso-puriform secretion which is stained with blood in bronchitis.

Cervical leucorrhœa is not uterine catarrh.

Labor, whether in abortion or at term, is indirectly one of the most powerful predisponents of cervical endo-metritis. The changes which the womb undergoes after delivery, and which are designed, through the process of involution, to restore it as nearly as possible to its original size and form, may occur so imperfectly, or so irregularly, as to leave that organ in a very unnatural state. In this condition of sub-involution, its various tissues, including the mucous membrane within the cervix, are prone to become inflamed. It is for this reason, as in the case before you, that endo-cervicitis often dates from delivery. When a patient tells you that, since the birth of her last child, she has suffered from symptoms which are the counterpart of those of which Mrs. —— complained, you will have a strong presumptive sign of her disorder. A careful examination locally will either confirm or disprove your suspicions.

Predisposing causes.

A sequel of labor.

The scrofulous cachexia also predisposes to this form of uterine inflammation. It could not be otherwise, when so important a part of the secretory apparatus is implicated. The same is true of the return of the menstrual cycle. The physiological afflux of blood to the uterine cervix, and especially to the vascular membrane lining its cavity, may develop into a state of hyperæmia, and so derange the process of nutrition as to establish a genuine inflammation. Dysmenorrhœa, too frequent, tardy, scanty, or irregular menstruation, tend in the same direction.

Scrofulosis.

Menstruation.

The tuberculous diathesis is also a powerful predisponent of cervical endo-metritis. Depraved nutrition, from whatever cause, too prolonged lactation, rapid child-bearing, hereditary feebleness of constitution, and habitual strain of the mental faculties, if it is of a depressing character, belong to the same list of causes.

Tuberculosis.

My observation leads me to remark that there is still another cause which should be included in this category. I allude to the influence of what is known as a "bilious climate." Wherever hepatic disorders prevail to any considerable extent, as in malarious districts, we find a strong tendency to this variety of uterine inflammation. Organic and functional diseases of the liver embarrass the circulation of venous blood through the pelvic viscera.* In a climate in which every kind of morbid state is stamped with the impress of "biliousness," this cause is constantly at work, and the step from congestion to inflammation of the cervix uteri is so short a step that it is very easily taken. Multitudes of women have cervical endo-metritis from this indirect cause alone. In confirmation of this view we find that, next to the large class of scrofulous subjects who suffer from it, women with dark hair and complexion, and black eyes, that is to say, who are of a bilious temperament, have this disease most frequently, and in its most intractable form. This is an item which those of you who are to locate in the South and West will do well to bear in mind.

Biliary disorders.

The exciting causes of this disease are very similar to those which often give rise to cervical metritis. A sudden arrest of the menstrual flow, dysmenorrhœa, cold wet feet and damp clothing, tight lacing and the wearing of heavy skirts that are hung at the waist, violent exercise at the month, too forcible and intemperate coitus, the retention of a portion of the secundines after a miscarriage, the use of harsh injections to prevent impregnation, or of harmful instruments to induce abortion, ungratified sexual desire, as in nymphomania; uterine displacements; obstinate constipation with paralysis or stricture of the rectum; ovaritis; gonorrhœa: rough travel in a carriage, the cars, or upon horseback, prolonged standing upon the feet, and the wearing of ill-adjusted pessaries, are the

Exciting causes.

*See page 144.

most common of these causes. Exceptionally, in corporeal endo-metritis, there is an extension of the inflammation from the cavity of the womb downwards into the canal of the cervix. This almost never occurs, unless it be in the puerperal state, in which case the endo-cervicitis is a sequel of the endo-metritis proper. In vulvo-vaginitis, whether it be specific or not, the inflammation may finally invade the cervical canal and extend as far as the internal os uteri. But these cases are comparatively rare.

From Epidemic Influenza.

A mild, and in many instances a self-limited form of cervical endo-metritis, is sometimes met with during the prevalence of an epidemic influenza. You have seen several cases of this kind in our Clinique during the present winter. Such attacks may be either primary or secondary. They sometimes alternate with catarrhal inflammation of other mucous passages, as, for example, the nares, the throat, and the bronchial tubes, and perhaps also of the alimentary mucous membrane. In women of a scrofulous, or tuberculous cachexia, as well as in those who are greatly debilitated from other causes, an incidental cervicitis of this kind is very likely to become chronic.

Symptoms.

The most prominent and persistent symptom (in a well marked case of this disease) is the leucorrhœa. It is the first abnormality to attract the patient's attention, and the one above all others which a majority of practitioners are most anxious to relieve and to remedy. It usually begins with a slight increase of the normal healthy mucus from the cervix, which is observed to be most abundant a day or two in advance of the menstrual flow. Or it may follow menstruation, and continue for some days after the cessation of the catamenial discharge. Sometimes it is intermitting in character, being brought on by violent exercise or excitement at any time during the intra-menstrual period. The more chronic its nature, the more copious and exhausting it becomes. It may be creamy, viscid, highly albuminous, and inspissated in character. After a longer or shorter period, which varies in different individuals, the discharge becomes habitual and constant. Whenever the patient assumes the upright posture there is a sensible escape of this secretion from the cervix uteri. When she arises in the morning, after lying in bed all night, this flow may even be profuse, as it was a little while ago in the case before you. If it is bloody you will remark that the blood is not thoroughly mingled, or incorporated with the mucus—as it would be in case of a muco-sanguineous discharge from the uterine cavity.

When the follicular inflammation within the cervix uteri is become deep-seated and chronic, more especially if it occurs in scrofulous subjects, the hyper-secretion is altered in character. Examination with the speculum discloses a string of tenacious, transparent, ropy mucus, hanging from the external os uteri into the vagina, and in exceptional cases, even from between the labia majora. Dr. W. Tyler Smith compares the appearance of this secretion from the cervix to that of soft soap. "It seems as if the alkali of the discharge combined with the fatty and albuminous element, to form a saponaceous compound."* Farther on in the course of the disease, and even although there may be no abrasion of the os uteri, and no ulceration, pus-corpuscles are added, and the discharge becomes muco-purulent. In most cases, however, it is puriform instead of purulent. It is seldom that the flow is acrid and excoriating in character, unless she has ulceration of the womb; or the inflammation is specific, as, for example, diphtheritic, or syphilitic, in its nature; or the tone of her general health is very low, by reason of debilitating diseases, such as stomatitis materna, hæmorrhage, inanition, and a consequent deterioration in the quality of the blood.

The puriform discharge.

All of which leads to the inference that this form of leucorrhœa should properly be regarded as a symptom, and not as a disease *per se*. In this respect it ranks with a cough, a hæmorrhage, a dropsy, or a diarrhœa. When you take the discharge directly from the os uteri, and examine it in the field of the microscope, it presents the appearance shown in this diagram. Here are cylindrical epithelial cells, mucus-corpuscles, pus-corpuscles, blood globules, and fatty particles. These are found floating in an alkaline plasma, which vehicle is furnished by the cervical glands. Dr. Tyler Smith observed that the clearness or the opacity, as well as the viscidity of the discharge, its creamy, soapy, gelatinous or ropy appear-

The leucorrhœa merely a symptom.

Varying characters of the flow.

* The Pathology and Treatment of Leucorrhœa, by W. Tyler Smith, M. D., etc., Philadelphia, 1855, page 64.

ance, and indeed all of its physical characters depend upon the alkalinity or the acidity of the secretion with which it is mingled. The acid mucus secreted in the vagina changes the quality of the leucorrhœal fluid poured out from the cervix uteri, as decidedly as it does that of the blood which escapes from the same channel in ordinary menstruation. I think it very important for you to remember this fact.

Cervical leucorrhœa from other causes.

You will not understand me to say that all cases of this form of leucorrhœa depend upon cervicitis. By no means. There are other causes, such as obliquities of the uterus, the presence of foreign growths, ulceration of the os uteri, granular degeneration, ovaritis and kindred affections even more remote, and which operate in a reflex way, that sometimes originate and perpetuate this discharge by stimulating an undue activity of the glands within the cervix. For the present I must defer their consideration.

Pelvic pains and suffering.

The dragging sensations about and within the pelvis are not always so marked and severe in this form of cervical inflammation as they are in cervical metritis. For in endo-cervicitis the neck of the womb is not necessarily so tumefied and tender; and we find that the contingent distress and pain in the sacral and lumbar regions vary with the quantity and quality of the leucorrhœal flow, rather than with the size of the cervix. Something depends, however, upon the state of the patient's strength, the duration of the disease, her ability to withstand suffering, or her tendency to exaggerate and overstate the kind and degree of her pain. She is very apt to complain of bearing down sensations, symptoms of prolapse, forcing of the pelvic viscera towards the vulva, and not infrequently of rectal aching and tenesmus whenever she stands upon her feet. Under these circumstances there is an aggravation of the symptoms from motion, pressure, coughing, or sitting down.

Burning sensations.

These patients frequently complain also of burning sensations, which are located either within the vagina, at the mouth of the womb, or in the ovarian region. Sometimes the cervix is so displaced and tender that intercourse is very painful. More rarely, however, the unnatural condition of the parts causes an increased sexual desire, which the patient feels must be gratified, even though it be at the cost of subsequent suffering. Straining at stool, or in urination, may cause a flow of mucus from the cervix, and even from the vagina. The bowels are almost always constipated, although in some cases there is an alternation of constipation and diarrhœa. The bladder is more or less implicated, and cystitis, vesical tenesmus, dysuria and retention are by no means infrequent.

Constitutional effects.

Either as a cause or a consequence of the local lesion, the digestion is impaired, the nervous system undermined, and the general health borne down. Among the lower orders especially, such patients are very wretched. They are martyrs to vice, ignorance and self-dependence, to their children and families, to their own improvidence, and not unfrequently to the incompetency of their doctors.

Weakness of the eyes.

A considerable proportion of cases of endo-cervicitis are characterized by impaired vision, or rather by weakness of the eyes and inability to use them. This is true not alone of inflammation of the cervical mucous membrane, but of other diseases of the uterine neck, and perhaps of the ovaries also. For there is an inexplicable sympathy between the inferior segment of the womb and the eyes. I have treated a case of incipient amaurosis which was entirely and promptly relieved by the removal of a small mucous polypus that was found hanging from the external os uteri. Women have in almost numberless instances complained to me of pain, aching and weakness of the eyes immediately after the application of even the mildest lotions directly to the cervix. It is not at all unusual for this symptom to follow copulation temporarily, and in case of immoderate indulgence of the sexual appetite, to become chronic and perhaps incurable. The patient before you had these symptoms in a marked degree, and just in proportion as the uterine irritation and inflammation have been relieved in her case, has the weakness of vision and its attendant symptoms improved. My friend Dr. Woodyatt, the oculist, informs me, however, that such symptomatic derangements of vision are apt to remain after the primary trouble with the uterus has been cured.

Upon making an examination with the speculum in a case of endo-cervicitis, if the woman has ever been pregnant, you will almost certainly find the cervix uteri somewhat swollen, the os patulous, and, if the leucorrhœal flow has been copious or long continued, the mucous lining of the canal of the cervix everted. In the virgin, however, and in those who have never conceived, as well as in very mild and recent cases, the tumefaction, the relaxed and open os uteri, and the hernia of the cervical mucous membrane may be lacking, and yet other equally reliable signs may lead you to diagnosticate the case as one of cervical endo-metritis. In other words, the inflammation in this case is limited to the cervical canal, bounded above by the internal os, and below by the external os uteri. I am convinced that endo-cervicitis is much more common among young unmarried women than it is generally supposed to be.

Examination with the speculum.

In the latter class the vaginal portion of the cervix is rarely inflamed. Its investing membrane is not congested, neither is it hot, dry, or especially tender. But in confirmed cases, occurring in women who have borne children, you will observe that the mucous membrane about and within the os uteri is in a state of hyperæmia and of evident inflammation. The nearer the menstrual period the more these parts will be congested, and the more open and dilatable the os tincæ.

Diagnosis.

In considering the diagnosis of this disease we are led to remark that the most mischievous results have followed the confounding of inflammation with ulceration and induration of the neck of the womb. Dr. Bennett, for example, believes them to be consecutive and inseparable, and, therefore, treats of them as synonymous, if not absolutely identical. Errors in diagnosis, confused ideas of disease, and the careless use of medical terms, are necessarily followed by harmful consequences. For they always reflect the treatment that will be adopted. If I were to teach you that inflammation, induration and ulceration are essentially one and the same disorder, my individual error as a teacher would react against the welfare of your patients and of the community, through you, because it would set you upon the wrong track in therapeutics.

Ulceration is incidental.

Remember, therefore, that the discharge from the uterine cervix of such products as I have described does not imply that there is necessarily any ulceration thereof. Take a pair of speculum forceps, such as I hold in my hand, wrap a bit of cotton about them in this manner, and pass them through the speculum as far as the os uteri. Let them approach the cervix very cautiously. Then turn them over and over, thus, very gently, and you will wind up and remove the stringy mucus just as if it were a spider's web. If this little manipulation is carefully performed, the free surface of the mucous membrane will be left exposed, and you will see at a glance whether you have a case of simple inflammation or of ulceration to deal with. But if you undertake to remove the mucus from the diseased part without this precaution, and mop it away roughly, the delicate vascular surface, more especially the hypertrophied villi will be wounded, and the part so bathed in blood that you can get no very definite idea of the lesion. For the same reason it is best to be careful in the introduction of the speculum, more especially the quadri-valve and cylindrical varieties, lest you injure the cervix and fail in your object.

A practical hint.

Now a simple abrasion of the os-uteri may be, and most frequently is, merely incidental to the endo-cervicitis. The leucorrhœal discharge does not come from the denuded surface, but is derived from within the canal of the cervix. If, however, the ulceration is deep-seated, and granular in character, and especially if the granulations are exuberant, and the patient is scrofulous, a large quantity of pus may be secreted from the surface of the sore.

The flow not from an ulcerated surface.

You will be able to diagnosticate endo-cervicitis from cervical metritis, by the absence of febrile action, and of local tenderness, which almost invariably accompany the latter; by the existence of a leucorrhœa, of congestion of the mucous membrane about and within the cervix, the open state of the os-uteri, the eversion instead of the retraction of its lining membrane, and by its relation to the scrofulous and catarrhal dyscrasiæ. Although these diseases are sometimes found to coexist, yet such a complication is not frequent.

Diagnosis from cervical metritis.

The prognosis should be guarded. If you promise to cure such cases in a given length of time you may be sadly disappointed; for they are by nature chronic and tedious. And there are so many causes which, directly and indirectly, modify the vascularity of the part that is inflamed, and derange and damage its glandular function, that your best inten-

Prognosis.

tions will be thwarted and your best prescriptions often rendered of no effect. Sometimes the sexual instinct and appetite of his patient is a sworn enemy of the physician, that overrules and overcomes his determination to cure her of this disease. Whether spontaneously aroused, or purposely stimulated, or whether it be gratified or repressed, the effect is to antidote and to counteract his efforts, to complicate the case, and to postpone the cure.

The return of the monthly crisis multiplies the contingencies with which this disease is beset. So also the central and dependent position of the womb, and more especially of its neck, and its relation to other organs, both near and remote, all of which tend not only to render the attack persistent and almost perpetual, but to bring on relapses when it has apparently been cured.

Of speedy cures.

Treatment.—Nothing is more common than for young physicians to claim that a few doses of this or that remedy have sufficed to cure a case of cervical leucorrhœa. And this independently of sexual excitement, the monthly exacerbation, and all the drawbacks which are but so many obstacles in the way of their superiors in age and experience. The fact is, their remedies may have been properly chosen, and most appropriate to the case in hand, but in the nature of things it is ascribing too much to them to insist that they are competent to cure such cases so promptly and decidedly. Merely to change the character or the quantity of the flow, or altogether to arrest it, is not to perform a radical cure. For relapses are the rule and not the exception. The doctor may plume himself on his skill in its treatment, and declare his patient well again, but the next day, the next week, or the next month, some exciting cause which is contingent upon her organization, or her position in the family, or in society, may upset all that he supposed he had accomplished, and consequently she is "as bad as ever again."

Remove the cause.

Most of the exciting causes of endo-cervicitis are avoidable. It will be necessary to remove your patient from under their influence. You will see to it that there shall be no sudden interruption or derangement of menstruation; that her clothing is suitable and sufficient; that her feet are warmly clad and dry; that her skirts are suspended from the shoulders; that there are no ligatures about her body or her limbs; that she is not the victim of excessive sexual indulgence (especially at or near the month), of uterine displacements, constipation, dysmenorrhœa, dysuria, ovaritis, blennorrhagia, rough riding, wearisome exercise, or the wearing of an *abominable* (not abdominal) supporter or pessary.

Both with reference to the prophylaxis and the cure of this complaint, an inherent tendency to scrofulous and catarrhal inflammation should receive your early and constant attention. If your experience shall correspond with my own, you will find that the prime indication with this class of subjects is to have them sufficiently nourished, to bring their assimilative functions and their blood up to the healthy standard. In other words, you must not only stop the drain, whatever it may be, which is exhausting their vitality, but also supply them with such available nutriment as shall more than compensate the waste that has been going on. It may be quite as difficult to select the proper diet, and to arrange all its details to suit each individual case, as it is to select the remedy, but, in my judgment, it is quite as requisite to the cure of the disorder.

The need of nourishment.

Milk in some form, bread and milk, cream, beef, mutton, oysters, fish, fowl, game, soups and broths of different kinds, if not too greasy, the whites of eggs, and malt liquors, may supply this need. Cod liver oil has benefited some of these cases amazingly. In others the digestion has been improved and the general strength fortified by the use of the acid phosphates. Brandy and whisky are usually interdicted, but sometimes a mild native wine, or the extract of malt, may be allowed. Condiments and coffee are often injurious, while acid drinks are not only grateful but useful also.

A proper diet.

Some of these patients will never get well while they remain within doors. Others need a change of scenery and surroundings, and they must travel. And yet another class must be kept in a passive state. But how to fill these indications without harmful consequences is the question for you to decide. When you have regulated all these incidental matters, which I assure you are much less trivial in their bearings than they seem in their recital, the case will be more than "half cured," and you will be prepared to study its special therapeutics.

Travel and exercise.

Excepting for the purpose of cleanliness, vaginal injections are of little avail in this disorder. For unless the mucous membrane that covers the vaginal portion of the cervix is also inflamed, or ulcerated, they do not reach the diseased part. And yet you will find that a majority of those who have already been under treatment for this disease have been in the habit of taking medicated injections of various kinds. With a view to clear the vagina of the unnatural discharges which come from the neck of the womb, to prevent their decomposition, and also, in case the endo-cervicitis is specific, to prevent the inoculation of the adjacent parts with the poisonous flow, we may prescribe injections of Castile suds, or of glycerine and tepid water.

Vaginal injections.

A better means of relief, however, consists in the direct application of pure glycerine to the inflamed cervix. This substance has the power of causing a free discharge of serum from its engorged capillaries, and thus of removing an incidental cause which not unfrequently serves of itself to perpetuate the disease. The determination of blood to the dependent cervix, and its stasis therein, is a prime cause of the excessive and abnormal secretion from the cervical glands. If we relieve this local embarrassment of the circulation, it is like extracting a splinter from the flesh in a case of irritative fever. Moreover, the expedient is simple, available and harmless. It neither interferes with the use of internal remedies nor antidotes them. It has no injurious effect upon menstruation, nor does it entail any reflex or remote consequences upon other organs, which may or may not be implicated. During the past six weeks this patient has had no other treatment. We have not given her a grain or a drop of medicine, and yet she is almost well.

The topical use of glycerine.

A good method of applying the glycerine is to make a firm tampon of cotton, tie a thread about the middle of it to facilitate its removal, saturate it thoroughly with pure glycerine, and introduce it into the vagina after the patient has retired for the night. It should be pushed up against the cervix and left there until morning, when it can be withdrawn. The removal of this tampon will be followed by a more or less copious discharge of a thin serum, which is the pro-

How to apply it.

duct of the "insalivation," as it has been termed. This little operation may be repeated, according to circumstances, from one to three times each week during the inter-menstrual period.

Another, and a more direct means of applying this substance is to take such an instrument as this, which is a flat uterine probe, armed with a bit of cotton-wool or soft sponge, saturate it with the glycerine, introduce it into the cavity of the cervix and pass it as far as the internal os uteri. Turn it about gently, and after a few seconds it may be withdrawn, freshly charged with glycerine, and again introduced. Fortunately the open state of the external os, in almost all of these cases, facilitates and even suggests a resort to this topical means of relief. The patient should remain for a time upon her couch, and should not go to ride or to walk for several hours after the application. In very rare cases the glycerine is poisonous to the mucous membrane, and can not be used in the manner directed. You should always be careful to select the best quality of glycerine for internal use.

Another method.

If the discharge is either purulent or puriform, the tincture of calendula may be added to the glycerine, in the proportion of one drachm to two ounces each of glycerine and distilled water, and applied locally. Or the hydrastis, hamamelis, arnica, or baptisia, may be used in the same way. In exceptional cases, occurring in strumous subjects, and which are very chronic and intractable, one drachm of the tincture of iodine may be mixed with two ounces of glycerine, and applied with a camel's hair pencil to the canal of the cervix. I have sometimes used the oleaginous collodion with the best possible results.

Calendula, hydrastis, etc.

Although, as I have already said, in endo-cervicitis the internal os uteri is in most instances closed, yet because it might possibly be agape, or readily forced open, it is not safe to resort to injections thrown into the cervix, lest the fluid pass into the womb, and even into the abdominal cavity.

Intra-cervical injections.

No matter what the variety or the degree of the uterine displacement in this disease, every species of mechanical support is more likely to do harm than good. The only pessary that I ever employ in these cases is the

Pessaries.

saturated tampon, of which I have just spoken, which some of my patients wear whenever they are upon their feet. Exceptionally the perineal strap or pad is palliative, and will permit of moderate locomotion and of riding out into the fresh air. But the ordinary supports, and especially the stem-pessaries, are absolutely harmful in the treatment of those uterine deviations which are incident to this form of endo-metritis.

Compression.

In very tedious cases compression of the inflamed mucous membrane exerts a salutary influence, not only in lessening the copiousness of the flow, but in curing the lesion upon which it depends. For this purpose the carbolized sponge tent may be introduced from time to time, and left *in situ* for some hours. Or the other varieties of tent may be preferred. Simpson's ebony bougies sometimes answer equally well. Medicated bougies and suppositories are not of any especial value in endo-cervicitis. Compression would, however, be harmful, excepting in chronic cases of this disease, and should always be used with caution.

Escharotics.

Concerning the employment of caustics in the management of this disease, they certainly are no better indicated than they would be in nasal catarrh, influenza, catarrhal ophthalmia, or a "cold in the head." It would be just as reasonable, and equally efficacious, to apply the nitrate of silver, or chromic acid indiscriminately, in the one case as in the other. Physicians succeed in curing bronchial, renal and intestinal catarrh without the topical use of alum, the acetate of lead, or even of carbolic acid, and why should they claim that a similar inflammation of the mucous membrane within the uterine cervix is not, and can not also be responsive to milder means of cure? Theoretically, the adherents of the Bennet school are certainly wrong in their deductions; practically, I believe, they are working more mischief (unwittingly, to be sure) than any equal number of physicians, of whatever denomination, the world over. For what excuse can there be for converting a case of simple endo-cervicitis into one of open ulceration of the os uteri, in order to cure it? And how shall the intelligent physiologist excuse himself to his own conscience for sealing a discharge from the neck of the womb, regardless of the consequences that may be entailed upon his patient?

I have long been of the opinion that, in the selection of the constitutional remedies for this form of leucorrhœa especially, the physical characters of the flow, as it is ordinarily obtained, have been considered more important and suggestive than the facts of the case will warrant. The usual mode of noting the peculiarities of the discharge which comes from the cervical canal is fallacious. An albuminous secretion, which is alkaline in its reaction, is subject to contact, succussion, retention and admixture with an acid mucus in the vagina, which changes its properties in many respects, if it does not alter it entirely, after which the product is recommended to be taken as a criterion of the actual lesion, and a guide in the choice of the remedy. Under these circumstances, nothing is more natural than that the flow should become white, watery, milky, opaque, cheesy, curdy, yellowish, brownish, flesh-colored, or even greenish. And, since the conditions which give rise to the varying qualities of the leucorrhœal flow (in endo-cervicitis, or uterine catarrh), are purely accidental, and contingent upon the passage of that flow through the vagina, I feel like insisting that they are not to be depended upon as therapeutical data.

A fallacious practice.

Take a parallel case. Suppose that, in nasal catarrh, the discharge were first subjected to the action of the vaginal mucus, or to any other acid mixture, and afterwards submitted to you as representing the proper pathological product itself, what kind of an idea would you form of the disease in question? And suppose, farther, that a physician should insist that, after such manipulation, the color and other characters of the discharge would indicate the remedy, what would you think of him?

Now, I propose, that in order to obtain a correct idea of the secretion which is poured out by the cervical glands in uterine leucorrhœa, we should not trust to the patient's version of the matter, neither to our own examination of the flow, when it has been mingled with the vaginal mucus, but that, in order to examine it properly, we should take the discharge directly from the cervix uteri itself, as well for curative as for diagnostic reasons. Then, as in nasal catarrh, we would have the original product unchanged, and whatever we could learn from it that would help us to differentiate between remedies would be much more satisfactory and trustworthy

Rule for examination of the flow in *cervical* leucorrhœa.

in every respect. And I do not know why a leucorrhœal secretion should not be thus carefully inspected from time to time, as we examine the sputa in pneumonia, or the urine in a case of Bright's disease. Moreover, it should be done in the same manner in making our provings.

Natural secretions and abnormal discharges.

I apprehend that the varying qualities of a natural secretion, as, for example, the menstrual blood, the urine, or the perspiration, as these fluids are influenced by disease, afford a much better criterion of the structural and functional conditions of the organ or organs involved, than do the physical properties of products which, like the sputa, diarrhœic discharges, and the cervico-leucorrhœal flow, are in themselves morbid. If this is true, they also supply us with a better guide in the selection of our remedies.

The physical properties of the flow in *cervical* leucorrhœa are many of them too fickle and varying to be possessed of the practical significance which has been ascribed to them. The leucorrhœa itself is but a symptom, and to divide and subdivide it, is perplexing to one's patience, and sometimes too transcendental to be of real use. If cures have been effected (and they undoubtedly have), when remedies for cervical leucorrhœa have been prescribed on these shadowy indications, the result must be attributed to the fact that they were accidentally suited to the relief of the more cardinal and essential conditions underlying those symptoms. We may, therefore, depend upon them only when we can not do better.

In *vaginal* leucorrhœa, however, the thickness, thinness, tenuity, color and peculiar character of the discharge, are more distinctive and significant. If it has acrid or corrosive properties, we should give this clinical fact its proper interpretation. For, excepting in case of malignant disease of the womb, as in medullary cancer, cauliflower excrescence, and the like, this kind of flow never comes from the cervix uteri. Where both these varieties of leucorrhœa co-exist, as they sometimes do, you will generally succeed in curing the vaginal form first, and that which depends upon endo-cervicitis afterwards.

If you can trace the origin of an attack of cervical endo-metritis to "taking cold," or to an epidemic influenza, no matter what length of time has elapsed since the disease set in, you will do well to prescribe the remedy or remedies that would have been suited to the primary disorder. Whatever remedy would have cured the "cold," the influenza, or the catarrhal fever, upon which the endo-cervicitis is secondary, may suffice to cure its remote effects and to help your patient out of her difficulty.

Practical hints.

Due notice must also be taken of the catarrhal dyscrasia, as it might be termed, and of the scrofulous and the syphilitic diatheses. So, likewise, of a predisposition to biliary derangements, whether it be chargeable to inherent peculiarities, or to the accidental circumstances of climate, season, an improper diet, or malmedication. In this climate the consideration and study of these utero-hepatic complications are indispensable. But above all, you will look for the most prominent and trustworthy indications for your remedies in those symptoms which are connected with and depend upon certain coincident derangements of ovulation, menstruation, and of the digestive, the respiratory, the circulatory and the nervous systems, and also of the bladder and the rectum. If you will adhere closely to this method of selecting the remedy in this class of cases, it will enable you to distinguish the true symptoms from those which are only incidental, and perhaps fallacious.

Thus, if the prominent symptoms complained of are referable to *ovarian irritation*, inflammation, or derangement, they might indicate belladonna, atropine, apis mel., colocynth, phosphorus, alumina, platina, china, hamamelis, pulsatilla, zincum val., lachesis, caulophyllin, lilium tig., conium, podophyllin, bufo, or some kindred remedy.

For reflex ovarian disease.

Or, if some *menstrual embarrassment* or difficulty gives a particular stamp, or character, to the symptoms, it may be indispensable for you to study the pathogenesis, and the published experience of the profession with bovista, secale cor., sabina, alumina, ferrum acet., calcarea carb., lilium tig., baryta carb., sepia, pulsatilla, ammonium carb., phosphoric acid, senecin, cocculus, helonin, cantharis, or xanthoxylum.

For contingent disorders of menstruation.

For the *digestive complications* the more common remedies are nux vomica, chamomilla, arsenicum alb., mercurius, graphites, lycopodium, colocynth, veratrum alb., aloes, opium, sepia, carbo veg.,

For utero-digestive complications.

collinsonia can., china, sulphur, hydrastis can., the citrate of iron and strychnia, kreasotum, plumbum, pulsatilla, alumina, natrum mur., podophyllin, æsculus hip., nitric acid, and nux moschata.

In utero-pectoral and respiratory ailments.

For those which implicate *respiration:* phosphorus, bryonia, sanguinaria, calcarea phos., calcarea carb., silicea, lycopodium, stannum, tartar emetic, lachesis, hyoscyamus, drosera or dulcamara.

In coincident disorders of the circulation.

For symptoms connected with the *local and general circulation:* veratrum vir., bryonia alb., stannum, apis mel., digitalis, cactus grand., aconite, gelseminum, veratrum alb., naja trip., or belladonna.

In utero-hysterical and nervous complications.

For the *nervous* symptoms, especially in those who are liable to Hysteria, almost any remedy in the Materia Medica might be required. Most likely, however, you will find what you want under the head of hyoscyamus, ignatia, coffea, moschus, caulophyllin, lilium tig., belladonna, atropine, cocculus, gelseminum, cimicifuga, causticum, chamomilla, agaricus musc., sulphuric ether, senecio, tarantula(?), scutellaria, or cypripedium.

For utero-vesical suffering.

If the *vesical* symptoms are the more painful and prominent, you should consult the class of remedies most frequently and commonly employed in the treatment of diseases of the bladder and urethra. This class includes cantharis, cannabis sat., dulcamara, belladonna, apis mellifica, mercurius, hyoscyamus, camphora, ferrum, chimaphila umb., and the eupatoreum purpureum.

For the utero-rectal symptoms.

When the *rectal* troubles predominate, we have aloes, podophyllin, nux vomica, sulphur, hamamelis, collinsonia can., and the æsculus hippocastanum.

Conclusion.

Do not understand me as recommending that these remedies shall be given consecutively, or without discrimination. In classifying them my object has not been to supersede the necessity for their differential study and adaptation, but to indicate the variety of symptoms which, in the treatment of this vexatious disorder, do really afford the most trustworthy guides in the selection of our means of cure. For almost every one of them has some especial relation to diseases of the uterine cervix.

LECTURE XXII.

THE DIFFERENTIAL DIAGNOSIS OF OVARIAN DROPSY.

GENTLEMEN:

I am privileged this morning to show you a case which is supposed to be one of ovarian dropsy. Two weeks ago this woman was sent to this hospital by my colleague, Prof. Pratt. The following is her clinical history:—

Case.—Mrs. H., aged 53, a widow, has four living children, the youngest of which is seventeen years old. In February, six years ago, she was seized with diphtheria, from which she had almost recovered, when, on March 1, she had a relapse. Her stomach became badly disordered, and she had violent vomiting. Up to that time her health had been good, although for three years and three months, or since 1863, she had not menstruated. With this relapse of the diphtheria the catamenia returned, at first moderately, afterwards copiously. The flow soon became almost continuous, averaging at least two days each week for some months following. Afterwards it was severe and profuse. Her physicians told her it was due to the "change of life," and one of them prescribed some barks and roots which arrested it for the space of two months, when it returned as before. She consulted other physicians, but they all were of opinion that it came from the same cause, and recommended her to rest and keep quiet.

About four years ago she consulted Dr. Pratt, at which time the flow was occasionally very profuse. In the spring of 1868, three and a half years ago, she had typhoid fever, and for three months the flow ceased. But, when she got well of the fever, it came on again. From that time until now, she has never passed a week without it. It is passive, with occasional aggravations, and always affords some relief, as also does a free diuresis.

In February last (eight months ago), she first noticed a swelling in her right side, which appeared as long as her hand, and about as thick. She can lie upon either side indiscriminately, but when, after lying upon one side for a time, she turns upon the other, she feels something move over to that side and settle down there. She can not eat with comfort while sitting, but must either stand up or lie down during her meals. Within two months the abdominal tumor has grown rapidly. It presses upwards against the diaphragm, and impedes respiration. Before that time she could feel the outline of the solid tumor through the abdominal parietes, but that is impossible now. The dyspnœa is worse on sitting than upon lying down. The largest measurement around the body and over the most prominent part of the tumor is forty-eight inches. Her weight is one hundred and sixty pounds, but she has lost flesh quite perceptibly since coming to the hospital a fortnight ago.

She still has occasional attacks of vomiting, which are usually, but not invariably, accompanied by increased hæmorrhage. Under these circumstances the flow is painless, but is apt to be preceded by more or less of nausea.

Mrs. H. has not had a cold during her six years' illness. She has formerly worked very hard in-doors and out. For ten years past she has acted in the capacity of midwife. She has had no swelling of the feet, the hands, or the face. About nine years ago, however, just before the change of life, she did have slight dropsical symptoms, but they soon passed away. During her early menstrual life the catamenia were free, but not copious. She always flowed a great deal in child-bed. Each of her children cost her a year's illness and indisposition. She has had three miscarriages, each of which was brought on by slight over-exertion, as from carrying a pail of water. There are occasional discharges from the womb, which are of a yellowish, and sometimes of a reddish cast.

This *verbatim* report is sufficient proof that the case before us is a complicated one. As such, it is a fitting representative of the class to which it belongs ; for in making out the differential diagnosis of ovarian dropsy, your skill will sometimes be put to the severest possible test.

While our patient is lying here so comfortably, I propose to teach you how to diagnosticate ovarian dropsy from ascites, from pregnancy, from uterine fibroids and fibro-cystic tumors of the womb, from physometra, distention and prolapse of the bladder, enlargements of the liver and spleen, and from tumors caused by a retention of the menses, or of fæcal matter.

I. *From Ascites.*—In the great majority of cases, abdominal dropsy is secondary upon some pre-existing chronic disease of the liver, of the spleen, of some portion of the digestive tract, of the kidneys, or, in rare instances, of the heart or lungs. In ovarian dropsy this rule is reversed, and the general ill health is the consequence of the development of the tumor.

In ascites, if the patient lies upon her back with her knees drawn up, the abdominal tumor becomes flattened anteriorly, and "bulges," or spreads out laterally. The sides and flanks, as well as the front surface of the enlargement, except directly around the umbilicus, are dull and flat on percussion. Around the navel, however, there is a resonant sound in ascites. If she turns upon either side, there will be dullness upon that side, and resonance upon the other. But in ovarian dropsy the contour of the tumor is not changed when the patient changes her position. It is not flattened in front when she lies upon her back. Its margin is easily mapped out. The flanks are not distended. There is no dullness or bulging in the lumbar regions, but a resonance which is quite clear and characteristic, and which assures us that the intestines lie behind a circumscribed sac, whatever its contents may be. This is so well shown in the case before you, that I am quite certain you will remember it as a chief means of diagnosticating ovarian dropsy from ascites.

Posture.

You will observe how tense and hard this swelling is. This also constitutes a diagnostic mark, for, in ascites the walls of the abdomen are either flaccid or elastic, and more or less relaxed; while in ovarian dropsy they are as tight as if there were an extreme degree of tympanites.

Consistence of the tumor.

In ascites the "touch" recognizes a fluctuation in the Douglas' cul-de-sac, which is lacking in ovarian dropsy. In ascites, also, the accumulation begins at the lowest and most dependent part of the abdomen, while in ovarian dropsy the tumor usually commences in the right or the left hypogastrium, or in one of the iliac fossæ. When it exists, extreme dropsy of the abdominal walls is almost always conjoined with malignant disease. Coincident œdema, especially of the feet, may exist from the first in ascites, but never occurs in ovarian dropsy except in the last stage of the disease.

The "touch."

Tapping is a final means of diagnosticating between these two affections. Having withdrawn the serum in case of ovarian dropsy, we find that the solid or semi-solid tumor does not float out of reach as before the operation,

Tapping.

but that it may now be quite readily examined and grasped by the hand through the abdominal parietes. After tapping, therefore, the size, shape and location of this tumor can be so well made out that we need not confound it with such hypertrophy of the liver, the spleen, or of the mesenteric glands, as might have attended upon ascites.

It is important for you to remember that in ascites, after paracentesis, the re-accumulation of water is slow, while, after the evacuation of an ovarian cyst, it is much more rapid and persistent. In one of my patients who had ovarian dropsy, from whom I withdrew many gallons of water, the abdominal tumor was quite as large as ever at the end of the first week.

Refilling of the sac or cyst.

In exceptional cases, however, ascites and ovarian dropsy co-exist, and both sets of symptoms are present at the same time in the same patient. The diagnosis between them is more difficult in case the cyst is unilocular than if it is multilocular, because in the former the abdominal enlargement is more rounded and uniform, and bears a closer resemblance to that of ascites.

May co-exist.

II. *From Pregnancy.*—Pregnancy is self-limited, and its general history is so well defined that you might suppose there would be little risk of confounding it with ovarian dropsy; but experience proves otherwise, for it has frequently happened to the surgeon to declare the patient ill with ovarian dropsy, when, in reality, she was pregnant, and upon making an abdominal section to find the fœtus in utero, instead of an ovarian cyst within the cavity of the peritoneum. So frequent is this error in diagnosis, that it would not perhaps be extravagant to say that at least one-third the cases of so-called ovarian dropsy, in which gynæcologists are consulted, prove to be cases of pregnancy.

Frequently confounded.

In ovarian dropsy menstruation is sometimes arrested. The reflex ovarian sympathies, which involve other organs, may simulate those proper to gestation. The digestive function is almost necessarily more or less impaired. The mammary glands may be developed and become tender, as in pregnancy. The breasts may fill with milk, and even the areolæ may become quite distinct. Usually, however, in ova-

Parallel symptoms.

rian dropsy, unless both ovaries are diseased, the menses return irregularly, or are too frequent and copious. Last year I was consulted in a case of ovarian dropsy occurring in a woman aged thirty-six years, who, by reason of a congenital absence of the vagina, had never menstruated. In the case before us we exclude pregnancy, because Mrs. H. is so very subject to hæmorrhage, which, if she were really pregnant, could only arise from mal-location, or partial detachment of the placenta. Moreover, her hæmorrhage is of too chronic a nature to pertain to the period of utero-gestation. The patient's age will sometimes assist in diagnosticating ovarian dropsy from pregnancy.

A rare case.

In general, we say that in pregnancy the abdominal tumor has some peculiarities of situation and growth which may perhaps serve to distinguish it from an ovarian enlargement. For example, it has originally been intra-pelvic; it ascends gradually or more rapidly, as the case may be, at about the fourth month, and its globular outline is easily recognized by palpation. If it deviates to either side of the median line, its margin is smooth and well defined. From the fourth until the eighth month it grows from below upwards. It assumes the form of a general swelling, and is never described by the patient as a "lump" in her side, or elsewhere.

Location and growth.

But we must not forget that both these affections may escape observation or suspicion until weeks or even months have elapsed before our advice is sought. Under these circumstances, we shall be compelled to rely upon other signs in order to separate them and to treat them properly.

The "touch" may aid very greatly in the diagnosis. In pregnancy, after the fifth month, and more especially in multiparæ, the uterine cervix is considerably softened, swollen, and compressible, and the external os uteri patulous. In uncomplicated ovarian dropsy its shape, size and cartilaginous character remain unchanged. In pregnancy, at or after the fifth month, you would expect to find the cervix at the superior strait, not far from the promontory of the sacrum. And, although it is frequently drawn up and either ante-flexed, or displaced toward the affected side in ovarian dropsy, still its location will in most cases not differ ma-

Changes in the cervix in both states.

terially from that of the unimpregnated uterus. If the internal os uteri were open, and the finger did not come into direct contact with the membranes, the placenta, or with some part of the fœtus, the woman could not be pregnant. The easy introduction of the uterine sound, and its ready passage to the fundus uteri, would also enable you to exclude pregnancy from the list of probabilities. But the sound should not be used unless it is manifest that, if the patient is pregnant, her "term" is very near.

The uterine souffle unreliable.

The uterine souffle is so equivocal a sign of pregnancy that, except as confirmatory, we can not place much dependence upon it; for it has been found that it does not arise, as was once supposed, from an increased development of vessels, and an augmented circulation of blood at the site of the placenta and through it. In other words, it is not necessarily connected with the utero-placental circulation. It may be present in fibroids, in uterine cancer and hypertrophy, in tumors within the broad ligament, in aneurism of the abdominal aorta, in case of a tumor pressing upon the iliac arteries, in sub-involution of the womb after delivery, and also in ovarian enlargement with or without dropsy.

The fœtal heart-sound unequivocal.

If you are fortunate enough to detect the fœtal heart-sounds, all doubt will be at an end. But, although this will afford you an unequivocal sign of pregnancy, if you can recognize it, it would not, however, be wise to conclude that your patient was not pregnant simply because, after repeated trials, you failed to find it; for it might be so distant, indistinct and obscure, or so modified, that you would not know it from other sounds. Or the position of the fœtus in utero might be such as to render it quite impossible for you to hear it at all.

May co-exist.

In advanced pregnancy, if the position of the child is favorable, and the abdominal walls are thin, it is sometimes possible to recognize the head, or the extremities of the fœtus, by palpation. Quickening, if it were genuine, would confirm this condition. And yet it has happened that the irregular outline of the proper ovarian tumor has been mistaken for that of the child; while the movements of the fœtus in utero are apt to be counterfeited in various ways.

It is, therefore, more difficult to diagnosticate ovarian dropsy from pregnancy than you would have supposed. Sometimes they co-exist. In very rare cases the dropsy is contingent upon gestation, and disappears after delivery.

Time as an element of diagnosis.

If you can not otherwise determine the diagnosis, it will be best for you to proceed as in other cases where pregnancy is possible, *id est*, to wait until the proper limit for that condition has passed, for, ordinarily, there need be no haste in deciding. If the woman is pregnant, the tumor will not sensibly increase in size, or develop in an upward direction, after eight and a half months. When ten or twelve months have elapsed since the swelling was first noticed, it is tolerably certain that there is some kind of a tumor present which is independent of pregnancy as a cause. The only exception to this rule would be found in case of extra-uterine pregnancy, in which the fœtus might be indefinitely retained. But this form of gestation is so rare as scarcely to deserve notice in this connection. In women, as you know, the natural limit for pregnancy is nine months, while the average duration of ovarian dropsy is about three years.

Hæmorrhage.

III. *From Uterine Fibroids.*—Although ovarian dropsy may be accompanied by irregular menstruation, in which the flow may be either too frequent or too copious, or both, nevertheless we can not properly say that patients having this form of dropsy are prone to uterine hæmorrhage. Indeed, the dropsical and the hæmorrhagic diathesis are at antipodes, and seldom or never exist in the same person. But the hypertrophy of the muscular structure of the womb, which is pathological and not physiological, or which, in other words, does not pertain to the development of the gravid uterus, but which follows abortion or labor, or an attack of metritis, is in the majority of cases attended by a more or less protracted and alarming menorrhagia. Statistics show that only *nine* per cent. of the cases of ovarian dropsy are accompanied by uterine hæmorrhage; while as large a proportion of cases of uterine fibroids as *seventy* per cent. are marked by this symptom. This estimate does not include those extra-mural or sub-peritoneal fibroids from which such a hæmorrhage would be impossible.

Whenever, therefore, you have a patient who is subject to considerable or continuous flooding, which begins and ceases without any especial relation to "the month," and more particularly if she is not pregnant, and there is present a pelvic or abdominal tumor of considerable size, you will have reason to suspect that she has one or more uterine fibroids. In that case the tumor will most probably be due to hypertrophy of the uterine muscular tissue, while the hæmorrhage is a species of critical outlet or safety-valve for the excess of blood carried thither.

Consentaneous mobility of the uterus and the tumor.

In uterine fibroids the tumor is hard and movable. Its mobility is diagnostic. When you can feel that a motion is imparted to the whole mass by a blow from the finger upon the posterior wall of the cervix-uteri, as in ballottement, or by introducing the uterine sound can lift the organ and satisfy yourself by the hand placed over the abdominal parietes that the entire tumor moves along with it, there can be little doubt of the presence of a uterine fibroid. Sometimes, however, it may happen in this form of neoplastic growth that the womb may be immovable, as it is in scirrhus of that organ.

Length of the uterine cavity.

The distance to which the sound will enter the womb is also significant. As a rule, if it passes in more than three inches the uterus is said to be enlarged; and enlargement of the uterine cavity is one of the most certain and constant signs of these same fibroid growths. In uncomplicated ovarian dropsy, if the womb is sometimes elongated it is in consequence of its displacement, and of the unnatural pressure of the ovarian tumor upon it. The manifest changes in the length and size of the uterus which are present in a case of fibroids, do not properly belong to the clinical history of ovarian dropsy. In the case before us, you will observe, I pass the sound into the womb to the distance of six inches, by actual measurement.

May co-exist.

Now this disclosure by the sound makes it necessary to remind you that, in very rare cases, these two affections also may co-exist. I am of opinion that they are both of them present in this patient. If it were otherwise, the symptoms elicited a little while ago by percussion of the abdomen would not be in accord with those just obtained by physical exploration of the womb. In our diagnosis of this form of dropsy from ascites, we recognized and settled the fact that this enormous abdominal tumor was due to the presence of one or more ovarian cysts. And now we find in the hæmorrhage to which Mrs. H. has so long been subject, as well as in the mobility of the tumor, and the distance to which the sound can be passed, that there is also a manifest hypertrophy of the womb. My colleague, the Professor of Surgery, will settle the question for us presently, when he comes to perform the operation of ovariotomy.*

Fibroids are of slow growth; and so, also, are ovarian tumors, in the early stages of the same. But ovarian tumors sometimes develop rapidly from the first, or having existed for some months and grown very slowly, they suddenly fill the abdomen and give rise to much suffering and discomfort. Uterine displacements and leucorrhœa form a natural and almost necessary part of the history of fibroids, while they are generally absent in ovarian dropsy.

Relative rapidity of growth.

IV. *From Fibro-cystic growths.*—Those fibroids which are attached to the exterior surface of the womb, and which lie beneath its peritoneal investment, sometimes undergo cystic degeneration. In this case the tumor, which may include a number of these degenerate fibroids, is likely to become of such a size as to fill the abdominal cavity, and to be mistaken for ovarian dropsy, ascites, and even for pregnancy. So close is this resemblance, that in many cases the most skillful practitioners of this specialty have been unable to diagnosticate a fibro-cystic from an ovarian tumor, before making an exploratory incision. Fortunately, however, this species of fibroid is comparatively rare.

Difficulty of diagnosis.

Dr. Routh's statistics show that in only three out of eighteen cases of fibro-cystic tumor was there any menorrhagia. Spencer Wells has several times diagnosed the presence of these fibro-cysts of the uterus by the escape through the trocar on paracentesis of a thin serum containing from five to fifteen per cent. of blood, with which it is so intimately mixed as not to separate from it until after standing for some hours.

Menorrhagia absent in this form of fibroids.

Without enlarging upon these and other points that will help you to diagnosticate ovarian dropsy from fibro-cystic growths, I

* Ovariotomy was performed in presence of the class by Prof. Danforth. The uterus was found to contain an intra-mural fibroid, and the abdomen a large ovarian cyst. The patient made a good recovery. See U. S. Med. & Surg. Journal, Vol. vii., page 191.

will refer you to a valuable classification of the more prominent symptoms arranged by Dr. Charles C. Lee, and published in the "N. Y. Medical Journal," vol. xiv., p. 474.

IN OVARIAN CYSTS.	IN FIBRO-CYSTS OF THE UTERUS.
1. Disease may occur at any period, even before puberty.	1. Scarcely ever occurs under thirty—generally from forty to fifty.
2. Development rapid—usually under two years.	2. Development slow—generally over two years.
3. Aspect of face unaltered, if the general health be fair.	3. "Facies uterina" generally marked; expression anxious and dejected.
4. Fluctuation equable over the whole surface of the tumor.	4. Fluctuation confined to certain regions—generally to upper portion, while the lower is hard and dull.
5. Vaginal examination shows little displacement of the uterus—the mass smooth and distinct from the uterus.	5. Vaginal examination shows the uterus high up or displaced. The mass either not detected or continuous with the uterus.
6. Mobility of the uterus independent of the tumor from the beginning—pelvic adhesions rare.	6. Independent mobility of the womb confined to the last stage of the disease. Pelvic adhesions common.
7. Tapping causes complete collapse of unilocular cysts; in polycystic tumors, it reveals the endocysts.	7. Tapping causes only partial collapse, leaving the base of the tumor firm and indurated.
8. The fluid is clear, straw-colored, serous; or viscid, clear, mucoid and albuminous.	8. The fluid is either brownish, bloody, sero-purulent, or muddy; or thin and yellowish, containing shreds of lymph or of cholesterin.
9. When exposed by gastrotomy the sac is pearly blue, or white and glistening; but rarely vascular.	9. The exposed sac is dark, vascular, thick, and frequently fasciculated with fibrous bands.

V. *From Physometra.*—Distention of the womb with gas is not very likely to be confounded with ovarian dropsy. If this abdominal enlargement, upon which I place my hand, was due to such a cause, the swelling would be tympanitic on percussion over its whole extent, instead of dull and flat as we find it. And then, too, the tumefaction could be very readily removed without a resort to such a severe operation as ovariotomy; for we could pass a male catheter through the cervix uteri and discharge its contents in a very few moments.

Empty the uterus.

Physometra is always attended by more or less troublesome hysterical manifestations, which do not pertain to ovarian dropsy, and which can be dissipated by means of an anæsthetic.

Anæsthesia.

VI. *From Distention and Prolapse of the Bladder.*—The skillful use of the female catheter and of conjoined external and internal manipulation, would enable you to decide between either of these affections and ovarian dropsy.

VII. *From Enlargements of the Liver and Spleen.*—Hypertrophy of the liver is almost invariably associated with chronic disease of that viscus. The form of dropsy that attends it is that of the abdomen. When effusion has taken place into the peritoneal sac, you will recognize the physical signs of ascites. The margin of the enlarged liver, which is well defined, the absence of uterine complication, which is suggestive, the digestive and constitutional disorder, which are significant from the outset, and the general contour of the tumor, will help you to differentiate between enlargement of the liver and the presence of one or more ovarian cysts.

Physical exploration.

So, also, with an abnormal development of the spleen. The constitutional symptoms which accompany it are characteristic. One or another of the forms of ague, and impairment of the quality of the blood, with leukæmia and perhaps anæmia also, will serve to identify this lesion. Physical exploration of the abdomen and of the internal generative organs will clear up the diagnosis between this species of tumor and ovarian dropsy. This patient's complexion, and the healthy color of her lips and alæ nasi, lead us to exclude hypertrophy of the spleen in her case.

Leucocytosis.

VIII. *From Tumors caused by retention of the Menses, and of Fæcal Matter.*—The former would depend upon an imperforate hymen, atresia of the vagina, or of the uterine cervix, or of both these passages, or upon obliteration of the neck of the womb by some flexion or deviation of the organ, or by some foreign growth which served to block up its outlet. In either case the "touch," and the introduction of the uterine sound, would discharge the menstrual deposit and remove the tumor. Such an expedient would be useless in real ovarian dropsy.

If there were excessive fæcal accumulation, the previous history of the case, and, more than all beside, a careful examination of the tumor, would disclose the difference between it and the disease we have before us this morning. The tumor would be hard and irregular, and nodulated to the feel, and could be traced along the course of the rectum and the colon. Emptying the bowel by enemata of oil, castile-suds, or of a similar solvent, would settle the question most effectually.

LECTURE XXIII.

AMENORRHŒA.

GENTLEMEN:—

During menstrual life, or between the ages of fourteen and forty-five, in this country, there are only two conditions in which the non-appearance of the menses can be considered healthy. These are during pregnancy and lactation. Under other circumstances, if this function is not properly performed the woman is not well. There is, therefore, a physiological and a pathological arrest of this function. I shall speak only of the latter this morning.

A physiological and a pathological arrest of menstruation.

The word Amenorrhœa is used generically. It signifies a class of affections which are characterized by an absence of the menstrual flow. It includes (1) *delayed* menstruation; (2) *suppression* of the flow; and (3) *retention* of the same. Let us consider these several conditions separately.

Definition and varieties.

1.—DELAYED MENSTRUATION.

This derangement consists in the non-performance of the menstrual function, in one who has arrived at the age of puberty. It is the *emansio mensium* of the old authors, and should not be confounded with a mere suspension of the flow in one who has menstruated before; neither with tardy menstruation in the case of women who are "irregular." The young girl has reached the age of fifteen, or perhaps of eighteen, or twenty, but this function is not yet established. For some reason the first appearance of the catamenia is delayed.

Emansio mensium.

Etiology.—This irregularity is often chargeable to defective development. The epoch of puberty has not really arrived. She is yet a child. Her eye lacks expression, her manners are less sprightly than they should be, and her movements do not indicate the graceful mobility of her

Delay of puberty.

sex. Her form and features, her carriage and bodily functions, do not assume their proper proportions and characteristics. She lacks individuality. She is masculine. Her womanly traits are not matured. Her health and her fecundity are implicated by this delay, and it becomes a serious matter to study into its causes and to treat it properly. For not only does her welfare concern her individual self, but also that of her relatives, of friends, and of society at large.

Delayed menstruation may be due to organic causes, as for example, to congenital absence of the uterus, the ovaries, the Fallopian tubes, or even of the vagina. Or it may be caused by inflammatory adhesions which have taken place at an early age in some portion of the generative intestine, or outlet. In some cases it constitutes an idiosyncrasy. In certain families the establishment of this function will in every instance be delayed until the subject is fifteen or twenty years old. Its first appearance is greatly influenced by external circumstances and surroundings, education, exercise, and associations. But more frequently its delay depends upon a depraved condition of the general health. In many cases there is a developing dyscrasia, as for example, tuberculosis, which interferes with and interrupts the coming on of the menses. Weakly, scrofulous, chlorotic girls are very liable to this form of amenorrhœa; and in the great majority of cases of this kind you will note that the effect is likely to be taken for the cause. In all of them the general tone and strength are lowered, the digestion impaired, the blood is vitiated or impoverished, and there is atony, debility, and torpor of the various functions.

Congenital defect.

The sequela of inflammation.

External conditions.

Cachexiæ.

Symptoms.—It is not unusual, in this form of amenorrhœa for the patient to complain regularly each month of the symptoms that usually attend upon the flow. She may have pain in the small of the back, dragging in the loins, aching across the hips, weariness of the limbs, severe and protracted headache, malaise, anorexia, and constipation. These symptoms may come and go with the regularity of the proper "period," but without the characteristic and necessary discharge. Sometimes they are followed by a vicarious hæmor-

Symptoms minus the flow.

rhage from the nose, the eyes, the ears, the lungs, the stomach, or the bowels. Or the proper flow may be substituted by a vicarious leucorrhœa.

Complicated with phthisis.

Delayed menstruation is especially significant in girls who are predisposed to any form of phthisis. In them it implies a depraved cachexia, a low state of nutrition, and a great liability either to hæmoptysis, or to the development of a harassing cough and hectic, which are the precursors of serious disease of one or more of the respiratory organs. If such an one who has passed her fourteenth year without ever having menstruated, has a cough, or dyspnœa, habitual or frequent sore throat, hoarseness, or pain in her side, it should be regarded as a sign of ill health, and of impending evil, and measures should be immediately taken for its relief. But, you should remember, that great harm may be done in these cases by the use of "forcing medicines," which are given indiscriminately, and are designed to compel the flow regardless of consequences and of the general condition upon which the disorder depends for its cause.

"Forcing medicines" injurious.

Diagnosis.—The diagnosis is not usually difficult. As a rule (to which, however, there are occasional exceptions,) conception before menstruation is impossible. You will, consequently, have less trouble in diagnosticating this form of amenorrhœa from pregnancy than in case of suppression or of retention. In delayed menstruation from organic causes there are no changes in the physical development of the person as in puberty. The mammæ are small and rudimentary, the figure is gaunt and not graceful, and, therefore, the chief presumptive, as well as the positive, signs of pregnancy are lacking. There are no changes in the uterine cervix, or in the size of the womb, and there is no abdominal tumor, as in gestation. The lapse of time does not alter the case, or relieve it by limitation. The incidental diseases are different. The monthly cycle may or may not be recognized in either case.

Negative signs.

Nevertheless, since it is possible that a girl may become pregnant before ever having menstruated, or, indeed, after her menses have been delayed for an unusual length of time, and before their final appearance, it will

Caution.

be best for you to qualify your diagnosis. Else it may happen, after all, that the cause of the delay in the catamenia has been a very natural and common one, and that she failed to menstruate because she was *enceinte*. A careful physical exploration would enable you to decide as to the presence or absence of the internal generative organs.

Prognosis.—The prognosis may depend upon the existence of organic defects. Of course, if the uterus were absent or only imperfectly developed, you could not promise a radical cure of this disorder of menstruation. And so also of a congenital absence of the ovaries, the Fallopian tubes, or of the vagina.

Where the amenorrhœa is attributable to general ill health, or to local disease, the prognosis will be that of the dyscrasia, or of the disorder, of which in reality the absence of menstruation is but a sequence and a symptom. We must weigh the chances of recovery from scrofulosis, tuberculosis, gastro-alimentary disease, pleurisy, and morbid conditions and alterations of the blood. In other words, both with respect to the prognosis and the treatment, we must remember that our patient "is not sick because she does not menstruate, but that she does not menstruate because she is sick."

An old and true maxim.

Treatment.—When you are consulted in a case of this kind you should not be inveigled into prescribing at random and indiscriminately. For many of these cases do not need any medicine whatever. If the patient is well in other respects, healthy, hearty, with a good appetite, and nothing to complain of, except that, as her mother or friend will tell you, she "has seen nothing," it is best to recommend fresh air and plenty of it, sunshine, cheerful society of a mixed kind, travel, a change of scene and surroundings, diversion, to take her from boarding-school, and afterwards to let Nature take care of herself. If she remains well, (and she may do so for months or years,) she will be better without medicine than with it. It is time enough to prescribe your pellets and powders for her when she can make a positive complaint of suffering and ill-health.

"Let well enough alone."

But if, on the contrary, the incipient signs of serious disease begin to crop out, you must anticipate and avert its full development. For by so doing you may, perhaps, ward off a threatening phthisis, or may save your pa-

Anticipative treatment.

tient much of suffering from other diseases, and really prolong her life. The more chronic and complicated the original affection, the more difficult will be the cure, and the greater the need of perseverance on your part.

2.—SUPPRESSED MENSTRUATION.

I have already said that a practical distinction should be made, and borne in mind, between suppression and retention of the menses.* This distinction is based upon the fact that menstruation, like other secretory and excretory functions, includes two distinct processes, *viz.:* (1.) the secerning, or exhaling, of the elements of a particular fluid from the blood; and (2) the pouring out, or escape of that product through a natural duct or outlet. Suppression of the menses concerns the former process exclusively. It relates to ovulation, and to its contingent secretion from the uterine mucous membrane. It is the *amenorrhée radicale* of Raciborski. When, after having been established and maintained for a longer or shorter period, this function ceases for other reasons than because the woman has become pregnant, is nursing her child, or has passed the climacteric, (unless there is an obstruction of the uterine cervix,) we say that she has menstrual suppression.

A practical distinction.

Here is an interesting case, the notes of which have been taken by our clinical assistant, Dr. Charles Adams:—

Case. — "About four weeks ago, Miss ——, aged 20, (late a resident of England,) applied at the College Dispensary for relief from the following symptoms: Cessation of the menses for the past four months, constant frontal headache, severe sacral pains, pains extending from the sacrum to the scapulæ, occasional œdema of the feet and ankles, pains occasionally running down the limbs, vertigo on going into the open air, and obstinate constipation. At times, also, she says that she has pains from one hip to the other. There is no leucorrhœa, and no epistaxis. She states that her mother died at the age of thirty-seven years of consumption, and that eight of her own sisters have died at about twenty-one years of age, after a short illness, presenting the same (or nearly the same) symptoms that she has detailed to me.

"As far as I can learn, there is no hereditary disease on the father's side. At the time of their decease, none of the eight

* See page 57.

sisters who died presented any obvious symptoms of consumption, but all of them seemed to drop off after suffering a short time as this patient suffers. One year ago she was cured in Bristol, England, of suppression of the menses of seven months' duration. I have prescribed for her three times without relieving anything more than the headache, and am led to believe that there must be a mechanical obstruction to menstruation (probably malposition of the uterus). Excepting a slight flush of the face, which is constant, this young woman presents no outward symptoms of internal trouble, and were it not for her strange story, I should, perhaps, be suspicious of pregnancy. The remedy which relieved the headache was apis mellifica, but after four days that had no effect."

Hereditary tendency to suppression.

This patient had menstruated before, and could not therefore be suffering from delayed menstruation, as we have just described it. She may have retention of the flow, in consequence of some uterine deviation, as the doctor suspects, but it is hardly probable that each of her eight sisters had amenorrhœa from this cause, and all at the same age. The very fact that their disease developed at this particular age renders it almost certain that they were the victims of tuberculosis, inherited from the mother, and that the menstrual suppression common to them all arose from this dyscrasia as a common cause. For it is not unusual for all, or nearly all, the daughters in a family in which phthisis is hereditary, to have this disease in a fatal form, when they are twenty to twenty-three years old. And amenorrhœa (*suppressio mensium*) almost always accompanies it.

Course and frequency.

Suppression of the menses is more common than either of the other forms of amenorrhœa. The busy practitioner has to prescribe for it every day. It may come on suddenly, or gradually and almost imperceptibly. The healthiest and most vigorous women, and especially those who are somewhat plethoric, are more likely to have it occur abruptly. Leuco-phlegmatic and fleshy women are prone to a gradual lessening and final arrest of the flow before the climacteric has arrived.

Avoidable causes.

Etiology. — The causes of suppression are numerous and varied. Perhaps the most frequent is exposure to cold, as in getting the feet wet, walking, sitting or sleeping in damp clothing, improper and extreme change of dress, as in leaving off the warm wrappings and flannels of winter, and substituting a thin party or ball dress. Taking a cold foot- or sitz-bath just before or during the flow is a very common cause of suppression. Emotional states often induce it. Among them are fear, fright, anxiety, mental depression, excess of mental application, the receipt of good or bad news, or solicitude for a sick friend, incompatibility in the marriage relation, the worry attendant upon being a witness at court, and confinement in prison.

Suppression is incident to attacks of fever, and of local inflammation, more particularly to ovaritis, endo-metritis, pleurisy, pneumonia and enteritis, to the presence of polypi, fibroids, hydatids and moles. It is often due to change of climate. One of my patients has had it for three months at a time while visiting the Rocky Mountain region. Another, and without any harmful consequences, every year at the White Mountains. Taking a sea voyage may have the same effect. A large proportion of the female emigrants arriving in New York have this form of amenorrhœa, which may persist for months after landing. It may also arise from chlorosis, anæmia and plethora. It is a species of idiosyncrasy with certain women, now and then to have the function of menstruation suspended for a longer or shorter time, and afterwards resumed again. The slightest forms of indiscretion at the month may suffice to arrest the flow. Taking a drink of ice-water, eating a little ice-cream, or indigestible food, or being too much upon the feet at the time, may cause it. Hewitt has had occasion more than once to observe "that women are liable to have the menstrual discharge suspended for one or two periods after first going to reside in a house, the staircases of which are of stone and uncarpeted, their previous residence having had a wooden staircase only.*

Incident to acute disease.

From change of climate and travel.

From an idiosyncrasy.

From trivial causes.

Chronic and habitual suppression is incident to advanced stages of consumption. In some cases, however, it characterizes the disease in its incipiency, and may be one of its first symptoms. You will be consulted for the

From chronic disease.

* The Diagnosis and Treatment of Diseases of Women, by Graily Hewitt. London, 1863, p. 44.

relief of this symptom in young women in whom it is supposed to be the chief and perhaps the sole cause of their ill-health. On proper inquiry, you ascertain that the patient has a slight, dry, hacking cough, without expectoration, but which is aggravated by exercise. She complains of stitching, lancinating pains in the chest, and dyspnœa from the slightest exertion, more particularly on ascending the stairs. She is easily fatigued, weak, and has lost all relish for substantial food. She has become emaciated, has lost in weight, and is more pale than usual.

Insidious complications.

These symptoms may have existed for a considerable time and developed insidiously, without creating any suspicion of disease of the lungs. But if you are observing, you will note the order in which they made their appearance ; you will learn that, in the majority of cases, the pectoral disorder has preceded the menstrual irregularity. In other words, the tubercular deposit, or the pneumonia, was idiopathic, while the amenorrhœa is secondary or symptomatic.

Essentially a glandular disease.

Under these circumstances, the blood becomes deteriorated in quality, in consequence of its imperfect aeration and of impaired nutrition. All the glandular functions are implicated. The ovaries, as well as the mesenteric glands, become diseased, and, if they perform their duty at all, do so but very irregularly and imperfectly. If the blood is too poor to furnish the proper elements for the gastric juice, for example, it may be unfit to stimulate the changes that should occur in the Graäfian vesicle, and which form an indispensable part of the function of ovulation.

Ovario-pectoral sympathies.

The intimate sympathy between the lungs and the ovaries, as well as the uterus, should not be forgotten. In every case of amenorrhœa, there is more or less liability to the development of pectoral disease. In the majority, the arrest of the menses predisposes to pulmonary hæmorrhage. This is the reason why hæmoptysis is more frequent among women than among men. And this also explains the more tardy convalescence of women from pneumonia, bronchitis, pleurisy, and even from pericarditis and endocarditis.

In many cases the pectoral symptoms and those of scanty or suppressed menstruation alternate. Or, with each return of the month, there may be a serious struggle, so to speak, between the lungs and the uterus. Here is a case in point, to which I was called last evening:

Case.—Miss ——, aged 20, has complained since leaving boarding-school, two years ago, of a harrassing cough, which never troubles her at any other time excepting at the month. Its coming on is the precursor of menstruation, and she is satisfied that, if she were to lose record of the time in which her catamenia were due, she would certainly be notified of the same by this cough. It anticipates the flow by some six to twenty-four hours, and subsides as soon as the discharge comes on. The longer the delay of the menses, and the more scanty the flow, the worse the cough.

Another cause of menstrual suppression was first recognized and described by the late Prof. Simpson. It consists in what he styled super-involution of the uterus following labor. This abnormality depends upon a species of marasmus, or excessive absorption of the uterine tissues after delivery, whereby the organ may be reduced to one-third of its natural size, and the proper exhalation of the menstrual blood from its mucous surface is rendered impossible. It is believed that in these cases the said textures undergo a fatty metamorphosis, and finally become atrophied and shrunken, as in the senile atrophy of those women who have passed the climacteric. Such an organic change would give rise to permanent arrest of the menses, and, although comparatively rare, might follow any case of labor, whether premature or at term. Sub-involution, or deficiency of absorption, following pregnancy and parturition, is, however, as I shall have occasion to tell you hereafter, much more frequently met with. It is intimately related to the clinical history of uterine obliquities.

Super-involution of the uterus.

Symptoms.—The most prominent symptom is the characteristic absence of the menstrual discharge, which is itself a symptom, and not a disease *per se*. All the attendant signs signify that some portion of the internal generative apparatus, more particularly the uterus and the ovaries, as well as the general nervous and vascular systems, are in an abnormal condition. Weakness, lassitude, aching, constant fatigue, lack of interest in family or social matters, indigestion, constipation, headache, cardiac oppression, palpitation, breathlessness, fickleness, peevishness, fugitive neuralgic

Nervous and vascular systems deranged.

pains, hysterical developments of various kinds, accompany this arrest of function. Some women suffer from ovarian neuralgia, others from a species of uterine colic, and not a few from cramps or spasms of one or of all the voluntary muscles whenever the month comes around and they do not flow. All, except those who are really plethoric, have symptoms of asthenia, sedation, atony, debility, and general torpor of the bodily functions. They become emaciated, bloodless, almost transparent, and go into a decline which develops itself more or less rapidly according to the original state of their health and vitality. In brief, a species of cachexia, which soon becomes chronic, and perhaps incurable, follows; and being complicated with general derangement and ill health, constitutes one of the most intractable affections to which women are liable. In exceptional cases, however, menstruation may be suspended for several months, and even for years, and finally restored without any harmful consequences whatever. One of the members of our college class last year cited the case of a woman whom he had known who did not menstruate from the age of 46 to 53—seven years. She then menstruated once, and afterwards became pregnant, and was delivered at term of a healthy living child.

The amenorrhœal cachexia.

Diagnosis.—You will have more trouble to diagnosticate suppression from pregnancy than from any and all other conditions. This difficulty is increased by the fact, that in forming a judgment in a given case, prior to the fourth month, we are left entirely at the mercy and caprice of the patient. She may tell us that she has incurred no possible risk of becoming pregnant, when such is not the truth. Or, if she is anxious to become a mother, may insist that nothing but conception could have caused the arrest in her case, for she was never irregular before. Too exclusive a reliance upon her word may mislead and deceive us; but in the first three months, there is little else upon which to predicate an opinion. The reflex and incidental symptoms, as nausea, loss of appetite, morning sickness, swelling of the breasts, are the same. Whatever changes occur in the uterine textures in consequence of impregnation begin in the body and fundus of the womb. We cannot reach or recognize them before the commencement of the twelfth or thirteenth week. Subsequent to that period, however the more unequivocal signs of

From pregnancy.

pregnancy begin to develop, and the diagnosis is more easy and certain. In doubtful cases, *time* will help you to differentiate between a physiological suppression of this sort, and one which is in every sense pathological. When complicated with retention, you may even have to wait until the fifth or sixth, or possibly the ninth, month before you can say with certainty whether the arrest of the menses was due to conception or to some accidental or morbific cause.

Time.

In simple suppression, however, there is no permanent and continuous abdominal development, no tumor, as in retention or in pregnancy.

It will sometimes be difficult to decide whether the non-appearance of the flow is or is not due to the "change of life." The age of the patient, and inquiries into her family history may help to settle this question. If she is past forty, the irregularity may be due to her age, although women do sometimes continue to menstruate much longer.

From "change of life."

One of my patients was "regular" until her death, which occurred in her sixty-second year. If the patient's mother and sisters ceased to menstruate as early as thirty or thirty-five, it might modify your diagnosis. Usually, if the suppression is from a morbific cause, it is preceded by a failure of the general health, and each month the patient complains of symptoms which pertain most decidedly to the return of the old habit. But, when the climacteric has been reached, and the arrest of the flow is chargeable to a physiological arrest of function, the ill health, if there is any, follows the change, and the monthly exacerbation does not recur.

Treatment.—You have, doubtless, drawn the proper inference with respect to the treatment for this form of amenorrhœa. Cure the original, idiopathic disease upon which this suppression is secondary, and, in the great majority of cases, if there be no organic obstacle, this particular function will be reëstablished. Or as Dr. William Hunter worded it in his Lectures, "With regard to the management of the menses, my opinion is, that you should pay no regard to them, but endeavor to put her to rights in other respects. If you cure the other disorders, you cure the irregularity of the menses, *which is the consequence and not the cause of her complaints.*"

A cardinal rule.

If the suppression is due to chlorosis, ovaritis, metritis, incipient tuberculosis, pneumonia, pleurisy, gastritis, hepatitis, rheumatism, or any other abnormal condition or diseased process, the indication presented is to cure the primary affection, after which we may reasonably expect the secondary one to disappear. Fortunately we find that remedies are possessed of corresponding relations to the various functions. For not only are the bodily organs linked in sympathy and susceptibility, but these sympathies and susceptibilities have their counterpart in the curative range of our remedies. The different sections of a correct and complete pathogenetic record are as intimately related as the several cantos of a grand old poem.

Emmenagogues.

If, therefore, you shall find that the remedy which is manifestly indicated for the cure of the complaint upon which the amenorrhœa is secondary, is also applicable in case of menstrual suppression, so much the better. But, as between prescribing pulsatilla, or senecin, or any of our medicines as emmenagogues merely, or iron, secale cornutum, and aloes in ponderous doses with the same end in view, there is really no difference. Both methods are unphysiological and harmful.

For pectoral complications.

Abundant experience has satisfied me that the calcarea carbonica is, perhaps, the most prominent and useful remedy for the relief of those menstrual irregularities which are incident to pectoral disease. It seems especially appropriate to complicated cases of pulmonary and uterine disorder in weakly, ill-conditioned females of a scrofulous diathesis, with amenorrhœa, an impoverished state of the blood, and a depraved condition of the nutritive system.

For suppression alternating with ophthalmia.

Pulsatilla is indicated in women with light hair and blue eyes, who are weakly, pale, and delicate, of mild and amiable disposition, and who are tearful and prone to melancholy. It is sometimes an excellent remedy in case of menstrual suppression complicated with ophthalmia. My attention was called to this fact some years ago by my excellent friend the late Dr. Lyman Kendall, of this city, who related the following

Case.—Mrs. ——, aged 32, had suffered frequent attacks of amenorrhœa, which persisted for from three to six months at a time. The suppression came without any apparent cause, and the return of the flow did not seem to be influenced in the least by any medicine which she could take. Her general health was good. She had never been sick in bed, and suffered no ill consequences of the amenorrhœa, excepting an intractable and troublesome inflammation of the eyes. Upon inquiry it was found that this inflammation came and went regularly, alternating with the amenorrhœa. When the catamenia were prompt and regular the conjunctivitis disappeared altogether; but when they were suppressed, the eyes became inflamed again. There was redness and swelling of the lids, lachrymation in the open air, and irritation and pressure as from sand in the eye. Pulsatilla[6] cured both these affections promptly and permanently.

From various causes.

I may give you an idea of the special indications for other remedies as follows:

a. In suppression from *mental causes* — Staphisagria or colocynth, if from indignation and chagrin; opium or coffea, sudden and excessive joy; chamomilla, from anger; opium, aconite or lycopodium, from fright.

b. From *check of perspiration* — Chamomilla, cuprum.

c. From *changes in the weather, cold and damp* — Dulcamara, rhododendron, nux mosch., pulsatilla.

d. Suppression with prominent *mental* symptoms — Stramonium, great loquacity, is tearful and supplicative at the month; natrum mur., for anxiety, solicitude, melancholy; ignatia, with sighing and hysterical sobbing; hposcyamus, singing delirium, spasmodic jerkings and twitchings, and excessive laughter; belladonna, with intolerance of light and noise, which make her head ache severely, and almost craze her; magnesia mur., for great excitement habitually, or accidentally, whenever the menses are due; aurum met., arrest of menses with inclination to commit suicide; macrotin, in rheumatic subjects.

e. If attended with *soreness of the throat* — Belladonna, magnesia mur., mercurius jodatus.

f. With *ophthalmia* — Pulsatilla, euphrasia.

g. With *swelling of the breasts* — Conium, zincum.

h. With *hæmorrhage* — Phosphorus, if from the lungs, the stomach, the bowels, or the urethra; bryonia, for incidental or vicarious epistaxis.

i. With *indigestion* — Kali carb., for sour eructations, with fugitive, shooting abdominal pains; nux vomica, arsenicum alb., podophyllin, lachesis, nux moschata.

j. With *cardiac* distress — Lachesis, apis mellifica, bryonia, aconite, lilium tig., macrotin.

k. With *abdominal tympanites* — Belladonna, phosphoric acid, chamomilla.

l. With *dropsy* — Apis mel., for incidental anasarca, swelling of the feet, puffiness of the cellular tissue; helleborus, for abdominal dropsy, with scanty flow of dark-colored urine; arsenicum. Dr. G. W. Barnes* reports "invariable success with apocynum can. in quite a number of cases of amenorrhœa in young girls, attended with bloating of the abdomen and extremities." He also had "good success with it at least in one case of this disease in which the latter symptoms were not marked."

m. With *chorea*, *hysteria*,† etc. — Belladonna, gelseminum, pulsatilla, macrotin, hyoscyamus, coffea, ferrum cit. et strychnia (in the 3d dec. trit.), cocculus, cuprum, causticum.

I am aware that these hints are more suggestive than satisfactory. Their chief value consists in the possibility that they may help you to decide between two or more remedies which, otherwise, might seem to be equally appropriate, and in this manner serve a good purpose. As a rule, however, in functional amenorrhœa, which is consequent upon different morbid states, whether they are acute or chronic, the symptoms proper to those conditions, and which would be your guide if there were no suppression, will indicate the remedy or remedies that are especially indicated.

A practical hint.

But if the suppression is idiopathic (which is comparatively rare), you will naturally seek to stimulate the functional activity of the ovaries, and of the uterine mucous membrane. This may be accomplished without the use of harsh emmenagogues. Pulsatilla, sepia, calcarea carb., podophyllin, apis mel., natrum mur., ferrum, china, phosphorus, sabina, sulphur, platina, or, among the newer remedies, senecin, collinsonia can., and the asclepias in., are sometimes given with excellent result. Dr. C. D. Williams reports some remarkable cures with xanthoxylum.‡

For idiopathic suppression.

* Hale's New Remedies, 1867, p. 83. † See page 56. ‡ United States Med. and Surg. Journal, October, 1871, p. 35.

The general treatment is sometimes even more important than the special. In the temporary suppression which frequently follows marriage, a single coitus, or change of climate and occupation, if you are careful not to overdo in the matter of dosing, and will take pains to correct the patient's habits, the function will regulate itself. In every case, she should take the fresh air daily. Walking, or riding in the sunshine, cheerful society, keeping the feet warm and dry, diversion, and a proper and nourishing diet, are useful auxiliaries towards a cure. They will help to restore the vital conditions which are inherent to this function, and indispensable for its proper performance. And they will also fortify the system against a degree of asthenia which is quite incompatible with ovulation.

General treatment.

In those who are predisposed to an arrest of the menses great care should be taken at the month lest a slight indiscretion or exposure induce it. With some women all that is necessary is for them to lie down and keep tolerably quiet and passive for one or two days. In others the flow will need prompting by appropriate internal remedies given in anticipation thereof; by the foot or sitz-bath; by an enema of tepid water thrown into the rectum; or by the introduction of the sponge-tent through the uterine cervix some hours, or perhaps the night before the flow is due. In some cases the passage of the uterine sound, or probe (which, if there is no uterine deviation, is not difficult at this period), may, by irritating the os uteri, produce the same effect. The habit of taking spirits, as gin or whisky, and hot drinks, herb teas and the like, should not be encouraged, for the indirect effect of such palliatives is to unhinge the nervous system and to increase the difficulty.

At the month.

3.—RETENTION OF THE MENSES.

In this form of menstrual irregularity there is a preternatural obstacle to the escape of the flow. Ovulation has been properly performed; the secretion or exhalation of the menstrual blood from the uterine mucous membrane has been poured into the cavity of the womb, but there is no outlet for it. Either the canal of the uterine cervix, or the vagina, or both these portions of the generative intestine, are closed, and there is no means of escape for the periodical discharge.

Etiology.—Menstrual retention may be caused by atresia of the cervix uteri, resulting from post-partum inflammation or from cauterization; spasmodic closure of the os internum; flexures and obliquities of the womb; the presence of polypi, or of coagula, which serve to obstruct the passage; atresia of the vagina; or closure of the same by an imperfect hymen. In exceptional cases it may be due to a species of uterine inertia. Here the flow exudes passively, but the condition of the patient's general health is so low, and the uterine fibre is so irresponsive to ordinary stimuli, that the peristaltic action of the womb is not aroused as it should be. The force that is designed to unlock the internal os and to expel the menstrual product is not called into exercise. The secretion is lodged, and there is no "show."

Accidental causes.

Symptoms.—In this class of cases, the menstrual molimen is more or less pronounced. The symptoms are those which accompany normal menstruation, always excepting the sanguineous flow from the vulva. Pains in the back and loins, around the pelvis, and down the thighs and limbs, bearing down and fullness within the pelvis, forcing pains, which are aggravated by standing or walking, headache, malaise, chills, nervous tension and perturbation, and sometimes dyspnœa, and diarrhœa or dysentery, recurring with some degree of regularity, may lead the patient to suppose the discharge is coming on. After a longer or shorter interval, however, these symptoms subside, and the effort to establish the flow has proved abortive. This state of things may continue for months, and even for years, to the manifest detriment of the general health.

The form without the flow.

Diagnosis.—Proper retention of this flow can only occur in those who have menstruated before. For this reason, it could not be readily confounded with, or mistaken for, Delayed Menstruation. The repeated efforts to expel the secretion, at each return of the monthly cycle, the kind and degree of suffering experienced, and the special clinical history of the case, would help you to differentiate between this form of menstrual derangement and a case of suppression, and also to diagnosticate it from "change of life," and from pregnancy.

Prognosis.—The prognosis will vary with the cause of the disorder, the age of the patient, and the condition of the general health. Other things equal, a recent case is more promising than a chronic one. If the blood has become deteriorated in quality, either from depraved nutrition or from the resorption of post-organic matters confined in the cavity ef the uterus, more serious consequences are to be apprehended. Or if, in consequence of the damming up of the discharge, the ovaries have become seriously diseased, we would not promise a prompt and radical cure to follow the restoration of the menses. For in exceptional cases the removal of the obstacle to the menstrual discharge, whatever it may have been, fails to re-establish this very important function.

Surgical means.

Treatment.—The prime indication is to remove the cause of the retention. Atresia of the cervix can usually be overcome by the careful and persistent employment of the uterine sound, or probe, Priestly's or Atlee's dilators, Simpson's ebony bougies, and the sponge tent. In rare cases the hysterotome may be requisite. I could cite many cases in which these means have cured retention of the menses due to atresia of the neck of the womb, occurring as a consequence of lying-in, and of excessive cauterization.

Dilatation, etc.

When the trouble depends upon spasm of the internal os-uteri, the same dilatation may be necessary, but it should be conjoined with such internal and hygienic treatment as is suited to overcome the tendency to local and general spasms. Here you will need to counteract the hysterical bias of the patient, and to place her under conditions which favor recovery. The topical and general use of electricity promises to be of great value in this particular class of cases.

Reposition of the uterus.

If the uterus is bent, or twisted upon itself, proper means must be taken to correct and cure the deviation. The most frequent of these displacements is retro-flexion, the womb being curved like a retort, and the canal of the cervix oblitated at the point at which the body of the organ is bent upon its neck. These cases are very tedious, but if you are really skillful, you will succeed in curing a large proportion of them.

Polypi and coagula are to be removed by excision, and by dilatation of the canal of the cervix. Atresia of the vagina will require a careful dissection of its adherent mucous surfaces, after which the freshened edges must be separated either by an oiled tampon or Sims' dilators, until they are healed. If the hymen is imperforate, it must be divided in order to discharge the contained fluid. The old plan was to make a crucial incision into this septum in such a case; but, serious results having followed the too rapid evacuation of the fluid, modern authorities advise that the cut shall be valve-shaped instead.

Incision of the cervix, and of the hymen.

If the retention is referable to uterine atony, the general health must be built up and fortified, and local excitation and stimulation of the womb secured by electricity, bathing, frictions along the spine, and the use of remedies suited to the especial and incidental symptoms, whatever they may be.

LECTURE XXIV.

OBSTRUCTIVE DYSMENORRHŒA.

GENTLEMEN:

One of my most intelligent and amiable patients has written the following history of her case, which, for the sake of the benefit that may accrue to others, she has consented that I may read to you:

Case.—I hardly know if I were a healthy child, but I was active, impulsive and sensitive. At eleven years of age the menses appeared, the result, perhaps, of the grief and excitement caused by my mother's death. For about one year they returned regularly, with little pain, and then *ceased*, owing, I think, to wetting my feet, and improper exercise. The result was a cough, dyspepsia, and other bad symptoms. My father employed a physician for me, who, after several months of medical treatment, brought on the menses again, but with much pain.

At seventeen years of age I was married, after which I resided four years in Boston. During these years, in which I experienced great mental suffering also, I suffered each month, resorting to such remedies as were prescribed in a domestic way by my friends, such, for example, as gin, injections of laudanum, chloroform, etc. About this time I was seized with "vomiting attacks," in which I would vomit a table-spoonful or more of clear green bile every ten or fifteen minutes for twelve hours, but never for a less time. As the vomiting, sometimes with purging, continued, the pain would lessen and finally disappear. The nausea and retching would leave suddenly and without apparent cause, for no medicine could be kept upon the stomach long enough to produce any effect. These attacks returned at intervals of three, five and eight months. I was treated for them by physicians in Elmira, N. Y., Boston, St. Louis and Chicago, and no one was able to relieve me, or to decide upon the cause of these paroxysms.

During the latter half of this period of ten years, my general health was much impaired, and I suffered greatly from gastric irritability and distress. From this irritation I have never found permanent relief.

After four years' residence in Boston I came to Illinois, seeking no particular medical aid for some years. At length I was induced to try a water-cure in New York, where I had the first vaginal examination. As a result, I was said to be suffering from "an irritation of the uterus and vagina, and nothing more." I remained three months under treatment, but still continued to suffer during menstruation.

A few years later I was placed under the care of a noted specialist in this city, who told me there was an "enlargement and retroversion" of my womb. He applied the caustic treatment for six months, and, although he declared that I "was cured," still I suffered as before at each menstrual period.

One year after this I went to another Hygienic Institution in New York. Here I was told that the "uterus was enlarged, indurated, retroverted, and fastened down, and had entirely changed its structure, and that the change must have been going on for many years." After having been pronounced "cured" only one year before, this was rather discouraging news. I remained at this institution four months, whence I was discharged, not as cured, but better. Still I suffered with menstruation.

In the winter of 1870, severe pain preceded the flow for several hours, and in addition to symptoms threatening a return of all my former difficulties, my bladder was much affected. At this time, and after a careful examination of my case, Dr. Ludlam decided the seat of my difficulty to be "in the neck of the uterus," which he found was "almost entirely closed." Under his treatment I experienced almost immediate relief, my general health improved, the bladder trouble disappeared, the gastric disorder became less annoying, and I suffered little or no pain during menstruation. Six months have now elapsed since I have finished his treatment, and the cure seems permanent.

Perhaps I should add that my pain was mostly in the abdomen, and of the nature of colic. Warm applications often produced fainting fits, and always had a tendency of that kind. Looseness of the bowels frequently accompanied the pains. I could only eat a very small amount of the simplest food. Eating always increased the pain. Finally, after nearly thirty years of painful menstruation, I have at last found relief!

Obstructive Dysmenorrhœa is a variety of painful menstruation, which depends upon a partial or complete closure or obstruction of the canal of the uterine cervix, whereby the menstrual flow can only escape, if at all, with great suffering and more or less irregularity. Although it is by no means a rare affection, the history of this case proves that it may

Definition of.

exist for months or years without being recognized and properly treated.

The causes of this disease are various. Sometimes it depends upon the original conformation of the uterus and uterine neck, in which case, from the very first the "periods," are always characterized by unusual delay and suffering. More frequently, however, it is acquired at a later stage of menstrual life. It may result from a flexure of the womb, in which that organ is bent upon itself like a retort. Opposite the lesser curve, in this case, the cavity of the cervix is obliterated.

Causes.

Versions, prolapsus, and other deviations in the position of the uterus are less likely to cause this form of dysmenorrhœa than flexions. And retro-flexion is more frequent in every form of painful menstruation than ante-flexion.

From uterine deviations.

In certain cases the cervico-uterine orifice and canal are mechanically obstructed by the presence of a foreign body, such as a polypus, a sub-mucous fibroid, or an old coagulum, and, notwithstanding the most violent efforts to expel the flow, it is partially or wholly retained within the womb. For this reason retention of the menses is often described by writers under the head of dysmenorrhœa, and *vice versa*.

From intra-uterine growths.

But a more frequent cause of obstructive dysmenorrhœa is a form of endo-cervicitis, in which the epithelial lining of the canal is exfoliated and lost, and, as a consequence, adhesions are formed between the opposite sides of the canal. These adhesions, whether traumatic, post-partum, or the result of a popular form of malpractice, that is of cauterization, cause an atresia which obstructs and practically closes the passage.

From cervical atresia.

As a rule, those women who have borne children, whether prematurely or at term, are supposed to be exempt from dysmenorrhœa. But this form of the disease is by no means a rare sequel to the abrasions and injuries consequent upon labor, as well as to the local inflammations which may occur about and within the cervix and the vagina during the puerperal state.

The harsh and indiscriminate employment of escharotics for the cure of uterine ulceration (against which I have so frequently cautioned you), is very mischievous in this respect. The actual cautery, or its potential substitute, the potassa cum calce, destroys the cervical epithelium, and there is nothing left to prevent the consequent adhesive inflammation from sealing up the outlet. Without their epithelium these surfaces grow together, just as your fingers would if the epidermis that separates and protects them were removed by a burn, and the surgeon who dressed it did not know enough to keep them apart until a new cuticle had formed. From considerable experience in this class of cases, I am persuaded that contraction, cicatrization, and even atresia of the cervix are frequent sequelæ of the milder, as well as of the more severe and reckless cauterization to which so many of our patients have been subjected before they come into our hands. The case just cited affords a good illustration of this fact. Mrs. — had already suffered from dysmenorrhœa for several years. The symptoms were sufficiently marked to suggest their own solution and significance, even to a first-course student. But, as if to render her menstruation not only difficult but impossible, she, too, must be cauterized!

From cauterization.

The symptoms of this disease are by no means limited to the site of the obstruction. Within the pelvis, and in the back and limbs, they are similar to those which ordinarily attend upon the menstrual effort. But in this case they are greatly exaggerated. When the patient is one who has never been pregnant, the uterine cavity is so small that the menstrual exhalation from its lining membrane soon fills it, and a feeling of distention and of extreme discomfort is induced. Aching and throbbing of the uterus, with uterine tenesmus are almost always present. In those who have borne children, and who have this form of dysmenorrhœa subsequently, the womb, if not really more capacious, is yet more tolerant of the retained fluid. These women therefore do not commonly suffer so severely as those who belong to the former class.

Symptoms.

In both classes, however, the presence and pressure of the blood, which has no adequate outlet, excites the peristaltic contractions of the uterus with a view to overcome the obstruction and to force the flow. The case then partakes of the nature of labor. The contractions of the uterus are much less powerful, because the fully-developed

Uterine tenesmus.

fibres of its muscular coat are lacking. But it often happens that they are more painful than in real labor. The antagonism between the body and fundus and the circular fibres about the internal os uteri is very apt not only to cause intra-pelvic suffering and agony, but to develop a train of reflex symptoms such as are met with in abortion and in labor at term.

Reflex disorders.

Of the functions which are thus indirectly implicated and deranged, that of digestion suffers most frequently. Obstinate and painful vomiting is almost always present with every return of the menstrual cycle, whether it be prolonged and complete or not. It depends upon a stricture of the os internum, and comes on in the same manner that it does in rigidity of the os uteri during labor, or at the moment that the presenting part passes through the ring that is made of the enormously dilated cervix. If there is ever so small a vent, and a portion only of the catamenial secretion escapes, the pain and emesis may subside. But, unless the flow comes on without any considerable delay, and pretty freely, the vomiting is likely to persist. And, what is a curious clinical fact, one that I am unable to explain, but which I have often observed, is that this vomiting is almost certain to continue for about twelve hours. Our patient says that she vomited "every ten or fifteen minutes for twelve hours, but never for a less time."

Indigestion.

Some cases of obstructive dysmenorrhœa are met with in which the menstrual arrest and derangement have given rise to very complicated disorders of digestion, which many physicians are incompetent to explain and to cure. The gastro-intestinal functions are involved just as they often are in the early months of pregnancy. Either through nervous or vascular connection between the uterus and the stomach, some portion of the small or large intestine, or the liver, or all these organs, the result is the various forms of indigestion, inanition, constipation and bilious disease that so frequently arise from painful and irregular menstruation.

Vesical and rectal complication.

In this, as in other varieties of dysmenorrhœa, it would be impossible for the bladder and the rectum not to sympathize with the uterus in its prolonged effort to empty itself of its contents. Consequently there is, sooner or later, in almost all of these cases, more or less of vesical and rectal tenesmus. This incidental suffering corresponds with that proper to the first stage of labor.

Nervous disorder.

Coincidently with the tenesmus of the pelvic organs there is often, and indeed usually, a train of nervous symptoms which are more or less pronounced and alarming. Headache, restlessness, insomnia, jactitation, spasms, and even convulsions are not infrequent, all of which, however, are relieved as soon as the flow begins, exactly as in labor when the rigid os uteri has yielded and the presenting part has passed the point of obstruction. A very painful and distressing form of spasm to which some of these patients are subject is one in which the muscles of the back part of the head, of the neck and of the superior portion of the spine are affected, resulting in opisthotonos. Painful, cramping, clonic spasms of the flexors of the fingers and toes often occur. Some women are liable to a temporary blindness at these times, and you will observe the pupil to be sometimes very much dilated and again contracted. In those who are decidedly hysterical, there may be, during the paroxysm, an evident disparity in the size of the pupils.

Menorrhagia infrequent.

In true obstructive dysmenorrhœa it seldom happens that the painful and persistent effort to restore the impeded flow finally causes it to become profuse. In this respect it differs from the congestive, the spasmodic, and the membranous varieties, which are all of them likely to be either accompanied or followed by menorrhagia. The amount of the discharge is not proportioned to the severity of the pain. The flow is scanty and intermittent, and, as in the case which I have related, the inter-menstrual period is generally lengthened and irregular.

Sterility from obstructive dysmenorrhœa.

If the obstruction is congenital, or has come on from any cause before marriage, these patients are sterile ; for the same mechanical obstacle which interfered with the menstrual exit, will prevent the ingress of the semen into the uterine cavity, and proper fecundation will be impossible. If the closure of the cervico-uterine outlet takes place in consequence of cauterization, or of post-partum inflammation in one who has borne a child or children, she also may afterwards become barren from the same cause.

If the dysmenorrhœa depends upon congenital mal-formation of the cervix uteri this condition can be readily recognized by the proper employment of a Sims' speculum and the uterine sound, conjoined with the "touch."

Diagnosis.

If it had its origin in puerperal inflammation; if it has followed the extension of simple or specific vaginitis into the canal of the cervix; if it depends upon some uterine obliquity, or the presence of a foreign growth; or if it is the sequel of cauterization, the previous history and treatment of the case will facilitate the diagnosis. The simple fact that at the first attempt you fail to pass the sound into the uterine cavity should not lead you to decide the case to be one of obstructive dysmenorrhœa; for in a healthy state of the uterine mucous membrane, and in the interval of menstruation, the internal os is in many cases so tightly closed that it requires considerable skill and experience to pass this instrument at all. But if the canal of the cervix is not absolutely impervious, a little patience and tact will enable you to succeed. You may sometimes insinuate a small Sims' probe, when a large sound, more especially a stiff one, could not be introduced without undue force and unnecessary suffering. I need hardly remind you that you will gain an entrance into the uterine cavity in this manner much more easily "at the month" than at any other time.

Physical exploration.

Passing the sound.

You should remember that in this form of dysmenorrhœa there is not necessarily a complete and entire retention of the menses. The distinguishing characteristic of the disease is that there is a mechanical impediment to the monthly flow, which may or may not amount to a positive obstruction and arrest thereof. The failure of the practitioner to get a correct idea of this fact explains the proneness to blunders in the diagnosis and treatment of this affection; for obstructive dysmenorrhœa bears as little resemblance to endo-cervicitis and to uterine ulceration as it does to perimetritis or to hæmatocele, and to confound them is both inexcusable and mischievous.

The flow, and what it signifies.

The prognosis will vary with the cause of the disease, and also with the consequences of the menstrual irregularity. If the original organic defect, whenever it exists, can be remedied or compensated by surgical means,

The prognosis.

recovery will follow. If the acquired or accidental obstruction, whatever it is, can be removed, the result may be favorable. Something, however, will depend upon the state of health, which is secondary, and which has been induced, directly or indirectly, by the persistent derangement of the menstrual function. If the dysmenorrhœa has existed for years, the patient may be so ill with symptomatic endometritis, gastritis, gastro-enteritis, ovaritis, cystitis, chronic hepatic and digestive derangements, tuberculosis, diseases of the nervous system, or a depraved condition of the blood, as to prevent her complete recovery. And this, although the ease and regularity of the flow have both finally been established. Therefore, you should be careful how you promise to perform a radical cure of this painful affection.

Treatment.—One of the most successful and satisfactory achievements of modern gynæcology consists in having supplied us with the means of cure for most cases of this disease. From the nature of its causes, you will infer that the treatment of obstructive dysmenorrhœa must be chiefly of a surgical kind. Internal remedies are suited to the relief, and possibly the cure, of other varieties of painful menstruation, but they are of little or no permanent avail in this. The cause of the suffering is physical and mechanical, just as in a case of stone in the bladder, or of biliary calculus, and although, by the use of constitutional means, we may mitigate the pain and other incidental symptoms, yet the cure will depend upon the removal of the cause.

Surgical treatment.

If the seat of the stricture is at the os externum, a slight incision may suffice to open the cervical canal. If, as most frequently happens, it is at the os internum, it will be most prudent to try the virtues of dilatation, and reserve the cutting as a *dernier ressort.* Dilatation is equally applicable to most cases of atresia of the cavity of the neck of the organ.

When the passage is very narrow you will begin with a small copper sound, or probe, which may be passed every third or fourth day until the canal is somewhat enlarged. This may be followed by the ordinary sound, small bougies, laminaria, or slippery elm tents, the use of Atlee's, Priestley's, or Nott's dilators, and finally by the sponge tent. And although (in order to take advantage of the natural tendency to

Dilatation.

expansion of the cervix), it is best to commence this treatment at the month, it must be continued during the inter-menstrual period also. As a rule, twice each week is as often as these operations can be borne, and sometimes this is too frequent.

Introduction of the necessary instruments.

As in passing the female catheter, so you will need to exercise considerable tact in the introduction of these instruments, more especially until, by repeated trials, you have learned the course and curve of the canal in each particular case. For its direction is so modified by the position of the patient, the fullness or emptiness of the bladder, the rectum, and even of the uterus itself, as well as by obliquities of the womb, that any rules which I might indicate would be of little practical service, unless you should modify them to suit the case in hand. As a rule, the copper sound is preferable to the stiff one ordinarily employed. Sims' probe is too flexible, and might stick fast in the rugæ of the cervix, or at the point of coarctation. If the womb is retro-flexed, the patient must be placed in the semi-prone, and, if needs be, in the knee-elbow position, in order that the fundus and body of the organ may gravitate into their normal relations, and so that, in passing, the point of the sound may take the natural direction with reference to the axis of the superior strait. The most difficult cases are those in which the cervical canal is tortuous and sinuous. You may or may not make use of the speculum to facilitate the introduction of the sound, or of the tents. In all ordinary cases I prefer to pass them without, instead of through the speculum; but perhaps you will do better with it.

Failure of dilatation.

Much has been said of the frequent failure of dilatation of the cervical canal as a cure for this disease, and also of the injurious consequences that sometimes result from it. My own opinion, which needs a word of explanation, and which is based upon experimental and not upon theoretical grounds, is that, if properly employed, dilatation is more successful and less harmful than is generally supposed. I am inclined to attribute its failure in the hands of some physicians to a lack of caution on their part in the choice and application of instruments; and also to too great haste to cure their patients, regardless of consequences.

That cervicitis, cellulitis, peritonitis, spasms, convulsions, and even hysterical tetanus, have sometimes followed the use of the dilators and of the sponge-tents is doubtless true, but there is little question that, if the correct and complete history of these cases were written, it would be found that either the tents were composed of improper material, were too large, or were pushed through the cervix uteri too forcibly, or that they were allowed to remain for too long a time before being removed. One of my patients suffered so severely that she could not tolerate a small ebony dilator, which was passed without difficulty, for more than ten minutes at a time. If I had not taken the precaution to remain with her and to observe the effect, but had left her with instructions that the instrument must be kept in place for some hours, she might have been dangerously ill from this cause alone.

Reported danger from.

It may seem incredible, to the more advanced members of the class especially, that any intelligent physician should be so careless as to introduce a slippery-elm or a sea-tangle tent at his office, and afterwards permit his patient to travel by stage or by rail for some miles to her residence, before it was removed! But this is not an infrequent occurrence, more particularly with those who practice most largely among the lower classes in such a city as this. The injurious effects of such a custom should be charged to the abuse and not to the proper use of the tent.

A barbarous practice.

Providing there is no acute inflammation of the endometrium, or of the mucous lining of the cervix uteri, no ulceration, and no extensive or deep-seated cicatrices to be broken up, I think that the whole or any portion of the neck of the womb may be as safely, although not so rapidly dilated, as the female urethra. In exceptional cases, where the obstruction has been relieved by dilatation, it returns after six or eight months.

Conclusions concerning dilatation.

Mischief sometimes results from a lack of care in the choice of the material of which the tent is made. The slippery-elm tents are useful and available, and answer a very good purpose when they are smooth and small enough to permit them to take the shape of the canal through which they are to pass. But when a larger tent is requisite, they are too stiff and straight to suit many cases. A large sea-tangle

Of the various tents.

tent expands so slowly as to be practically useless, and to try to introduce several small ones at once, or, rather into the same cervix, that they may expand simultaneously, is a blundering and unsatisfactory operation. The hard rubber bougies are of various sizes, and can be bent into the desired form by heating them over a lamp, which items are much in their favor; but they are too blunt for use in the early stages of treatment, when the passage is very narrow. If the sponge tent is an old one, it is apt to be hard and unsuitable. Moreover, when kept in contact with the cervico-uterine fluids, such a bit of sponge will more readily decompose. Now that our sponge tents are carbolized, however, it is quite probable that some of the evil consequences attributed to the use of this instrument will be omitted in future.

Precautions in practicing dilatation.

The rashness and injudicious haste with which dilatation has sometimes been practiced, have excited a prejudice against it in the minds of many. There are physicians who undertake to dilate the contracted cervix in obstructive dysmenorrhœa with the same dispatch with which a surgeon would amputate a limb, or excise the tonsils. The whole operation must be performed at once, and the unfortunate results that may follow are almost invariably attributed to the instruments used, instead of to the lack of discrimination and judgment on the part of the operator. The proper plan is to "feel one's way," as the phrase is, and to take plenty of time in order to overcome the obstruction without any serious shock to the patient's system, or any risk of the diseases which I have named as contingent upon this operation. If you cannot succeed in one month, it is better to take two or three, or six, if need be, and to make gradual progress towards a cure, than to be precipitate and finally to bring yourselves to condemn this expedient altogether. The cautious and persistent dilatation of the cervix was the only means employed in the case cited at the opening of this lecture. I have resorted to it in many other instances with equally good results.

Incision of the cervix uteri.

When, however, you have made a faithful trial of dilatation, and it has failed to bring the hoped-for results; or, if after having afforded temporary relief, there is a serious relapse, and you are satisfied that a radical cure is not possible by this means, incision of the cervix is a final resource. I do not say that you should never have recourse to this latter expedient before having tried the method by dilatation, but only that I think it more prudent and preferable to hold this operation in reserve, both because it is beset with more real danger, and also because, if it will answer, the simpler means is the safer of the two. There are cases, undoubtedly, in which the incision or slitting of the cervix is indispensable.

Concerning the method of performing this operation, I cannot do better than to call your attention to the remarks of my friend Dr. T. G. Comstock, of St. Louis, upon this subject.*

"The patient is placed before a good light, in the left semi-prone position, a little inclined upon the chest, with the knees well drawn up against the abdomen, and the hips on the edge of the mattress, when the speculum is introduced (we usually employ Cuzco's), and the uterus exposed between its blades. By means of a wire tenaculum, the uterus is seized and drawn down a little, and fixed by slipping one of the loops of the tenaculum over the brim of the speculum; then with a pair of Sims' curved or angulated scissors (one blade of which is carefully introduced within the os, just far enough to cut through to the junction of the cervix with the vagina, the handles of the scissors being closed), the section of the cervix is made first on the right side, and then in the same manner on the left side. Now the whole operation is half completed. The scissors being withdrawn, the metrotome is to be introduced. The instrument we employ is Dr. White's, and it looks not unlike the ordinary uterine sound, but is armed with two concealed cutting blades, which are regulated by a screw in the handle. This instrument is passed within the uterine canal, an inch and one quarter or more, above the incision already made; then the cutting blades are carefully expanded and the instrument is to be withdrawn, cutting its way out, so that the os internum is incised on each side. It has been advised to introduce the instrument again, and make sections of the os internum, exactly at right angles with the preceding, but the utility of this last recommendation is doubtful. After the incision, there will be a little hæmorrhage (occasionally a very severe one, although, fortunately, in over thirty operations we have never

*U. S. Medical and Surgical Journal, vol. vii, page 134.

seen it), which may be stopped by washing the blood away with ice-water, or by applying persulphate of iron solution, diluted in three parts of glycerine, then, by means of a pyramidal-shaped piece of cotton, saturated with the preparation spoken of, the cut surfaces are to be well packed by introducing the same, and then below this is to be placed a second large piece of wetted-cotton, so as to maintain *in situ* the cotton between the cut surfaces of the uterine canal. The patient is then carefully placed on her back, and required to keep still, and take a plain diet. I usually leave the dressing quite undisturbed for about thirty-six hours, then the speculum is introduced, and the cotton all removed. The uterine sound is carefully introduced, and the cut surfaces touched with it, so as to prevent union, then cotton saturated with carbolic acid one drachm, in solution with one ounce of glycerine, is introduced, and pushed up as high as possible between the cut surfaces, and this is packed with a good supply of cotton saturated in pure glycerine.

"In order to make the operation a success, the dressing should be changed every second day, for fourteen days, and the uterine sound occasionally carefully passed. Sometimes the canal will seem to contract in spite of the operation; in such a case a sea-tangle tent may be introduced and maintained in place some twelve hours or possibly longer, by packing cotton in glycerine below it.

"This operation should always be undertaken just after the patient has menstruated, so that she may be well before the next menstrual period. It requires seventeen or eighteen days after the incision for the parts to entirely heal. The operation may be made with or without the inhalation of chloroform. We usually prefer to give the chloroform."

Instead of Cuzco's speculum, I use Sims'; and for the wire tenaculum, recommended by Dr. Comstock, I would substitute this little uterine tenaculum, which is Nott's.

Qualifications.

For making the incisions, I have always employed Simpson's hysterotome, and this most frequently to the exclusion of the primary slitting with the scissors, which, in ordinary cases, where there is no especial induration, hypertrophy, no uterine hæmorrhage or intra-uterine fibroids, and no conical enlargement of the cervix, appears to me to be unnecessary. It may be requisite to repeat the operation two, or even three times.

Without great care in its performance, there is danger of sudden and fatal hæmorrhage, hæmatocele, peritonitis, cellulitis, or endo-metritis. The risk of these accidents is in ratio with the extent and depth of the incisions which are made through the os internum, and also in the abdominal portion of the cervix uteri, at a point superior to the insertion of the vagina. Something will likewise depend upon the predisposition to surgical fever and inflammation which the patient may possess, as well as upon accidental circumstances that may favor or retard her recovery. After the operation she should be kept in bed for a number of days. Fatal peritonitis has been known to occur from a lack of care in this regard, as late as the tenth day after the incision.

Dangers attending.

Precautions.

In every case the patient and her immediate friends should be made acquainted beforehand with the nature of the proposed operation, the dangers with which it is beset, and the possibility that it may need to be repeated before the cure can be considered complete.

NEURALGIC DYSMENORRHŒA.

Case.—I was called September 16, 1860, to visit Mrs. ——, aged 21, of tall, slender habit, nervo-sanguine temperament, and a most amiable disposition. Found her suffering from intense neuralgic pains in the uterine, lumbar and ischiatic regions. Her period had passed as usual more than a fortnight before, and for ten days previous to my first visit, these paroxysms of neuralgia had taken on an intermittent type, recurring every afternoon.

My patient had first menstruated at the age of thirteen. She has never had any retention of the flow, but has always suffered extremely. Has been married about six months, but has not been pregnant, nor has she experienced the least change in her menstrual symptoms since her marriage. In February last, while residing in Western New York, she had a severe attack of diphtheria. This was followed by rheumatism, or rheumatic neuralgia of the left arm. When the menses returned at the next month, there was a metastasis of this pain to the lumbar and uterine regions. From that time until the present the "period" has been characterized by the most intense suffering. Indeed there is no very decided remission of her suffering excepting for about one week in advance of the flow. For the day and night immediately preceding the appearance of the catamenia her sufferings are almost intolerable. She becomes exceedingly nervous, and restless, or wild with excitement, delirious, or has cramps and spasms of the most frightful kind.

For the relief of the neuralgia, I prescribed, in turn, arsenicum, cocculus, coffea, hyoscyamus, and, with the return of the scanty flow, apis mellifica, and caulophyllin. These remedies were repeated at reasonable intervals, — each of the two latter palliating somewhat the severity of the symptoms at first, but subsequently proving of no effect.

On the afternoon of the third day of the flow she had severe hysterical convulsions, which were controlled by moschus in the third decimal trituration. This remedy, however, only made her the more sensible of her sufferings.

After treating her most assiduously through the next menstrual interim — during which time she experienced but partial relief from the neuralgia, — the recurrence of the catamenia, on the 25th of October, was marked by precisely the same symptoms as before. It was impossible to discover that a single point had been gained by some six weeks' faithful trial.

Convinced of the existence of a local cause for the mischief, I proposed an examination per vaginam. Passing my finger carefully towards the external os uteri, — the vaginal walls being almost as closely contracted as in vaginismus, and the patient in intense pain, — I found the womb *in situ*, and the lower extremity of the cervix quite normal to the touch. On going a little higher, in order to ascertain the condition of the upper portion of the neck, my finger fell into a groove which extended all the way around the organ at the junction of the vaginal portion with the lower segment of the womb. This very marked constriction led me to infer that there was a decided spasm of the circular fibres of the neck of the uterus, or in other words a stricture of the cervix, leaving it in much the same condition as if it had been ligated at that point.

Simpson's sound was passed without difficulty as far as the os internum, but by no manipulation could I succeed in carrying it into the uterine cavity. A smaller probe, made expressly, was afterwards introduced, then the sound, and finally this little silver instrument, which resembles one of Simpson's intra-uterine pessaries, was passed completely through the cervico-uterine canal.

This instrument was carefully adjusted at nine in the evening, one day in advance of the expected flow. She was instructed to lie quietly upon the back as long as possible, in order that it might not be displaced, or drop away. It was retained until twelve o'clock — three hours — when it came away of itself. After this she enjoyed a tolerably good night's rest. The next morning the flow came on, and more freely than usual, and with less of suffering than she had experienced for years before. Once only during this period the flow became scanty, when a few doses of apis mellifica3 brought it on again, but without any return of the neuralgia.

Contrary to my expectations, the relief seemed permanent. During the next inter-menstrual period she appeared to be quite well; rode out almost daily, attended evening parties, danced and sang (for she was a favorite singer), and was indeed the happiest woman in the city. The only subsequent trouble experienced was six months later, when she had a slight attack of uterine colic, which was promptly relieved by ignatia3.

The importance of physical exploration.

There are several points of interest connected with this case, the practical relations of which may interest you. Apart from its chronic nature, and the degree of suffering involved, the fact that she had been treated by several eminent physicians in different parts of the country with such a signal want of success, leads one to inquire into the reasons for their failure. The more obvious of these reasons evidently was the lack of a correct diagnosis. The husband assured me that but one of the doctors had ever proposed an examination of this case per vaginam, and that one was not permitted to make it. For this reason,—because they did not pursue this investigation as they should have done,—the whole corps, embracing distinguished practitioners of both schools, failed to bring relief. Indeed my immediate predecessor had told the patient's friends that nothing could be of more than temporary benefit, and accordingly prescribed the free use of the sulphate of morphia, which I found her in the habit of taking *ad libitum*, and in incredible quantities.

Such an oversight is scarcely excusable upon any grounds whatever. As physicians we should respect the delicacy of the sex, and the cautions enjoined and practiced by the profession against all unnecessary and unwarrantable officiousness in trivial cases, where a manual examination is uncalled for; but to allow any squeamish scruples to be in the way of the patient's recovery, or to fancy that constitutional remedies given in the dark, are capable of removing a mechanical difficulty of this kind, argues both a criminal and a crazy neglect of duty on the part of the doctor.

It is worthy of remark that by proper means the diagnosis was not difficult, and that the relief afforded by the single introduction of this dilator was complete and permanent. I saw my patient three years later, and she had had no return of the difficulty. In this operation there was no cutting of the contracted cervical fibres, for, as you perceive, this instrument has no edge with which to divide them. The mere passage of the smaller sound, and then of the larger one, did not accomplish the result, for their use in the first instance did not lessen the pain and suffering in the least. There were no evidences of existing or of previous inflammation; and if there had been, we can not suppose that so simple and transient a means could possibly dispose of them so instantaneously almost, and so entirely.

Entire relief through a simple operative expedient.

This case was evidently one of neuralgia, a pure neurosis, dependent upon permanent contraction of some of the circular fibres of the upper portion of the cervix uteri, unaccompanied either by inflammation or its consequences, but presenting its symptoms both during the monthly flow and also in the interval between the periods.

A neurosis.

In most cases of neuralgic dysmenorrhœa, the pain and suffering are limited to the monthly return. Any undue determination of blood to the uterus, or even a slight delay in the appearance of the discharge, incidental irritation or displacement of the organ, or ulceration or inflammation thereof, may be the exciting cause of the attack. The pain may be limited to the pelvic or the ovarian regions, or it may assume the form of neuralgia located elsewhere, as in neuralgic headache, neuralgia of the face, the teeth, the eyes, the fingers, the toes, the mammæ, the intercostal spaces, the stomach or bowels, or even of the heart. In such cases the suffering commonly subsides when the "period" has passed. But, exceptionally, as in the case of which I have spoken, where the local spasm or irritation of the cervix is perpetuated, the remote pain and suffering do not subside, but persist throughout the month. You should remember this fact, else the continuance of this form of secondary neuralgia may lead you to suppose that it has no possible connection with the uterus.

Symptoms of neuralgic dysmenorrhœa.

In those who are predisposed to this form of dysmenorrhœa, and who are generally of a neuralgic tendency, the slightest exciting causes may induce it. One of my patients, a very observing and truthful person, who had had this disease for many years, remarked that when she ate very lightly, on the advent of the menses, the suffering was very much lessened. Her habit was to diet herself strictly the day before the flow came on, and to eat sparingly of light food until it appeared freely. A hearty meal at the beginning of the period would increase the suffering in a ten-fold degree.

Causes of dysmenorrhœa.

All those habits of mind and body, which induce prostration and perturbation of the nervous system, are likely in those who are impressionable, to bring on this form of painful menstruation. The incidental suffering, as in neuralgia, is always periodic and paroxysmal. A predisposition to this peculiar kind of nervous derangement, which implicates menstruation and involves great suffering, runs in families, and, during the first few years of their menstrual and sometimes of their married life, every daughter will be the victim of these functional derangements. Not unfrequently the most aggravated cases of neuralgic dysmenorrhœa occur in the experience of those women whose married life is an unhappy one, and who, either from a physical inaptitude for, loathing, or an excess of venery, suffer the evil consequences of forcible, frequent or incomplete intercourse.

When the flow commences, the pain usually remits. And this is true however remote its location. But sometimes the relief is more direct and positive. Only yesterday a lady told me that she always felt light of heart and buoyant immediately the flow began, although but a few minutes before she had been in real agony, and was peevish, irritable, and extremely sensitive to any little slight or injury. The relief sometimes re-acts in such a way as to bring on a hysterical fit of crying or weeping, or of both these together; or it may be followed by tranquil and refreshing sleep. In very rare cases it is followed by inordinate sexual desire, amounting to temporary nymphomania.

Relation of the flow to the degree of pain.

You will sometimes, but not always, find the distinctive and characteristic indications for the remedy in the kind, degree, location, and especial peculiarities of the pain, wherever it may be seated. These details are so varied, and so insusceptible of classification, that

Indications for internal remedies.

you will be compelled to select from a list of remedies which are suited to the cure of every shade and form of neuralgia.

Acting upon the hint that so slight a cause as the swallowing of a teaspoonful or two of cold water may cause a spasm of the uterine cervix, with scanty and painful flow, my friend, Dr. M. F. Page, has sometimes given gelseminum [1], fifteen drops in half a teacupful of warm water, one teaspoonful to be taken every five minutes until relieved, then less frequently with the happiest results. In this form of dysmenorrhœa, at or near the climacteric, he has great confidence in veratrum viride [1], five drops in the same quantity of warm water, and the same dose repeated every ten or fifteen minutes. Yet, it often happens, that what will relieve one case will in another case seem to be without effect, even where the symptoms are very similar.

Warm instead of cold water.

Gelseminum.

Veratrum viride.

There are some cases of this disease which can be cured most promptly and satisfactorily, and without any harmful consequences, by the use of local means. Careful dilatation may suffice — as it did with my patient — to paralyze and overcome the morbid spasm and hyperæsthesia of the uterine cervix, upon which the whole mischief really depends. In neuralgic and spasmodic dysmenorrhœa, I think it better to perform this operation with solid than with sponge tents. Indeed, in some cases of this kind, I have remarked a singular aggravation of the suffering from the use of the latter, especially when introduced in advance of the flow.

Dilatation.

LECTURE XXV.

UTERINE SURGERY *versus* UTERINE THERAPEUTICS.

GENTLEMEN:

The line of demarcation between sanity and insanity, animal and vegetable life, and this world and the next, is not more indefinite than that which separates surgical from therapeutical indications in the cure of many diseases. This is especially true of the treatment of the Diseases of Women. What reliance shall be placed on manual operations, and what upon medicinal influences in curing them, is an unsettled question. There are those who insist that, in this specialty, surgery is almost omnipotent, and *per contra* those also who claim that constitutional remedies alone are adequate to the end in view.

Value of uterine surgery.

The attentive student of gynæcology is aware that within the last quarter of a century, Uterine Surgery has developed from a rudimentary to an almost perfect branch of medical science. It has furnished us with the most approved and available means of diagnosis, and with a multitude of resources for the relief and cure of certain diseases that were the opprobrium of medicine. It has fulfilled old indications with new and approved instruments, reconstructed the special pathology of sexual disease, and re-organized our aims and purposes and expedients in such a manner as to add very greatly to the comfort and welfare of woman. It has added another chair to the medical curriculum, augmented and improved our literature, and developed a new and most useful specialty, which already is more popular than any other, and which, at no distant day, bids fair to engross the attention and to appropriate to itself a large share of the medical talent of this and other countries.

It was a very natural consequence of this rapid growth in the professional and popular favor that the claims set up for Surgery, as applied to the treatment of the Diseases of Women, should be somewhat exclusive and extravagant. Dr. Bennet frames his formula that ulceration and induration of the uterine cervix lie at the bottom of nearly all the diseases peculiar to the sex. Local cauterization will frequently remove these conditions — which he has been shrewd enough to confound in his writings, and therefore escharotics are specific. The generalization is the bait, the manipulation attracts, and the parade causes a premium to be placed on the operation. Forthwith his experiments and deductions are the text and the theory for an indiscriminate local treatment designed alike for all kinds of uterine affections and utero-visceral derangements.

Extravagant claims.

Sir Jas. Simpson incised the cervix as a remedy for obstructive dysmenorrhœa. Sims adapted his scissors as a uterotome, and improved upon the operation. The same operation was soon recommended for the cure of sterility, and retro-flexion of the uterus. Then it was applied to the relief of the intractable uterine hæmorrhage, and as a means of exploration and of facilitating excision in uterine fibroids. Now, in multitudes of cases, the uterine cervix is slit open, with every possible kind of result. The operation is a favorite one, for blood is shed, and there is some cutting in the dark,—which is always attractive in ratio with the risks that are taken.

Illustrations.

The various modifications and varied uses of the uterine speculum, the sound, the probe, the sponge and other tents, the exploring needle, the endoscope, and physical exploration by palpation, auscultation and percussion, have engaged the almost exclusive attention and confidence of uterine pathologists. Armed with these instruments, and *au fait* in using them for purposes of diagnosis and of treatment, it is not at all strange that they have come to place an almost exclusive reliance upon them, and that the claims of a coincident and conservative therapeutics should have been either overlooked or disregarded. They esteem the proposal to unite a course of medical with the surgical treatment of uterine ulceration, cervicitis, or endo-metritis, for example, as altogether superfluous — a species of superfœtation. When their resources are sufficient, and their work is substantially done, why propose to add anything, or to substitute it with what is less attractive,

Uterine therapeutics practically ignored.

flashy, seductive and sensational? For, with all our boasting, it remains that, in this class of diseases, the operation of the best chosen internal remedies, is not and cannot be instantaneous. The relief they bring in chronic uterine and ovarian affections especially, comes only "after many days." They do their work quietly, and without any of the *ad captandum eclat* of a surgical exploit, or a sanguinary battle from the possible effects of which the patient may never recover. It is an axiom in midwifery that, whether natural or induced, the most rapid cases of labor are not the safest. In uterine surgery the risks are in ratio with the boldness and dispatch of the operator, which qualities are almost inseparable from its employment.

It is equally obvious that the disproportionate development of uterine surgery is due to causes that can be explained, and which are avoidable. Let me call your attention to a few of them.

1. *The growing scepticism in the minds of specialists concerning the effects and efficacy of internal medication.* Providing he is educated and thoughtful, the pursuit of a medical specialty invariably inclines the physician to place less reliance, than does the general practitioner, upon constitutional treatment as a means of cure. The oculist and the aurist are not given to the common weakness of dosing their patients. Those who treat the diseases of the respiratory organs exclusively and most skillfully have more confidence in hygienic measures than in medicine. With every class of specialists, the higher the grade of their qualification, and the broader their field of observation, the lower their estimate of general treatment. For these men are sufficiently educated to discriminate and to differentiate. Their knowledge of physiology and of pathology assures them that, not only does every part suffer with the sick organ, or member, but that for the same reason, whatever lowers the general vitality will lessen the chances of recovery.

Scepticism respecting medication.

Uterine pathologists necessarily reach a similar conclusion. Unless their ideas of medicine, and of its capacity to cure, or to injure, are stereotyped and more or less antiquated, they gradually abandon the old therapeutics, and learn to place an increased trust in modern surgery, with its topical expedients and its manifold resources. The

Abandonment of old ideas.

cultivated gynæcologist of our day would as soon think of resorting to general blood-letting in hysteria, as to the use of emmenagogues in amenorrhœa. When Dr. Thomas counsels that the bowels shall be left in a constipated condition in endo-metritis, it implies not only that he has a clear idea of the indications that are presented for the cure of that disease, but also that, in proscribing cathartics, he is interested in removing a fertile source of mischief in uterine complaints.*

Without pausing to elaborate this idea, it must suffice to call your attention to the fact that the cultivation and practice of this specialty, as of every other, has had a two-fold result; (1) it has stimulated a development of a special branch of surgery: and (2) it has impaired the general confidence in wholesale medication for the cure of limited functional and organic disease.

Surgery more popular.

2. *The natural preference which physicians, and their patients also, have for operative interference instead of internal treatment, whenever the former is possible.* As compared with the surgeon, the physician labors at a great disadvantage. And the reward of his skill and patience are often disproportionate to the time and care bestowed on the cure of intricate and dangerous diseases. Although they may be equally skillful, each in his own department, my friend the professor of surgery will most likely gain more *eclat* by cutting off a limb, or excising a tumor, than my colleague in the chair of theory and practice will from curing a case of cerebro-spinal meningitis, Bright's disease, or of angina pectoris. All of which implies that we involuntarily place a premium on the manual operation, while it is such an ordinary affair for the physician to tide his patient over his difficulties in a more quiet way, that but little relative stir is made concerning it.

Therapeutics ought not to be neglected.

We do not criticize this propensity, although it has sometimes led to deplorable results. For it is impossible that such a large number of earnest and able workers should devote their lives to the study and practice of uterine surgery without bringing it to a certain degree of perfection. And the more popular, the larger the field of experience, the greater the number of those who are competent to

* A Practical Treatise on the Diseases of Women; by T. Gaillard Thomas, M. D., etc., etc., Philadelphia, 1872, page 227.

practice it, the older the study, the more thorough its literature, the greater, better and more lasting will be the benefits conferred by it upon the profession and upon the race.

But an evident result of this bias toward surgery is a neglect to cultivate and develop the curative sphere and relation of our remedies to the class of diseases under consideration. We study the special therapeutics of other ailments most carefully. It is not permissible to transfer them to the domain of a different branch of the healing art. Every species of clinical enquiry and analysis is entered upon and prosecuted with a view to the proper selection of the remedy or remedies. The symptoms are balanced, the signs are translated into a familiar language, everything is made available, medically, to effect a cure through the operation of the vital forces.

Study them.

If we could point to therapeutical results in gynæcology which compare with those of uterine surgery, results which were as carefully obtained, as accurate and trustworthy in every particular, as critically analyzed and as readily available, our usefulness would be doubled, and the little world in which we now work as specialists would consist of two hemispheres instead of one.

Why.

3. *The comparatively limited opportunities and skill of those who have labored especially to develop uterine therapeutics.*—The allurements to surgery, and its very general practice among physicians and specialists, diminishes the number of those who are laboring to define and determine the special therapeutics of uterine and kindred diseases. And the tendency of patients who are thus afflicted to estimate what is done for their relief and cure by the scale of suffering and risk at the hands of the doctor, lessens the number of those who are willing to trust and to wait for the results which might often be obtained by fitly-chosen remedies. Add to this that those of our physicians who are most competent to do this work are usually engaged in general practice, and it is really no reflection upon their popularity, or their ability, to say that one reason why uterine surgery has outstripped uterine therapeutics in the race, is because the opportunities and skill of those who practice the latter are comparatively limited.

Disadvantages of the specialist.

4. *The bias towards harsh and harmful remedies whenever internal means are employed.*—There is a current idea which holds that when the internal generative organs of the female are diseased, they require that stronger medicines should be given than in case of a similar disease which is seated in another organ or apparatus. This view is entertained by many who do not hesitate to acknowledge the wonderful delicacy of the nervous and vascular sympathies of the uterus and its appendages. And yet they insist that it is sometimes necessary to medicate these patients very thoroughly before any benefit can be derived from remedies that have been taken internally.

A great error.

The consequence is that, becoming disgusted with such treatment, or afraid of it, these patients put themselves in the care of such doctors as will not dose them at all, but who will rely exclusively upon other means of relief.

5. *The theory that constitutional treatment is destined altogether to supersede surgery in the management of these sexual disorders.*—Surgery is the complement of therapeutics as one hand is of the other, or the right eye of its fellow. To assume that it is possible in all respects to substitute, or to supersede the necessity for either of them, would be like limiting the obstetrician to the use of but one hand, or the microscopist to that of one eye exclusively, and denying them the privilege of using the other under all circumstances. The practical accoucheur is ambidextrous. And, if the microscopist uses but one eye at a time he alternates them. Each has its own sphere and function, and they must share the duty that is to be performed; for, although one may be preferable to the other, according to idiosyncrasy, habit, education or circumstance, still it remains that this dual arrangement is a part, and an indispensable part, of our organization as individuals.

Surgery and therapeutics.

The same is true of the curative relations of medicine and surgery. Both are requisite, each in its proper place, but which shall be the more prominent will depend upon the peculiarities, habits and education of the physician, and also, as we have shown, upon a variety of circumstances. To declare that either of them is superfluous, and to declaim against its employment, very naturally excites a pre-

Both essential.

judice against those who talk and act so unreasonably. It is a question of boundary lines merely, and since the whole field belongs to us, we can shift the fences from time to time and cultivate the crop of expedients that will prove to be most valuable and useful.

To compensate for this lack of interest in medicine as applied to the treatment of the diseases of women, it will be necessary,

1. *To have a series of new provings, on women, which shall be made with the greatest possible care and discrimination.*—The health of woman is beset by so many contingencies, and she is subject to such crises as to render it very difficult to find one who, both in herself and her surroundings, is suited to become a prover; and the physicians who are really competent to superintend such a proving are perhaps equally rare. For, if such an index to the remedial relations of a drug shall be trustworthy, it implies that the physician who undertakes this labor is fully conversant with the whole range of uterine pathology; that he has subjected his medicine to the test of a most searching examination; eliminated all the symptoms which are naturally incident to menstruation, maternity, puberty, the climacteric, and also to her relations as wife and mother, to the church and to society, as well as to the distinctive susceptibilities that pertain to her sex, and which are so perplexing to all of us, and retained and classified only those symptoms which were unmistakably due to the action of the drug.

New provings by woman a necessity.

The fact that this labor has not already been perfected, and that it is a task of no small magnitude, should not deter those who hope for better things of uterine therapeutics, from its faithful and persistent prosecution. And I urge it upon you as members of this class to determine that you will add something to the common stock of knowledge on this subject, something tangible and available, something that will be of service to those who are suffering, and which will prove that the pains you have taken in the study of special pathology and therapeutics have not been lost either to yourselves or to the profession at large. For, suppose that we had a full and complete proving of calcarea carbonica, or of sepia, or of any other remedy, made with particular reference

Also, combined effort to increase our knowledge.

to the female organism, and under the eye of a skillful specialist; there is no question that its influence for good would outweigh that which attaches to the invention of a new instrument, even if that instrument were as useful as the uterine sound.

2. *The most painstaking study of the differential diagnosis of the diseases of the female generative system.*—This condition is requisite not only because it concerns the skillful treatment of these affections, but also because it bears a vital relation to gynæcological literature. If he keeps them to himself, the physician's short-comings are self-limited; but if he publishes his blunders, he perpetuates their remembrance and ensures their repetition. Therefore, he should know what he has done, as well as what he is doing.

Study diagnosis.

With all due respect to those who have directly and indirectly contributed to our knowledge of materia medica, as it is applied to the diseases of women, it must be confessed that their labors would have been more fruitful of good if they had been better versed in uterine pathology and diagnosis. The clinical history of hundreds of cases that have been reported confirms the truth of this remark, and shows the need of culture in this direction. If every woman who takes a drug with a view to its physiological effects, were carefully examined, both physically and otherwise, before, during and after making the "proving;" if she could be removed from all the vicissitudes which are certain to derange her sexual sympathies and to upset her health, the symptoms evolved and collected would be a better criterion of the range of action of the drug than we can otherwise obtain. And if every physician were fully posted in the matter of diagnosticating the contingent symptoms, or deviations from perfect health, which occur in most women (which are necessarily transient and self-limited), and such as are really pathological and persistent, those which do not get well of themselves, and are not often cured, as well as those caused by emotional states, independently of our remedies, the value of our clinical record would be increased a thousand fold.

Also pathology.

This opens an avenue for usefulness and distinction; for it is left for our school of practice to develop the *medical* side of this question. We need such a chart of the remedial action, both pathogenetic and clinical, of medicines that are suited to the female organism, as we do not at present possess. This is a *sine qua non.* It can not be obtained by the *exclusive* study of symptomatology after the old method, (1), because many of the resources of surgery are necessary as a means of determining whether or not the prover is in good health beforehand; (2), without these facilities, we could not know the variety, extent, nature or seat of the lesions present in a given case, whether they are functional or organic, and therefore our testimony concerning their cure could not be depended upon; and (3), it must be true of the tissues which compose the generative intestine, as it is of other textures, that they have their proper pathological and therapeutical, as well as their anatomical, physiological and surgical history and relations.

And pathogenesis.

And symptomatology.

MENORRHŒA — CERVICAL EPISTAXIS.

Case. — Miss M——, 19 years of age, has been an invalid for four years past. She is not confined to her room except at irregular intervals, but is active and able to ride or walk, and to some extent enjoy the society of her friends. She began to menstruate at fifteen. The first period came on with a great deal of pain and difficulty, but when the flow was finally established it continued for three weeks without cessation. After five days' intermission it commenced again, but without any considerable suffering. Again it continued until almost the end of the month, and again it returned with the regularity of the normal monthly discharge. In this manner, for four years, the flow has been almost constant. The longest interval in which she has ever been free from it, in all that time, is seven days. There is no dysmenorrhœa, the loss of blood is not excessive, but the flow is passive and painless, and continues when she is sleeping as well as during her waking hours. Sometimes under strong mental excitement, as when she is at a concert or in company, and her mind is diverted, it ceases temporarily, and afterwards returns as before. The same effect has been observed in consequence of a carriage ride and of a journey by rail; but it is of very short duration.

If the flow is arrested, she suffers no inconvenience excepting a "rush of blood to the head," accompanied by more or less vertigo, headache, flushed face, dimness of vision, and a heavy, dull feeling, with disposition to sleep. At other times her mind is clear and her spirits are good. And yet she feels somewhat weakened and enervated by the constant loss of blood. Her appetite is good. There is no intra-pelvic pain or distress, no hæmorrhoids, no constipation, and no urinary derangement. The only suffering noted is a feeling of aching and weariness in the region of the ovaries, more especially of the left one, at the month and after unusual exercise. During her whole menstrual life her mother was subject to a similar hæmorrhage.

This patient's general appearance does not indicate that she is ill. She has walked several squares to the Dispensary this morning, with less fatigue than you would have supposed possible. Her color is somewhat heightened by the exercise in the open air, for her sister says that she is usually more pale than now, excepting only when her hæmorrhage has ceased and the blood rushes to her head.

It is sometimes very important, in cases of this kind, to discover the relation which a passive uterine hæmorrhage bears to the catamenial function. If the flow dates from the first establishment of this function at puberty, as in this instance, or if it habitually ceases a short time before the "period," and then recurs regularly, you may conclude that it is essentially a menstrual disorder. There are some exceptions to this rule, as in case of medullary carcinoma, and sub-mucous polypi, and perhaps in syphilitic endometritis also; but, in most instances, the manner and time of its advent, and its regular periodicity afterwards (even although the period may be longer or shorter than natural), are to be taken as evidence of its connection with the process of ovulation.

Relation to menstruation.

A diagnostic rule.

Nor is it difficult to explain this result. The physiological injection of the endometrium, which is a condition of the menstrual secretion, is relieved and removed when the healthy woman has menstruated. But, if she is not well, that extraordinary fullness of its vessels may continue, even although the menstrual flow has been discharged; and there will remain a passive congestion of some portion of the uterine mucous membrane. This engorgement may relieve itself by a profuse and copious hæmorrhage, as in menorrhagia, or even in metrorrhagia; or it may pass away by a sort of cervical epistaxis,

A physiological reason.

or passive flow, in which the local excess of blood oozes out and escapes more leisurely. In the former case the critical and alarming hæmorrhage is sudden, and of short duration ; in the latter it is a mere prolongation or continuation of the menses, without any very serious symptoms, until the month is nearly or quite spent, and it is time that they should return again. One is acute, active, and irregular in its recurrence ; the other chronic, passive, and distinctly periodical.

Peculiarity of the flow.

There is another reason why this woman's hæmorrhage, although so long continued, must be classed as menstrual — a real case of menorrhœa. It is that the amount of the flow is not influenced by the exercise which she takes, or by other circumstances, more decidedly than it is in ordinary menstruation. If that hæmorrhage depended upon the presence of a sub-mucous or interstitial fibroid, a polypus, ulceration, cancerous degeneration, or venous engorgement, the quantity of blood lost would vary with her habits. Above all things, it would not be lessened by riding and active exercise.

Its critical nature.

Viewing this species of hæmorrhage as in a sense critical, and remembering the "habit" which has grown out of its continuance, with brief intervals only, for years, we should naturally expect that the arrest of the flow would occasion more or less of suffering and disorder elsewhere. Hence the "rush of blood to the head," of which this woman complains whenever the flow has ceased, and which subsides as soon as that flow is restored. The same cause will sometimes induce a violent attack of facial neuralgia, or sick headache, vomiting, delirium, hysteria, spasms, coma, or even convulsions.

To show that this disease is not infrequent, and that the case before you is a typical one, I will read you some extracts from a letter received a few days ago from Dr. R. C. Sabin, of Wisconsin, a member of the class for 1871-72:

Case. — "My patient is now eighteen years of age. She commenced menstruation at fifteen, and the flow has been almost constant ever since. The longest time in which she has been free from it is two weeks, when the interruption was caused by a journey by rail. The discharge is of a bright red color, thin and watery, and has no odor. After continuing for a month or six weeks, the flow becomes stringy and thick, and then ceases for two or three days. Her health is always impaired at the time the flow stops, and there is giddiness, sudden flushes of the face, blindness, etc. These symptoms pass off as the flow returns. The urine is high-colored, and of a strong nauseous odor.

"She is of scrofulous habit, short and fleshy, and is troubled with frequent moist eruptions. The constant drain does not seem to have the least effect in reducing her weight. She was extremely fleshy as a child. Her general health seems good, she goes to school, and has a gooda appetite

"She has taken, at different times, sepia, pulsatilla, calcarea carb., china, hamamelis and ferrum. The latter benefits her general condition, and, temporarily, lessens the amount of the flow. Hamamelis will also check it in a few days, but then she feels wretched until the discharge comes on again."

Necessity of physical examination.

In these cases you should not fail to make a careful vaginal examination before you venture an opinion concerning the nature of the disease, or the proper course of treatment to be pursued. You may find the cervix uteri tender, swollen, congested, or in a state of areolar hyperplasia; or a small mucous polyp may have sufficed to perpetuate the mischief. Bi-manual examination, and the double touch, may discover such a state of ovarian irritation and inflammation as will account for the symptoms and give you a hint toward their relief.

Modifying circumstances.

It is sometimes important to know whether this or other menstrual disorders have been hereditary in the patient's family. Especial inquiries should be made concerning the hæmorrhagic diathesis, or if the patient has ever had chlorosis or anæmia. The clinical history of the case might also be modified if the woman had ever borne children, or been pregnant and suffered an abortion, and in some cases by her having nursed an infant. And so also by marriage, intemperate coitus, residence in a mountainous, a marshy, or an aguish district, by high living, and the free use of alcoholic drinks. For all these are so many avoidable causes of the disease under consideration.

The hæmorrhage may persist without manifest injury.

The fact that in this woman's history, as well as in Dr. Sabin's case, the hæmorrhage has persisted for several years is proof that it may continue indefinitely, and without any very serious impairment of the general health. Its duration may even extend from puberty to the climacteric, and then expire by limitation. Usually, however, such persons survive the change of life with difficulty, for the arrest of the accustomed discharge is apt to induce disease of a more serious character elsewhere.

Sterility from.

One of the most troublesome consequences of this form of uterine hæmorrhage is sterility. Whatever the state of their general health, in women whose pelvic circulation is being thus constantly drained, the vitality of the internal generative organs is low. And even if ovulation is properly performed, the lining membrane of the generative intestine is not in a condition to favor conception. Moreover the sanguineous flow itself would be very likely to interfere with a fruitful intercourse. Hence you will be consulted for the cure of barrenness which, directly or indirectly, is due to such a hæmorrhage as this woman has had for the past four years.

Medicine *versus* Surgery.

Treatment. — In the whole range of medical practice, I scarcely know of a class of cases which is better suited to illustrate the efficacy of properly chosen internal remedies, conjoined with suitable hygienic regulations, than this. Here is a case of hæmorrhage which depends upon a pathological disorder of one of the most prominent of all the bodily functions. It has a definite clinical history. Its symptoms are significant. Its causes are obvious and avoidable. Its diagnosis and prognosis are not difficult. Its treatment is similar to that of other diseased conditions. And it can be cured by therapeutic means exclusively.

Not to be confounded with "unavoidable hæmorrhage."

In all these respects such a case as the one before you differs from uterine hæmorrhage accompanying or following labor or abortion, or from habitual and excessive losses of blood in consequence of intra-uterine growths. In them the hæmorrhage is accidental and more or less dangerous. It is a mere contingency, and must be relieved at once, or the patient's life may be sacrificed. The simple expedient of emptying the womb and securing its contraction may be sufficient. But in the passive form of uterine hæmorrhage, connected with menstruation, surgical appliances are either powerless or harmful, and no such very general indication is presented. We are forced to depend upon uterine therapeutics.

In the selection of a remedy, or remedies, we should not overlook the significance of certain incidental states or conditions, for example, the different dyscrasiæ, each of which is possessed of its own clinical bearing. Thus:

General therapeutics.

If the patient is predisposed to hæmorrhage, such remedies as china, ipecacuanha, sabina, platina, secale cornutum, ferrum, nux vomica, natrum mur., hamamelis, trillium, rhus tox., calcarea carb., belladonna, crocus, carbo veg., phosphorus, arsenicum alb., and sulphuric or nitric acid may be indicated. She should be put upon cool acidulated drinks, and enjoined to keep as quiet as possible during the first week or ten days of the period especially.

For the hæmorrhagic diathesis.

If she is in a state of chloro-anæmia, the remedy must cover the symptoms which are most prominent. Among them you will observe such as signify a profound impression of the nervous and circulatory, as well as of the digestive and menstrual functions. And, whether the hæmorrhage is the cause or the consequence of the impaired quality of the blood, the case will have to be treated as one of chlorosis with serious complications.*

For the chloro-anæmia.

In case of confirmed scrofulosis with menorrhœa, I apprehend it to be of the utmost importance to attend to the physiological needs of the organism in advance of medication. First, select a suitable diet, one that can and will be assimilated. It should consist of a proper and available proportion of the oleo-albuminous elements. These should be cooked and presented in a pleasant and palatable form, and at a suitable time of the day. The appetite should be encouraged by mental diversion and suitable exercise in the open air. For the function of hæmatogenesis, or blood-making, to which the lymphatic glandular apparatus is especially devoted, must proceed properly, else the quality of the blood will become so seriously impaired that hæmorrhage will almost certainly follow.

For the scrofulous cachexia.

The most prominent remedies suited to this cachexia, and the symptoms that are likely to spring from it in this form of cervical epistaxis, are calcarea carb., calcarea phos., hepar sulphuris, silicea, baryta carb., jodium, phytolacca, carbo veg., mezereum, merc.

* See page 103 of this volume.

sol., merc. jod., sulphur, and the nitric, muriatic or sulphuric acids.

For the syphilitic cachexia.

In some obstinate examples of this form of passive uterine hæmorrhage (if your experience accords with mine), you will find that when the most carefully selected remedies have failed, as they sometimes do, you will succeed in curing it by giving medicines which are anti-syphilitic in their character. In this way the kali jodatum, kali hyd., thuja, merc. præcip. ruber, and nitric acid, in such potencies as you shall select, may help you out of the difficulty. Of course, if you succeed by giving them upon the theory that there was a slight taint of syphilis in the lesion, it will not be either prudent or necessary to tell the patient or her friends why this particular class of remedies was chosen.

For ovarian complications.

Ovarian disease is so frequently at the bottom of these hæmorrhagic complaints that you should be very careful not to overlook it. For, as a rule, the ovaritis precedes the hæmorrhage, and is the cause both of its long continuance and of its periodical return. This is especially true if the chronic and unnatural flow dates from puberty. The remedies which are best adapted to the cure of this complication are belladonna, colocynth, hamamelis, lilium tig., lachesis, carbo veg., conium, veratrum vir., platina, mercurius corr., and pulsatilla. In a word, the cardinal symptoms that properly belong to the lesion of the ovaries, when the ovaritis and the hæmorrhage co-exist, are a more trustworthy guide in the selection of the remedy than the quantity, or even the quality, of the sanguineous flow itself.

Change of climate.

Since it is possible that a change of climate may aid in the recovery, one who has lived in a mountainous region may be sent to a different section; or one who has resided in a low, marshy district, may be transferred to the mountains. Sometimes a cure will follow a change from the prairies to the sea-side, or *vice versa*, the object being to bring about an entire renovation by a change of external conditions. Or a sea-voyage, or salt-water baths, may prove very beneficial.

Suitable exercise.

While it is requisite that such patients as Miss —— should take sufficient exercise, it is equally important that they should not overdo. Horseback riding, or running the sewing machine, skating, or dancing, for example, would aggravate or increase her disorder. The exercise should be more gentle and passive.

I have more confidence in nitric acid, in the second decimal dilution, than in any other single remedy in these cases. It is not, however, specific. She will take it four times daily, and report the result.

Nitric acid.

FIBRO-CYSTIC TUMOR OF THE UTERUS.

I will close this lecture with a few remarks upon the case of fibro-cystic tumor of the uterus, which I had before the class in the hospital last week.

Case.—Mrs. C. D——, aged 31 years, English, first observed an enlargement in her right inguinal region of about the size of an orange, ten years ago. This tumor did not appear to grow at all until after her marriage, which was two years since. She very soon became pregnant, and the tumor increased in size in proportion with the development of the gravid uterus. After her delivery at term, the growth was observed by the physician, who expressed his surprise that a second child did not follow the first. She weaned her baby when it was thirteen months old, since which time the enlargement has increased more rapidly, until the abdomen is enormously distended.

Mrs. D. has menstruated regularly and normally since weaning the child, and has never been subject to hæmorrhage. The uterus is *in situ*, the sound passes to the depth of three inches only, and the mobility of the organ, independent of the abdominal tumor, is clearly recognized. The wave-line is observable, and all the signs are those of an ovarian cyst.

This case, you will remember, was diagnosticated as one of ovarian dropsy. The next day my colleague, Prof. Danforth cut down upon the tumor in your presence. Adhesions were found upon all sides, and throughout its whole extent. When these were finally broken up, its separation effected, and the tumor turned out, it was found to be attached by a slender pedicle to the right side of the body of the uterus, very near its fundus. You remember that tapping the mass with a Spencer Wells' trocar failed to bring away any fluid. The pedicle was ligated, and the tumor, which weighed twenty pounds, removed as in the cases of ovariotomy which have been performed before the class during this session.

Here, then, was an error in diagnosis, for which I am responsible. I confess the fact, and, contrary to the custom of most teachers, propose to tell you how it happened to be made, and how you can avoid such a mistake in the future.

An error in diagnosis.

When I found that the uterine cavity was not enlarged, and that the sound, although it reached the fundus uteri, would pass only three inches; and was assured by the patient that she had never been subject to hæmorrhage, it was very natural and proper to exclude the possibility of the growth being either a sub-mucous or an interstitial fibroid: and when, with the sound in utero and my hand over the abdomen, I found that it was possible to move the womb considerably without changing the position or relations of the tumor in the least, I felt warranted in deciding that the growth was not uterine at all. For, even if it were a sub-peritoneal fibroid, its mobility should be consentaneous, or synchronous, so to speak, with that of the uterus; while in this instance the uterus was moveable, but the tumor was not.

Deceptive symptoms.

The fact that this unusual state of things existed, and the reason why this important differential sign between uterine and other tumors failed in this instance, was easily explained after the operation. The pedicle was three inches or more in length, slender, and well defined. The tumor was firmly bound by adhesions on all sides. The length, form and location of the pedicle would have allowed the uterus to be moved quite freely without moving the tumor, even if the adhesions had not glued it so securely to the neighboring parts.

Dr. Atthill, in speaking of the diagnostic value of the mobility of the uterus independently of the tumor in these cases, says, "Still even here error is possible, for if a fibrous tumor spring from the uterus by a moderately long pedicle, or even by a short one, we may be able to move the uterus to such an extent as to lead to the conclusion that it is free, and on the other hand it is possible that in a case of ovarian disease the uterus might be so bound down by adhesions as to be immovable.*

In most fibro-cystic tumors of the uterus the cysts are small.

* Clinical Lectures on the Diseases Peculiar to Women, by Lombe Atthill, M. D., etc., Dublin, 1871.

The fluctuation felt through the abdominal parietes is therefore deceptive. The wave-line is not pathognomonic of ovarian dropsy, for you are witnesses that it existed in this case, and yet there was no ovarian disease of any kind. Its occurrence was also explained by what happened during the operation. When my colleague opened the peritoneal sac, it was found to contain a layer of ascitic fluid, which could not gravitate from the anterior parietes of the abdomen on account of the adhesions. Subperitoneal fibroids are seldom single, and when there is more than one the margin of each can be more readily mapped out, and the probable character of the growth determined beforehand.

Differentiation sometimes impossible.

In review of this case, therefore, I do not see how it would be possible for one to say positively that the symptoms present were those of a uterine fibroid and not of ovarian dropsy. In other words, the differential diagnosis between these two affections (especially in case of a single fibro-cyst) is, in the present state of our knowledge, imperfect and impossible. In exceptional cases we can not tell one from the other, until after the exploratory incision is made.

An interesting case of this kind was related to me by Dr. B. R. Westfall, of Macomb, Illinois. I will read you from his notes:

Case.

"November 30, 1868.—Was called to see Mrs. S——, aged thirty-two years, then in her second labor. Noticing that the abdomen seemed unusually large, I placed my hand over the abdominal parietes, and found two distinct tumors of about equal size, which, during the contractions of the uterus, were sufficiently separated to enable me to trace the boundaries of each. Supposing the one to be an ovarian tumor, I questioned the patient to ascertain if *she* had discovered it. She said she had discovered both tumors in a few months after conception, and supposed that she would be delivered of twins. She had never felt any pain or other discomfort to lead her to suspect any disease. The labor progressed and terminated successfully. Recovery was as rapid as usual. I examined the tumor frequently afterward, and found each time that it was rapidly shrinking. After three months I could find no trace of it.

"In October, 1870, I was called to examine my patient again, as she was satisfied she was *enceinte*, and that the tumor was again being developed. I found it situated to the left of the uterus as before, and of about equal proportions with it. It continued to grow in the same ratio with the fœtus. No inconvenience was felt, except that the weight was unpleasant when she was upon her feet. Her subsequent labor and convalescence were as satisfactory as before, but the tumor did not decrease in size as rapidly as it had done before, and never entirely disappeared. The smallest it became was about the size and shape of a goose-egg. It remained for some time *in statu quo*.

"October 20, 1871.—Nine months after parturition, menstruation returned, and the tumor began to enlarge, and at each period to grow perceptibly. The growth was sudden, being most marked a few days before the menses were due. Fifteen months after its birth the child was weaned, and from this date the enlargement was still more rapid, until she has attained the size of a woman at the seventh month of gestation.

"January 10, 1872.—It being determined to resort to ovariotomy, the attending surgeon, who had diagnosticated the presence of a cyst, made the incision, and, upon inserting a trocar, failed to bring away any fluid. The tumor proved to be a fibroid. The woman died thirty hours after the operation."

If this same error had not been frequently committed by men of large experience and professional acumen, I should have felt a greater annoyance with the result in Mrs. D.'s case. Spencer Wells says: "It is very difficult—perhaps impossible—to distinguish between a multilocular ovarian cyst and a fibro-cystic uterine tumor when the cysts are large and the connection with the rest of the uterus is elongated. I removed one such tumor, which some men of great experience took to be ovarian. The cyst held twenty-six pints of fluid. The seat of pedicle connecting it with the uterus was three to four inches long, and the uterus moved quite independently of the tumor. Indeed, it was not until I came to divide the pedicle that I knew what I had to to deal with."

Dr. Charles C. Lee cites a case of fibro-cystic uterine growth which was mistaken for ovarian dropsy, in which the womb "*was perfectly movable on the sound, without imparting the slightest motion to the abdominal tumor.*" Indeed, in Dr. Lee's essay on the Diagnosis of Ovarian Tumors from Fibro-cystic Tumors of the Uterus,* you will find the particulars of eighteen cases, which although they had been diagnosticated as ovarian, proved, upon the section and separation of the growth from its peritoneal attachments, to be extra-uterine.

Spencer Wells has, in some cases, been able to diagnosticate a fibro-cyst of the uterus from ovarian dropsy by obtaining on paracentesis a thin serum which contained from five to fifteen per centum of blood. These were so intimately mixed that they would not separate until the fluid had been allowed to stand for some hours. But this particular fluid is not always or often obtained upon tapping. For according to Kœberlé, in the uterine fibrocyst it may be either yellowish, thin, serous and rich in lymph, or cholestrin, or brownish, muddy, sero-purulent or bloody. All of which signifies, that, as a distinguishing symptom, and separately considered, this sign is of no more value than the others.

* New York Medical Journal, vol. xix, p 452.

LECTURE XXVI.

APHTHOUS ULCERATION OF THE OS AND CERVIX UTERI.

GENTLEMEN:

This patient's clinical history will afford a good text for some remarks upon a form of uterine ulceration which, although it is not a very common, is nevertheless a very troublesome affection.

Case.—Mrs. S——, forty years of age, the mother of four children, has been ill for eighteen months past. She is pale, and has the worn look of one whose strength has been exhausted either by a drain of the vital fluids, or from inanition. She has a slight leucorrhœa, but the discharge bears no relation to the month, and from her description appears to be exclusively vaginal. There is at times much burning in the vagina, and at the neck of the womb. This is aggravated by standing a long time, or by riding. It is also apt to be worse in the evening. Sometimes there is strangury, but it is of brief duration and not very severe. There is not a great deal of inter-pelvic pain and distress. Her appetite is poor and capricious. Her food "does not appear to do her any good." Her nervous system is shattered. She cannot sleep, is exceedingly anxious about her children, and, in short, "nothing goes right any more." On examination the vagina is found to be considerably inflamed, hot and dry, and the anterior lip of the uterine cervix to be the seat of an aphthous ulcer, which is twice the size of the thumb nail. The only treatment she has had was a four months' course of bi-weekly cauterizations, from which her health became so bad that she was obliged to stop taking them.

This form of uterine ulceration begins with a slight vesicular, or herpetic eruption, which is located upon the cervix. The vesicles, which are as delicate as those of varicella, soon burst, the epithelium becomes detached, and small curd-like spots appear. With a pencil-brush these spots can be easily removed, and the denuded surface remains a *bona fide* ulcer. If a number of these vesicles coalesce,

The eruptive stage.

they finally develop into an extensive patch of ulceration. Sometimes the ulcers are small, yellow and of regular outline; again they are much larger, with an inflamed base and an irregular ragged outline. Now and then the serum discharged from the vesicles is so acrid and excoriating as to inoculate the neighboring surfaces.

Symptoms.

The chief characteristics of the aphthous ulcer, however, are its shallowness, its being preceded and accompanied usually by the herpetic eruption on the cervix uteri, and the repeated attempts and failures to reproduce the proper investing epithelium. The surface of this ulcer, as seen through the speculum, is half concealed beneath an abnormal investiture, which is constantly being exfoliated and reproduced. In this respect it resembles the aphthous ulcer of stomatitis, and like it, is an evidence of a depraved state of nutrition, a kind of scorbutic cachexia.

Diagnosis.

The diagnosis is very important, for it has very much to do with the treatment and conduct of the case. The only forms of uterine ulceration with which this is liable to be confounded are the diphtheritic and the syphilitic. From the diphtheritic ulcer it may be known by the delicate and imperfectly organized structure of the membrane that covers the ulcer, which in respect of its color and thickness, is very different from the wash-leather deposit in diphtheria. The attendant constitutional symptoms are much more grave in diphtheria than in an ordinary case of aphthous ulceration.

The syphilitic ulcer is of a dark, red hue, and never bright or yellow, and the general constitutional symptoms are wholly different from those which are incident to the aphthous form of uterine ulceration.

Causes.

The principal causes of this disease are defective nutrition, an impoverished state of the blood, chlorosis, tabes mesenterica, chronic gastritis or gastro-enteritis, and the exhausting processes of gestation and lactation.

Treatment.

The treatment is very simple, and if properly chosen, very successful. Much depends upon the correct diagnosis of the difficulty. Such cases are sometimes cured unwittingly, and neither the doctor nor the patient knows what has been done. More frequently, however, they are made worse by the treatment adopted. This result may often be ascribed to the fact that physicians do not always discriminate as to the particular variety of ulceration with which they have to deal, and that the means chosen are inappropriate, too harsh, and therefore harmful. It is not at all unusual for the simplest cases of this kind to run along for months, and finally, for them to be nearly or quite sacrificed upon the altar of a promiscuous cauterization.

Let me tell you, gentlemen, that in the whole range of our art, I do not know of any temptation to compare with that which sometimes prompts and permits the physician to diagnosticate and to pretend to cure the most serious uterine diseases when they have no real existence. Patients not unfrequently declare themselves ill with some particular "weakness," and, whether they are mistaken or not, will insist upon being treated therefor, either at our hands or by another. The fashion is to gratify them, and to put a premium upon every kind of local expedient especially.

Reprehensible practice.

Thousands of women have thus been cauterized for uterine ulceration which, before the application of the escharotic, had no existence. Multitudes of them have done penance by wearing pessaries, and supporters of every description for luxations of the womb that could not be found, except in their own imagination, or in that of the physician. They have been bed-ridden and abused until the weakness of the sex has become a by-word and a reproach, mainly because the doctors have been too anxious to "make out a case;" and afterwards, because they have seen fit to persecute them with the most harmful appliances.

The doctor who treats a broken leg or a case of small-pox must be skilled in diagnosis, and measurably honest. His selfishness may prompt him to make his patients as many visits as possible, and to extort a fabulous fee for his services; but, concerning the nature of the accident, or of the ailment in question, there is little relative opportunity for him to deceive the sufferer or the friends. But when he is consulted in the case of a woman who is supposed to be ill with a sexual infirmity, the conditions are changed. He makes his diagnosis in the dark, as it were, and who shall disprove it? His professional opinion is not open to criticism, nor his skill to a healthful competition. And hence the peculiar temptation, in this department of our calling, to those members of the profession who have a bias towards dishonesty, and who seize upon every opportunity to make the most out of a class of cases which are often obscure, intricate and tedious at the best.

Bennett and a host of lesser lights have decreed the uterine cervix to be the center of pathological interest in woman. Too many physicians make it the focus of pecuniary interest, and therefore punish it through personal cupidity and a lack of conscience, as well as of knowledge.

Here is a poor woman whose local disease is the sign and seal of a constitutional cachexy. She is ill from her head to her feet. Her whole organism is deranged. A few little vesicles were developed upon the neck of her womb. Their investing tunic was ruptured, and an aphthous ulcer was the consequence. That ulceration has perpetuated itself, because the general condition from which it came has not been cured. A moment's reflection will satisfy you that cauterization is contra-indicated. For even if its effect were locally beneficial, and not injurious, it could do no good in a general way. The cause would remain, and the consequence would repeat itself.

A constitutional and not merely a local disease.

A more skillful, and successful method of cure in these cases, is to set about correcting the vitiated condition of the system, precisely as you would in a case of stomatitis materna.* You may order a diet consisting chiefly of the nitrogenous principles. Beef, in the form of steak or broths, oyster-soup, the whites of eggs, and milk, are preferable. To correct the strumous habit, the vegetable acids are also necessary. Baked apples, peaches, grapes, oranges, or lemonade, are almost always grateful, and, I believe, useful in such cases. Where patients have foresworn tea and coffee, I have sometimes prescribed that they should resume their use, with a view to arrest the too rapid metamorphosis of tissue which is going on.

Improve the general health.

For the first or vesicular stage of this disorder, and in old cases where a new crop of vesicles appears from time to time, cantharis, rhus tox., or aurum muriaticum, are usually sufficient.

For the vesicular stage.

* See page 218.

If there is also an aphthous condition of the mouth and of the alimentary mucous membrane, you may find it necessary to prescribe arsenicum alb., hydrastin, nux vomica, belladonna, mercurius jod., or the nitric or sulphuric acid.

For the aphthous condition.

Locally, I think it a good plan, in this form of uterine ulceration especially, to use the same remedy that is administered internally. It can be applied with water, or glycerine, or both these substances as a vehicle. A very simple and available injection consists of adding a tablespoonful of glycerine to as much castile suds as will be needed for one application. In addition to the medicines already named, the coptis trifolia, borax, kali bichromatum, and of late years, the carbolic acid in weak solution, deserve to be mentioned in this connection. If the suppuration is very considerable, as it sometimes is, calendula injections may be used with advantage. Where there is chronic vaginitis, with profuse leucorrhœa, and desquamation of the vaginal epithelium, whatever variety of injection is chosen, may be brought in contact with the entire mucous membrane of that canal through such an instrument as this, which is a cylindrical speculum, that is perforated with numerous holes of the size of a large shot. For the herpetic form of this disease, Leadam recommends the injection of a weak solution of the thuja oc., to be repeated two or three times daily.

Local treatment.

The objection to the topical use of astringents, as for example, tannic acid, alum, and the acetate of lead, in cases of this kind is that they do not possess any especial and specifically curative relation to the disease itself; and also that they are extremely liable to cause such a modification of the circulation as shall tend to involve the menstrual function, and thereby to complicate the case.

Objections to astringents, etc.

We will give Mrs. S—— arsenicum alb. 3, a dose three times daily. Her diet will consist of bread and milk with beef, potatoes and tomatoes, for dinner. Once each day she will drink a glass of good fresh lemonade; and she will not let the day pass without going to walk or ride a little in the open air. She will also use the injection of castile suds and glycerine every night and morning.*

Prescription.

*In four weeks this patient was well. She took no other remedies.

DIPHTHERITIC ULCERATION OF THE OS UTERI.

In this variety of uterine ulceration the constitutional symptoms correspond with those which are present in diphtheria, affecting other portions of mucous membrane, as for example, the nasal and respiratory passages. There is the same evidence of blood-poisoning, the same prostration and attendant phenomena, and the same sequelæ that occur when the throat is the seat of the abnormal deposit.

Constitutional symptoms.

Examination per vaginam reveals an ulcer upon one or both lips of the cervix, which is covered, or nearly so, with a heterologous deposit. This deposit or pseudo-membrane is a foreign growth, which, in due time, exfoliates. In some cases instead of one or two large-sized ulcers, there are a number of small, whitish, shining patches, which vary in size from that of a split pea to half a hazel-nut. These patches may, or may not, coalesce. To the "touch" they impart a rough or dry sensation that is quite peculiar, and very different from the feel of other ulcers.

Physical symptoms.

The pseudo-membrane which covers the diphtheritic ulcer, or patch, is at first very adherent, and cannot be detached without more or less injury and consequent hæmorrhage. After a little while, however, the friction of the parts during the motion of the body, as in walking or sitting upright, or a careless introduction of the finger, or of the speculum, may separate them. Their removal leaves a raw, bleeding, painful, intractable, suppurating ulcer, which may, or may not, extemporize another wash-leather covering for itself. According to Becquerel, in the order of their coming, the formation of these false membranes precedes the development of the ulcer, or diphtheritic chancre. It is only while something of the covering remains that these ulcers can be diagnosticated with absolute certainty.

The pseudo-membrane.

As a rule the larger the surface of the diphtheritic ulcer, the more superficial it is; and *per contra*, the smaller its dimensions, the greater its depth. The deeper the ulcer, the more profuse the discharge. Sometimes the flow therefrom is acrid and corrosive, and as in

The depth of the ulcer, and the discharge.

nasal diphtheria especially, it destroys, or perhaps inoculates the adjacent tissues. This discharge is always fetid, and, when it is obtained directly from the ulcerated surface, emits the peculiar diphtheritic odor. True diphtheria may be produced in other persons by inoculation with this virus.

Diphtheritic ulceration of the os uteri is rarely an idiopathic affection. The throat and other parts are generally first attacked, and afterwards the vulva, vagina and neck of the womb. As in syphilitic ulceration, the superior vagina and cervix are less frequently the seat of the lesion than are the inferior vagina and the vulva. It has been remarked that, as in other forms of diphtheria, this species of uterine ulceration is especially liable to occur during the epidemic prevalence of variola, rubeola and erysipelas. Many obscure affections of the generative system have undoubtedly resulted from prolonged exposure to diphtheria, and the fatigue of nursing those who were ill with that disease. In these cases the utero-vaginal mucous membrane has probably been the seat of diphtheritic inflammation and ulceration, where nothing of the kind was suspected.

A secondary disease.

If the diphtheritic ulceration of the os and cervix uteri takes place during pregnancy, it is very likely to cause abortion; if during the lying-in state, it may invade the uterine cavity, in which case pseudo-membranous patches have been found at post mortem lining the uterus itself.

Dr. Tilt reports a case in which he claims that a patient had a diphtheritic ulcer of the os uteri from leech-bites. But, in order to produce a generic ulcer of this kind, it is necessary that the specific cause should be at work. For this specific agency, whatever it may be, is just as requisite in this case as it is in diphtheritic angina or conjunctivitis. The only cases of diphtheritic ulceration of the os uteri and the vagina which I have seen have occurred in the persons of those women who, from watching and taking care of those who were ill with diphtheria, became predisposed to this form of the complaint and took it in this way. It is possible, and even probable, that some previous disorder of the generative system, in each of these cases, may have caused the lesion to locate itself upon the uterus rather than in the throat. During the prevalence of an epidemic

Cause.

of diphtheria you should examine this class of patients very carefully with the speculum.

Treatment.

The treatment need not differ essentially from that proper for other forms of diphtheria. If any one remedy deserves more prominent mention than another, it is cantharis. And this not only because of its frequent indication in the treatment of other varieties of diphtheria, but also on account of its special curative relation to the cervix uteri. Mercurius jod., kali bich., kali brom., phytolacca, nitric acid, jodium and hepar sulphuris may be of great service under their especial indications.

Local treatment.

Locally, injections of the tincture of hydrastis, or calendula, or of any of the aforenamed remedies, diluted with water, or glycerine, or both, are sometimes very serviceable. If the discharge is very fetid and offensive, the chlorate of potassa, in the proportion of half a drachm to four fluid-ounces of distilled water, and used in the same manner, answers a good purpose as an antiseptic. And so also does a weak solution of carbolic acid, of kreasote, or of the permanganate of potash. The objection to the potash salt is on account of its color. My friend, Dr. W. H. Holcombe, has made use of the kali bichromicum, in the strength of half a grain of the crude drug dissolved in a tumbler of water, "as an injection for ulcerated os uteri, and even for leucorrhœa, with good effect." This may also be used for the relief of diphtheritic ulceration and of vaginal diphtheritis.

PELVIC CELLULITIS.—PERI-METRITIS.—PELVIC ABSCESS.

I will now show you a case of pelvic cellulitis. This patient comes from the woman's ward of the hospital, where she has been under my care for a week past. The following is her clinical history, as it was noted by the Resident Physician, Dr. Chas. Adams:

Case.—Mrs. S——, æt. 30, was delivered by forceps of a dead child twelve weeks ago. Following this her physician said that she had puerperal fever. When she entered the hospital she complained of acute pain in the right iliac region, which was aggravated by touch and motion. There was a tumor (for which she had been blistered) in the right iliac fossa, which was of irregular outline, and could be very plainly felt above the brim of the pelvis. The corresponding limb was retracted. She could not lie upon that side. She had diarrhœa, with black, shiny stools. She complained of cramps in the uterine region on going to stool. Burning during micturition. Emaciation. Pulse 85, and weak. Tongue coated. Yesterday she commenced to have a pretty free discharge of pus from the uterus, and her symptoms are already somewhat relieved. Until then the vagina was hot, dry and very sensitive. The tumor could be recognized by the "touch," located at the right side of the cervix uteri in the roof of the vagina.

Synonyms.—This disease has received several names which only serve to confuse the mind. Thus, among its synonyms are pelvic cellulitis, peri-uterine cellulitis, perimetritis, parametritis, pelvic abscess, intra-pelvic abscess, abscess of the uterus, inflammation and abscess of the broad ligaments. The term peri-uterine cellulitis, proposed by Dr. Thomas, as locating the lesion more definitely, and implying that this is one of the sequelæ of uterine disease or accident, is perhaps least objectionable.

You are aware that the pelvis is lined with a fascia which is reflected over the muscles contained within it, and over the pelvic organs also, and which serves to shield, to strengthen and to separate them. Now between the layers of this pelvic fascia, when they come into contact with each other, and also between the fascia and the organ which it covers or separates from another organ, there is interposed a quantity of loose cellular tissue. This tissue is particularly abundant between the folds of the broad ligaments, about the abdominal portion of the uterine cervix, between the uterus and the bladder, about the urethra, in the recto-vaginal septum, and in the recto-sacral space. There is considerable discrepancy among authors concerning the presence of this areolar tissue between the peritoneum and the uterus itself, a majority insisting that there is so little of it there as scarcely to be worth mentioning. Hence there are those physicians who insist that peri-uterine cellulitis proper is a kind of mythical disorder—one of the refinements of uterine diagnosis.

The pelvic cellular tissue.

But I apprehend that there is no real conflict between the authority of the anatomist on this point, and the experience of the gynæcologist, when he finds that attacks of inflammation are sometimes seated in the areolar tissue about the uterus. For this form of the disease is especially incident to the puerperal state. And when we remember the changes that take place in the other uterine textures in consequence of conception, I can see no reason to doubt that there is, during pregnancy, a corresponding growth and development of its cellular tissue also. Authors have not, in so far as I am aware, said anything on this subject. Nevertheless it may be true that this particular tissue, like the muscular coat of the womb, is produced and then removed to answer certain very important physiological ends; and that this consecutive development and decline constitute a predisposing cause of cellulitis as one of the contingents of labor, whether premature or at term. At any rate, I give you the hint as one that contains something practical.

An important suggestion.

Peri-uterine cellulitis, therefore, is an inflammation of the connective tissue about the uterus and within the pelvis. As I have said, when it is not traumatic, it rarely occurs except as a sequel or contingent of lying-in. Gestation and labor are, therefore, its most powerful predisponents. The disease is less frequent than puerperal peritonitis and phlebitis, but is probably more common than many practitioners have supposed. (*Exit the patient.*)

Frequency of.

Authors divide this disease into three, but I shall specify four stages. The first is that of congestion, the second of effusion, the third of absorption or resolution, and the fourth of suppuration. I add the stage of resolution, because I believe that appropriate treatment will sometimes enable us to cure our patients without allowing the disease to pass on to the suppurative stage.

Its four stages.

The First or Congestive Stage.—The congestion may set in abruptly a few hours after delivery, or it may be delayed until some days or even weeks have passed, and then may come on insidiously. The symptoms are such as mark the onset of inflammatory fever. There is a more or less decided chill, which may or may not be repeated. If the chill is lacking, it will be substituted by rigors, which are sometimes painful and persistent in ratio with the exhausted and debilitated condition of the patient. The febrile re-action is very decided. The heat of the skin is often intense, the pulse full, strong and

Symptoms of.

rapid, or, in weak subjects, quick, frequent and irritable. The tongue is furred, and not unfrequently there is nausea with disposition to emesis.

Intra-pelvic pain.

These symptoms are accompanied, or followed almost immediately, by intra-pelvic pain and distress. The location of this pain varies with the seat of the inflammation. If the cellular tissue between the broad ligaments is attacked, the pain will be referred to the corresponding side of the pelvis, in which it will be deep-seated and very severe. If the same tissue surrounding the uterine neck is the seat of the lesion, the suffering will be in the upper part of the vagina, and contact with this organ, even by the exercise of the most delicate "touch," will be insupportable. If the peritoneum is also inflamed, the pain will be acute and lancinating in character. Most of the pain experienced, however, is ascribed to the pressure of the effused fluid (which has escaped into this tissue) against the neighboring organs. In many cases the bladder, and in others the rectum, are thus mechanically pressed upon, giving rise to strangury and tenesmus, which are not relieved by the usual remedies. Very often, more especially after the tumor caused by the effused serum has been formed, the pain is described as throbbing and paroxysmal. It is usually not diffuse, but local and circumscribed in its extent. In acute cases the congestive stage is limited to a few hours.

Formation of the tumor.

The Second or Stage of Effusion.—As in peritonitis or pleurisy, the period of effusion generally follows in pretty rapid succession. The serum escapes from the capillaries into the meshes of the areolar tissue, infiltrates it, and solidifies as if it were out of the body, or just as it does in the pulmonary air-cells when it causes a hepatized state of the lung in pneumonia. The resulting tumor varies in its shape and size according to circumstances. If the space between the fasciæ is limited and of a particular shape, the "swelling" cannot be larger, and must be of the same configuration. It grows rapidly until it has attained its maximum size, becoming more and more firm and dense, or perhaps softer, in its structure. If the patient is in a weak, adynamic state, however, the clot will not be firm, and the tumor will remain flaccid, or become softer, in some such manner as it does in pelvic hæmatocele. In many examples the tumor is exquisitely tender to the touch, but again it is not so.

In the majority of cases of peri-uterine cellulitis, the tumefaction is situated in the lateral portion of the pelvis. You may find it in one or the other of the iliac regions. And its presence is best made out by means of the bi-manual exploration. The index finger of the right hand being introduced into the vagina for the purpose of examining the os and cervix uteri, as well as the cul-de-sac of Douglas, the iliac region is examined at the same time through the abdominal parietes with the other hand. Between the two the size, shape and consistence of the tumor, whether it be above the pelvic brim or below it, can be pretty accurately determined. If there are any remaining doubts, the finger may be introduced into the rectum, and so much of the posterior and lateral walls of the womb as are within reach may also be examined. As a rule the uterus is fixed, or but slightly movable.

Location of.

One of the first symptoms indicative of this effusion is a local heat, swelling and tenderness of the vagina, which is apt to be felt at one side of the canal, and limited to one spot. Later the vaginal wall covering the tumor becomes thickened and indurated. It may, or may not, remain sensitive.

Symptoms.

If the tumor develops in either iliac fossa, the corresponding limb will usually, but not always, be flexed. This retraction of the thigh relieves the pain by relaxing the muscles in the immediate vicinity of the tumor. It is involuntary, and more or less complaint will be made when the leg is distended.

In puerperal women the milk and lochia are usually suppressed. This complicates the case, and implicates the nervous system more especially. Delirium, insomnia, unrest, spasms, convulsions, and even mania have followed from this cause. In rarer cases there is retention of urine, and still more rarely an almost total suppression thereof. Vomiting is a frequent accompaniment of pelvic cellulitis, possibly, as Dr. Atthill suggests, because of the endo-metritis which generally coexists.

Incidental symptoms.

This stage of effusion, with its resulting tumor, may continue unchanged for a variable period ranging from one week to a month. There is no fixed limit to its duration. Sometimes, in consequence of a relapse, the congestion is again established, and the resulting effusion following, there is an increased pouring out of serum and a marked and sudden growth of the tumor. Again the inflammation being passive, the tumor becomes insensibly larger. Or it may develop in the right iliac fossa, and when some considerable time has elapsed, commence to grow and finally attain a marked development in the left one. Successive tumors of this kind occurring in the same locality, are by no means rare.

Course and duration.

The Third Stage, or that of Resolution.—The stage of absorption, or of resolution, is that in which the tumor may remain for some time at a stand-still, and finally pass away without ending in suppuration. As you will infer, if for any reason, as for example because of a depraved cachexia, great debility from previous illness, inanition or excessive medication, the patients' vitality is very much reduced, the resolution of the swelling would be impossible, and suppuration would almost inevitably follow. Under the circumstances, therefore, in which we are likely to find these patients, this third stage of the disease will frequently be lacking altogether.

May be wanting.

But when her strength has previously been good, her gestation and labor have been accomplished without too great a draught upon her nutritive and nervous resources; when she has been well nursed and properly fed, medicated and otherwise cared for; and above all when there is no prevalent epidemic erysipelas, or puerperal disorder, we may observe the tumor gradually and quietly resolving itself away under appropriate treatment. If the swelling consists of effused serum, and not of coagulable lymph, it may be more readily absorbed.

Conditions that promote resolution.

The Fourth, or Suppurative Stage.—If left to itself, however, or mal-treated, and in a majority of cases almost inevitably, the tendency of this disease is to terminate in suppuration. With the commencement of this process the symptoms vary as in the case of abscesses located elsewhere. If the pain and tenderness have subsided, they are very apt to return. The tumor may become extremely sensitive again, and motion, or the pressure upon the tumor caused by an attempt

Symptoms of.

to stand upon the feet, to urinate, or while at stool, may occasion extreme suffering. The limb cannot be extended. The patient's body is flexed in the bed. A species of hectic fever, of a remittent type, sets in. There are rigors alternating with great heat, and evening exacerbations of fever, which sometimes mislead the physician. When she sleeps there is a profuse and exhausting perspiration, as in the worst cases of phthisis. The face and skin are pale. The countenance assumes the expression which surgeons recognize as characterizing that pus has been formed somewhere in the body, and is awaiting its discharge. The pulse continues rapid, although it has lost in strength. There is anorexia and great debility, with or without diarrhœa.

Accompanying hectic.

Even although the tumor may have been firm and like fibro-cartilage, or almost like scirrhus, to the touch, it now begins to soften. This softening may be recognized either by abdominal or vaginal palpation, or by both combined. It may occur gradually, or develop itself more rapidly. The weaker the patient the less the resistance to this process, and the more speedy the resulting fluctuation. This fluctuation is in most cases observable at the upper part of the vagina at one side of, or directly behind the cervix uteri, in the posterior cul-de-sac. "From some peculiar arrangement of the layers of the pelvic fasciæ, when pus is formed in the course of a pelvic cellulitis, occurring in the upper half of the true cavity of the pelvis—and this, you must remember, is the most frequent seat of the disease—it has a tendency always to point in this direction and to find an exit for itself, either at the lower base of the broad ligaments, or in the posterior cul-de-sac of the vault of the vagina; and it is at these spots, where the fascial layer seems to be unusually thin and weak, that the feeling of fluctuation is ordinarily first detected."*

Seat of the fluctuation.

Now this fluctuation may be due to the presence of effused liquor sanguinis, or of pus. But if the disease has persisted, as in the case before us, for a considerable time, and been attended by the inflammatory fever, followed by the hectic, the copious perspiration after sleeping, and the frequent, irritable pulse, you may be reasonably assured of the presence of pus in the tumor.

Diagnosis of the presence of pus.

*Clinical Lectures on the Diseases of Women, by Sir J. Y. Simpson. D. Appleton & Co., New York, 1872, page 72.

Concerning the means of escape for the pus, when it has been formed, it is important to remember that it may extemporize an outlet for itself through the bladder, the uterus, the vagina, or the rectum. If it forms at the superior strait, it may gravitate, and, running down along the course of the muscles, may pass beneath the pelvic fasciæ, and escape with the femoral vessels, so as to point near the groin. Sometimes it passes backwards through the great ischiatic foramen, and forms an abscess in the region of the hip; or it may even point at the great trochanter of the thigh bone. In rare instances it perforates both the uterus and the bladder, and leaves a fistula between them. Still more rarely, perhaps, it discharges into the cavity of the peritoneum. In seventy cases of puerperal pelvic cellulitis, Dr. McClintock, of Dublin,* found that thirty-seven ended with suppuration and the discharge of pus. Of these twenty-four were opened externally, or burst, of which twenty were discharged from the iliac region, two above the pubis, one in the inguinal region, and one beside the anus. Six others found an outlet through the vagina, five through the anus, and two burst into the bladder.

Its varied means of escape.

With respect to the essential nature of this disorder, I have long held and taught the idea set forth by Virchow, that, in reality, it is a species of erysipelas. Its clinical history, its epidemic prevalence, and its special therapeutics, correspond with those of erysipelas, more closely than with any other disorder. It is quite probable that many cases of this disease have been mistaken for puerperal peritonitis, and that the propagation of this latter malady by certain fomites is really to be explained upon the theory of the inoculability of the erysipelatous poison as in the case of phlegmonous erysipelas.

Essential nature of pelvic cellulitis.

Is probably allied to erysipelas.

Causes.—I have already reminded you that pelvic cellulitis is one of the contingencies of lying-in. It may follow in consequence of injuries sustained in natural unassisted labor. One of its most frequent causes is the traumatic injury of the cervix uteri by pressure of the presenting part, especially of the head, during delivery. In abortion

Parturition.

* Clinical Memoirs on the Diseases of Women.

it may follow a similar injury to the neck of the womb. For this reason it is comparatively frequent where abortion has been induced by means that are almost necessarily harmful. Women have sometimes brought it on themselves in this way.

A sequel to dystocia.

Puerperal cellulitis is one of the sequelæ of instrumental delivery, more especially when the resort to the forceps and other instruments has been unwarrantably delayed, when they have been ignorantly or carelessly used, and when the patient has not received the proper attention and nursing after their employment. These causes are more efficient in proportion with the debilitated and depraved condition of the patient's system, and also with her proneness to scrofulosis, phthisis, and even to certain acute diseases, as, for example, pneumonia and erysipelas.

A contingent of uterine surgery.

The non-puerperal cellulitis may result from the forcible introduction, or the prolonged retention, of the sound and the sponge or other tents. The wearing of intra-uterine pessaries, even the best of them, is very apt to induce it. Incision of the cervix uteri, whether for the cure of obstructive dysmenorrhœa, for the removal or arrest of development of fibroids, or even for the arrest of uterine hæmorrhage, is not an infrequent cause. It has followed amputation of the cervix, ovariotomy, the ligation of polypi, the excision of hæmorrhoidal tumors, the operation for vesico- and recto-vaginal fistulæ, and also that for ruptured perineum. It has also resulted from the use of very severe escharotics, as the potassa cum calce; the wearing of vaginal pessaries for a long time without removal; excessive and too forcible coitus; and the extension of corporeal metritis and ovaritis to the areolar tissue about the uterus, and between the layers of the broad ligaments.

Coincident Diseases.—Peri-uterine cellulitis rarely runs its whole course without being more or less complicated with other diseases. This is true, indeed, of most of the ailments for which you will be called upon to prescribe. The lines that separate pneumonia from pleurisy, or rheumatism from neuralgia, for example, are much more distinct and clear in the books than you will find them to be at the bedside. So you will most frequently observe that this form of cellulitis is more or less confounded with pelvi-peritonitis, ovaritis, and endometritis, in which case its clinical history and symptoms will be modified accordingly.

Diagnosis.—This fact complicates its diagnosis. If you are not more skillful than your predecessors, you will sometimes be puzzled to differentiate between pelvic peritonitis, pelvic hæmotocele, uterine fibroids and pelvic cellulitis. Let me beg your earnest attention therefore, while I tell you how you may know them apart.

Sometimes very difficult.

The pelvic areolar tissue being between the layers of the broad ligaments, and beneath the outer coat of the uterus, both of which structures are composed of reflections of peritoneum, it may be supposed that in case of inflammation of either of them, the symptoms must necessarily be very distinct, not to say pathognomonic, in order to be recognized. As a rule, the pain in the first stage, prior to effusion, is less acute in cellulitis than in pelvi-peritonitis. In the former, if the exudation of the liquor sanguinis is copious, the suffering is increased by it; while in the latter, as in pleurisy or synovitis, the effusion is followed by a mitigation, if not by an entire remission of pain; which may return, but which, from that time forward, is less acute and altogether changed in its character.

From pelvi-peritonitis.

In most cases of cellulitis the tenderness, pain and local heat are referred to and commence in the iliac fossæ. The same is true of puerperal ovaritis, in which the peritoneal investment of the ovary becomes inflamed during lying-in. But in the former the pain does not change its location, nor does it incline to become diffused over the abdomen, both of which symptoms are proper to ovaritis occurring in puerperal women.

I have copied Dr. Thomas' table, giving the differential signs between peri-uterine cellulitis and pelvi-peritonitis, upon the blackboard:*

PERI-UTERINE CELLULITIS.	PELVIC PERITONITIS.
1. Tumor easily reached, generally found to one side of the uterus, and may be felt above the pelvic brim;	1. Tumor, if discoverable, very high, only in vaginal cul-de-sac, does not extend above the superior strait;
2. Tendency to suppuration;	2. Suppuration less common;
3. Abdominal tenderness chiefly over one iliac fossa;	3. Abdominal tenderness excessive above brim of the pelvis;

* A Practical Treatise on the Diseases of Women. By T. Gaillard Thomas, M.D., etc. Third edition, 1872, page 461.

PERI-UTERINE CELLULITIS.	PELVIC PERITONITIS.
4. Tumefaction generally noticed laterally in the pelvis ;	4. Generally noticed near or upon the median line ;
5. Tendency to monthly relapses not marked ;	5. Tendency to relapse every month very marked ;
6. Retraction of thigh not rare ;	6. Retraction of thigh rarely occurs ;
7. Pain severe and steady ;	7. Pain excessive and often paroxysmal :
8. Facies not much altered ;	8. Facies very anxious ;
9. Nausea and vomiting not excessive ;	9. Nausea and vomiting often excessive ;
10. Does not necessarily displace the uterus ;	10. Displaces the uterus as a rule ;
11. Uterus fixed to a limited extent ;	11. Uterus immovable on all sides.

The statement of some of these signs needs to be qualified. If, for example, the inflammation in cellulitis were always limited to the broad ligament on either side, the tumor could invariably be reached without difficulty by downward pressure in the corresponding iliac fossa. But the fact is that it has no such constant seat. It may happen that the connective tissue surrounding the inferior segment of the womb, or about the cervix uteri, shall be inflamed, while that which separates the layers of the broad ligament escapes altogether. In this case we should fail to find the tumor at the superior strait, but might detect it per vaginam or by the rectum. In exceptional instances of pelvic cellulitis; it is impossible to locate the tumor at all.

Peritonitis is more directly related to disorders of menstruation, and to the return of the monthly cycle, than cellulitis. The commencement and brief continuance of the peritoneal pain in the median line, and the absence of a marked tendency to suppuration, will generally enable you to separate this disease from pelvic cellulitis. Owing to the extension of the inflammation in this form of peritonitis, the induration, if there is any, is not always located in the median line, as the pain was at the beginning of the attack. When gonorrhœal, or, indeed, ordinary inflammation, extends from the uterine cavity through the Fallopian tubes, and invades the abdomen and the pelvis, it is more likely to give rise to peritonitis than to cellulitis. You should not forget that, while pelvi-peritonitis is quite a common affection with non-puerperal women, pelvic cellulitis almost never occurs excepting among those who have recently been confined.

It must be acknowledged, however, that the lines which separate these two diseases are not always distinct. For, whether it be due to the fact that the textures involved are contiguous, and that these lesions frequently co-exist, or that our present means of differentiation are imperfect, it remains that they may be combined without our knowing it, and that we are liable occasionally to mistake one for the other.

They may co-exist.

Although pelvic cellulitis and pelvic hæmatocele are both of them most frequent after delivery, yet the conditions of the patient's general system upon which they are prone to occur are very different. Thus, pelvic hæmatocele takes place in consequence of a weak, adynamic state in which the blood has become of bad quality by extreme losses, as in uterine hæmorrhage, or from the rupture of one or more small vessels during labor. It is also incident to the hæmorrhagic diathesis. Neither of these conditions pertain to the etiology of pelvic cellulitis.

From pelvic hæmatocele.

In pelvic hæmatocele the formation of the tumor is not preceded by local congestion, and symptoms proper to the first stage of an acute inflammation, as in cellulitis. It comes on suddenly, and is accompanied by signs of prostration, sinking and collapse. The tumor in hæmatocele varies in its consistence, but is never hard and ligneous to the feel, like that of cellulitis. The more impoverished the blood, the softer the tumor. In cellulitis, the tendency toward suppuration causes the swelling to become softer as it grows older. The opposite change occurs in the hæmatomatous tumor, which gradually becomes harder than it was originally.

Uterine fibroids come on insidiously and grow very slowly. Until they occasion trouble mechanically they are neither sensitive nor do they cause pain in the womb or the adjacent parts. If sub-mucous, or interstitial, they are characterized by the frequent occurrence of metrorrhagia, and inter-periodic hæmorrhage, which is not a contingent of cellulitis. The tumor, in case of fibroid, is firm and not œdematous to the feel, and there is no tendency in it toward suppuration. Fibroids do not render the uterus immovable, as the tumor in cellulitis often does.

From uterine fibroids.

In case, however, that you can not otherwise decide as to the nature of the pelvic tumor, you may pass the exploring-needle into it from its vaginal surface. If you bring away a drop or two of pus upon the instrument, it is a positive sign of abscess; if blood only, and that of a dark, purplish color, it may be a case of hæmatocele; and if no specimen of any kind of abnormal product is obtained, the negative symptom will satisfy you that it is probably a case of uterine fibroid. This is an excellent means of diagnosis and may really be a great blessing in your hands. For the safety of your patient, as well as of your own reputation, will depend upon your skill in diagnosis.

Relapsing abscess.

Sequelæ.—The most common sequel of this form of cellulitis is pelvic abscess. It often happens that the evacuation of the tumor a single time will not suffice. In many cases these abscesses continue to discharge for months and even for years. The accompanying symptoms vary with the location of the tumor and its means of outlet. Incredible quantities of pus are poured out, and the patient's strength and vitality are so undermined that her health may be ruined thereby.

Sterility.

Another result of this disease, which is frequently entailed upon those who have had it, is sterility. It is not unusual for a woman to lose her first-born in consequence of a difficult labor, to have cellulitis in child-bed, and to recover her health in every respect, except that in future she remains barren. In this case the cellular inflammation has caused the function of reproduction to be suspended. This frequently happens as an indirect result of criminal abortion.

Menstrual disorders.

Menstruation is sometimes most seriously implicated, either because of ovarian complications, with cellulitis, or from some partial or complete obstruction of the Fallopian tube or of the cervix uteri.

Other sequelæ include certain uterine displacements, and the vesico- or recto-vaginal fistulæ which are sometimes caused by sloughing of the septa between the bladder, or the bowels and the vagina.

The general conditior and concurrent disease.

Prognosis.—The prognosis should be cautiously made. If it is possible to secure the resolution of the tumor, and to prevent serious relapses, the patient will probably recover. Much will depend, however, upon the general strength and vitality. If these shall be very much reduced, the case is less promising. So also with the chronic and incurable disorders of digestion with which it may be complicated. But you should not despair of curing even the worst attack, provided the patient is not already moribund, and you can supply certain physiological requisites for her recovery.

If the disease is epidemic, the prospects are less favorable. If it occurs in the winter or spring months, during stormy and inclement weather, when erysipelas, diphtheria, scarlatina, or dysentery, and kindred diseases are prevalent, it subtracts so much from the chances of recovery. Those cases which arise from traumatic injury are generally more grave than such as are referable to more ordinary causes.

The epidemic tendency.

If the disease invades other organs, as when the pus that has formed finds an outlet through the uterus or the bladder, it may prove fatal through the serious complications that follow. If the abscess discharges into the cavity of the abdomen, the patient will be very apt to die suddenly.

The janitor's bell, which is as inevitable as one's shadow, has overtaken us. I will speak of the treatment of pelvic cellulitis at my next lecture.

LECTURE XXVII.

PELVIC CELLULITIS (CONTINUED).

GENTLEMEN:

At the close of the last lecture I had finished my remarks on the special pathology of peri-uterine cellulitis. In illustration of the fact that this disease may run an erratic course, and finally develop into pelvic abscess, and that physicians are prone to err in its diagnosis, I will read you the notes of a case which is still under treatment. The report was taken verbatim from the patient's mouth:

Case.—I am twenty-eight years old, and was confined two years ago with my first and only child. I had enjoyed perfect health during pregnancy, excepting a soreness of one of my breasts, which was occasioned by my own imprudence. My labor began at seven o'clock in the evening, and lasted until one o'clock the next morning, when I was delivered of a dead child. I was under the care of a midwife who gave me some powders, a little wine, and free draughts of cinnamon tea, in order to hasten the pains, which she thought were too slow. From ten P.M. to one o'clock A.M., I had one continual pain, and was finally delivered in the standing posture. The child which, two hours before its birth had been alive, was a very large one.

For some days after delivery I lost a great deal of clotted and very offensive blood. I had pains low in the sides and groins almost immediately, and, five days afterwards was taken with a very severe chill, which was followed by a burning fever. The milk disappeared twenty-four hours later. The flow became yellowish and watery, instead of bloody. A physician was called, who decided that I had puerperal fever. He prescribed medicines to control the fever, and ordered vaginal injections of water containing carbolic acid. At first I seemed to improve, but in a few days the pain in the sides returned. The doctor examined me internally (with a speculum), and said that I had ulcers on the neck of the womb. He burned them twice a week for about six weeks with the nitrate of silver, but, before they were cured, I was taken one morning with severe cramps in the bowels, which lasted the whole day, and were followed by chills and fever. These cramps came every two or three days, and were very painful. The doctor ordered paregoric, and afterwards laudanum.

In the middle of the following May I was compelled to change my residence. My ride in the carriage was a very painful one, and in a few days I was worse than ever. I began to have a severe and steady pain in the left side of the bowels, low down (iliac region), and the doctor, after another examination, declared me to be threatened with an ovarian tumor and hardening of the left ligament. A greenish ointment was applied over the whole side of the abdomen, and the swelling gradually disappeared, but the ligament (Poupart's) has always remained hard. I took at that time a great deal of iron, and of the iodide of potash, continuing it until my stomach could support it no longer.

In the summer a diarrhœa, with straining, and a pain which continued after each passage, set in. This lasted for many months and left my bowels in a very weak state. I, however, improved gradually, and finally the doctor ordered me to go out of doors. Walking was difficult and painful. In August, while in the open air, I caught a severe cold, and became very sick again, with cramps in the stomach and bowels, vomiting and diarrhœa, with dreadful straining. Another physician was called in counsel, and I was said to be in great danger. They said I had a commencing peritonitis, with great swelling of the womb and general inflammation.

The end of September came before I was able to be up again, but the diarrhœa and pains continued, and made me so weak and wretched that, in the following January, I resolved to try Homœopathy, and accordingly sent for Dr. S****. Within a month the diarrhœa and pain ceased entirely, my appetite returned, and I gained flesh and strength. I felt so much better, indeed, that I accepted a proposition to go to Europe. But toward the middle of March, I began to feel considerable pain in the right side (iliac region), which, until that time, had been well. These pains soon became so severe that I lost all rest. Nothing unnatural could be seen or felt in that locality. The pains were of a tearing character, and extended from the right hip through the groin to the knee. All the pains which I had suffered before were as nothing compared with these. For six weeks I never slept without taking the hydrate of chloral, a very little of which sufficed.

Dr. S. thought my suffering was due to neuralgia, and, believing that the sea-air would most probably cure me, advised me not to abandon the idea of going abroad. Consequently, although I had noticed two small lumps in my left groin, as they were not painful, I paid no attention to them, and left Chicago for New York in the latter end of May. The journey proved very hurtful, the lumps increased in size, and I was compelled to take to my bed almost immediately after my arrival in New York.

The first of June Dr. F***** came to see me, and after a thorough examination told me that I had no sign of ever having had an ovarian tumor, that the glands were swollen, that my sickness would be tedious, but that, with proper care, he thought I would recover. He did not wish to frighten me by saying that I already had one or more abscesses.

The first of these abscesses was opened by the doctor on the eighth day of June, and the second a week later. Even after they were discharged, moving in the bed was very difficult, and walking quite impossible. The flow of pus continued profusely for about a month, and, having given up the proposed voyage, I was not well enough to return to Chicago until the twelfth day of July. Dr. F. feared lest the journey by rail might determine another abscess, but it did not seem to do as much harm as it had done before.

Arrived at home, I placed myself under the care of Dr. R. Ludlam, and although I still suffered severely at times, I was able to get up and to sit in an arm-chair before the fire. Walking was still difficult, and I abstained from it. The Great Fire came early in October, my house was burned up, and it was expected that it would prostrate me entirely; but in this we were agreeably disappointed, for I never felt so well as for about six months afterwards. One abscess (orifice) closed entirely, and the other almost ceased to discharge.

At the end of March I began to experience a return of the old pains in the left side, which were attributed to my having walked too far in making an excursion down town. I had chills and fever, and the doctor feared that another abscess would form. Three weeks later an abscess pointed just beneath the scar formed by the first one. It was lanced, and discharged, but less freely than before. In all other respects, excepting this local trouble, I am well.

In addition to the symptoms which this patient has detailed so intelligently, others were elicited on physical examination. While this last abscess was forming, the "touch" revealed a swelling of about the size of a pullet's egg in the left vaginal cul-de-sac. This tumor was somewhat soft and very sensitive, so that when I pressed upon it my patient felt inclined to faint. The left border of the uterus and of the cervix were tumefied and puffy, or œdematous. The

Further symptoms.

Douglas' cul-de-sac felt thickened, indurated, and less supple than natural, giving the impression that (probably at the time she experienced the severe tenesmus of the bowel) there had been a retro-uterine tumor also. The vagina was hot and dry. Conjoined manipulation, with pressure in the left iliac fossa, could not be borne. The peri-rectal tissue was also indurated. The bladder and urethra appeared to have escaped implication. Abdominal palpation was not painful. The uterus was forced to the opposite, or right side of the pelvis (right latero-version), a displacement which might explain the prolonged and severe attack of neuralgia from which she had suffered more than a year before.

I must not omit a reference to the fact that in this case the two first abscesses discharged above, and the last one below Poupart's ligament. She is taking calcarea carbonica[3], morning, noon and night.

Treatment.— It has been said that practically it is not a very serious matter to be able to form a correct diagnosis between pelvic cellulitis and the diseases which so closely resemble it. But, gentlemen, I am of a very different opinion. For, suppose a physician should tell you that it was of very little consequence to him whether his patient had the pleurisy or the erysipelas, and that the treatment was substantially the same, no matter what the name of the disease, what would you say of him, and what would be the measure of your trust in him as a skillful and successful practitioner? And if we expect him to discriminate between pleurisy and erysipelas, why should he not also, when it is possible, separate peritonitis from erysipelas? In other words, if there is a difference in the morbid anatomy of inflammation which varies with its seat in particular tissues, and if these differences are always characteristic of the disease in question, why should they not modify the treatment accordingly? Since the symptoms, course, and mode of termination of the diseases are really so unlike, is there any good reason why an inflammation of a serous membrane should be treated as if it were identical with an inflammation of the cellular tissue? I think not.

Inferences based on correct diagnosis.

I know that it is possible, and that there is a strong temptation so to refine and to rarify the symptoms by which diseases are differentiated as to leave no particular meaning in them, and to exclude a more practical idea of disease and its treatment. But this is the other extreme. We must, and will always have, a theory of the disease which we undertake to cure. And, good or bad, true or false, that theory stands in our minds as a chart of its special pathology. Other things equal, the clearer and more correct our views on the subject, the fuller will be the measure of our success and usefulness; for the physician who knows as definitely and accurately as possible what it is that he wishes to cure, will usually exercise the greatest care in the choice of the means which he employs to that end.

Pathological deductions.

Now our clinical knowledge of the nature, peculiarities, complications, and tendencies of cellulitis enables us, not only to treat the symptoms that are present in the earlier stages of the disease, but to forecast and avert such as might and would otherwise follow. When we are called to a patient like either of those of whom I have spoken, and whose case is the groundwork of these remarks, we must cast about to see if we can not terminate the inflammation, or at least avoid some of its more serious consequences.

And what are the consequences that we wish, if possible, to turn aside? They are (1) to prevent the exudation of the liquor sanguinis, or serum, into the meshes of the intra-pelvic areolar tissue; (2) if it has been already poured out, to promote its absorption and removal, and (3) to prevent suppuration, or abscess. These general indications, therefore, correspond with, and concern the three last stages of pelvic cellulitis, viz.: effusion, resolution and suppuration.

General indications.

If we consider these enquiries in the order named, you will perhaps be able to obtain the best idea of the special therapeutics of pelvic cellulitis. It is as reasonable to suppose that we have remedies which are capable of acting in such a manner upon the congested cellular tissue as to prevent effusion therein, as that we have those which are known to produce a similar effect in the first stage of serous inflammations. There is no reason why, if we begin in season, many cases of threatened cellulitis should not be prevented from progressing beyond the stage of congestion. We ought to be able to cut short

To prevent effusion.

this disease as we sometimes do pleurisy, peritonitis, synovitis, and pneumonia.

Of course, if the patient is peculiarly susceptible, and the internal conditions, as well as the external circumstances, conspire to produce it; and more than all, if we are not called in the incipient stage, or what is equivalent, do not know what disease we are prescribing for, the chances are that effusion will not, or can not be prevented. But our duty is plain. If there are remedies that are capable of removing and relieving the accumulation and stagnation of red and white corpuscles in the vessels of this same connective tissue, and of thus averting the consequences that might follow, we should be prepared to prescribe them intelligently.

Aconite.

The well-known effects of aconite in allaying the fever, in equalizing the circulation, in promoting a critical perspiration, or diuresis, and putting an end to threatened local inflammation, renders it very useful in this stage of the disease. The disease being consecutive to parturition, and allied as it is in most cases to surgical fever, the earlier this remedy is used the better. My own preference is to give it in the second or third decimal attenuation, and, under these particular circumstances, to repeat the dose as often as every fifteen or twenty to thirty minutes.

Arnica.

If the patient suffered extremely during labor, if labor was very prolonged, or if it was completed by instrumental aid, arnica may be used both topically and internally. There is no valid objection against alternating aconite and arnica for the relief of these symptoms. The arnica should, however, be given at longer intervals than the aconite, and, if you prefer it, in a higher potency.

Belladonna.

Belladonna has a specific relation to cellulitis, especially if it is of an erysipelatous type or character. In the outset of the attack it may even be preferable to aconite, providing there is not a very high degree of fever, and the nervous symptoms predominate. Given early and rapidly, it may suffice to avert the inflammation, particularly in the case of nervous and delicate women, with arrest of the lochia, meteorism of the abdomen, throbbing headache, delirium and photophobia. Many experienced and reliable practitioners prescribe aconite and belladonna in alternation for the relief of these symptoms, and are of opinion that, thus given, they do most excellent service. Whether or not the same prompt and desirable results could, in this instance, be obtained by the remedies given singly, my experience will not enable me to decide. Nor will the experience of any single practitioner settle this question for you.

Veratrum viride.

There is another remedy which I believe to be of incalculable service in the incipient stage of puerperal cellulitis, as indeed it is in puerperal peritonitis also. That remedy is the veratrum viride. Those of you who were present at the meeting of the Chicago Academy of Medicine, held last month (February, 1872), will remember the excellent report of Dr. W. H. Burt, of this city, on the physiological and toxical effects of this poison.* Its wonderful power to control and regulate the vascular movements, to equalize the circulation, and, as it were, to stamp out a local congestion that would almost inevitably result in inflammation, is being recognized by physicians of all schools.

My experience, as stated before the Academy during the discussion on Dr. Burt's paper, has satisfied me that this remedy holds some specific relation to the female generative system. Precisely what that relation is, I can not say. But it appears to be especially adapted to the relief and removal of puerperal inflammation. For many years I have been in the habit of prescribing it whenever, in a lying-in woman, the first symptoms of pelvic, or peritoneal congestion show themselves; and, when my directions have been faithfully followed, the result has been most happy. It restores the milk and lochia, when these have been suddenly suppressed, quiets the nervous perturbation, relieves the tympanites and the tenesmus, whether vesical or rectal, and frequently cuts short the attack. When called in season, I have seldom failed to set aside a threatened cellulitis by the same means. My custom is to give it in the second or third decimal dilution. In an urgent case, the dose should be repeated every twenty minutes or half hour, for four or five times successively, and afterwards less frequently.

You will find the particulars of some very interesting cases of

* See the U. S. Med. and Surgical Journal, Vol. VII, page 268.

erysipelas cured by the local and general use of the veratrum viride in Prof. Hale's work on Materia Medica.*

In addition to the faithful employment of one or more of these internal remedies, it may serve a good purpose, and can do no possible harm, to resort to the local use of dry heat by means of hot flannels, or of a dinner plate that has been immersed in hot water, wrapped in flannel and then placed directly over the seat of the pain. Sometimes great good can be effected by applications of towels or cloths wrung out of hot water, and frequently repeated. But best of all is the simple, old-fashioned bran poultice that I have so frequently recommended you not to forget in cases of threatened puerperal inflammation of whatever variety.

Local adjuvants.

For the stage of effusion, which in many, and perhaps in a majority of cases (as you will be called to them in private practice), can not be averted, a different class of remedies are certain to be indicated. Prominent among them are apis mellifica, arsenicum alb., bryonia, rhus toxicodendron, digitalis, cantharis, mercurius sol., stibium, helleborus niger, colchicum and sulphur, which may be given according to the particular symptoms, or group of symptoms that are present.

For the stage of effusion.

Concerning the use of the apis mel., which is an invaluable remedy at this stage of the complaint, I am of the opinion that many physicians have failed with it because the preparation which they have given has not been trustworthy. In 1868, my friend, Dr. J. D. Craig, of Niles, Mich., sent me a trituration of the remedy which he had prepared and prescribed with excellent effect. His method was to extract the sting of the honey-bee, and its poison-bag also, with a pair of forceps, and then to triturate these with the saccharum lactis in the proportion of two grains of the sugar to one sting. This he called the first trituration, from which others could be made in the usual manner. I have prescribed this preparation in the second stage of cellulitis, and in dropsical disease, with good effect, and can therefore recommend it to you.

Apis mel.

But, if you desire to facilitate resolution, and to counteract the

* The Hom. Mat. Medica of the New Remedies, by E. M. Hale, M.D., etc., second edition, 1867, page 1053.

tendency to suppuration (which indications are identical), it is indispensable for you to put your patient upon a good diet. If the digestion is impaired, and food can not be taken, or tolerated, that disorder should be corrected as speedily as possible. And, when it is remedied, you must see to it that your patient is not starved into the very condition that you wish to avoid. For in most cases of this kind, the quantity of serum effused, the size of the tumor, and the risk of abscess bear a proper relation to the impaired quality of the blood, and to the too rapid destruction of tissue that is going on in the system. And, unless the patient's strength is fortified against it, you will learn when it is too late, that either a passive, but very extensive, infiltration of serum has taken place, or that pus has already been formed and is seeking an outlet.

A good diet.

Under these circumstances, therefore, do not permit the febrile condition to mislead you. If such a result were desirable, a rigid diet would be the very best means of inducing a hectic fever and its attendant symptoms. For the weaker your patient, the greater the liability to fever and to the non-removal of the tumor, excepting through the process of suppuration. In puerperal women, especially, whose strength has been taxed during gestation, and who have survived the martyrdom of labor, there is a strong predisposition to the *diathèse de suppuration* of Trousseau. If you persist in keeping them upon an insufficient aliment, the best chosen remedies will not help you out of the difficulty. Indeed this is one of those conditions in which good food may be worth more than medicine. I firmly believe that the patient who was before you at my last lecture, would have died during her first week in the hospital if she had not been properly nourished.

Caution.

Nor do I know of anything that is more beneficial in some of these cases than certain preparations of alcohol. There is no danger of exciting inflammation or fever by the proper use of the best brandy, or whiskey. Stimulation will be well borne, and may bridge over the chasm. The alcohol acts most beneficially if mixed with some nutrient, as for example, with milk, the whites of eggs, or beef tea. Two or three table-spoonfuls of milk punch may be given every one to four hours, according to circumstances, and continued until the

Stimulants.

crisis has passed. Wine will not suffice. The malt liquors will answer a better purpose farther on.

Emollients.

Certain external means may conduce to the same end. I have great confidence in the bran poultice already recommended. It may be applied day and night for an indefinite period. Where the induration, or rather, the tumor is above the brim of the pelvis, an excellent expedient, designed to facilitate its resolution, is the local application of the camphorated oil, which consists, as you know, of gum camphor dissolved in olive oil. The inflamed region should be thoroughly anointed with it, and then covered with a thick layer of cotton batting. If the pain is very acute, and more especially if it is ovarian, one part of the tincture of hamamelis may be added to four parts of hot water, and applied topically by means of a compress. If the cellulitis is of traumatic origin, arnica may be used in the same way. A blister would de-vitalize the tissues and do positive harm, and so also would the tincture of iodine. Absolute rest is indispensable to the cure.

To promote suppuration.

The best general rule for the treatment of the suppurative stage is to avert it if you can, but to promote the discharge of pus if you must. If you find that an abscess really is forming, no matter where the fluctuation may first be observed, give the patient hepar sulphuris, calcarea carb., mercurius sol., sulphur, or such other remedies as the symptoms may require. Or, if the discharge has already been too copious and long continued, silicea may be prescribed with a view to its arrest.

Emollients of linseed meal, slippery elm, or bread and milk, hot fomentations and the hip-bath will sometimes afford relief to the pain and hasten the formation and discharge of pus. Or you may apply warm water per vaginam by means of a syphon, so as to facilitate the same process internally.

How to open the abscess.

If the abscess points externally (and it is most desirable that it should do so), it may and should be lanced so soon as it is ready to discharge. Wait until the integument covering the tumor has softened and become thin; and be careful to make the puncture as low down as possible in order not to open the cavity of the peritoneum. It is safest to cut close to Poupart's ligament, more especially from the middle portion of that ligament outwards, in order to shun the sheath of the femoral vessels. Some authorities recommend to make a valvular incision in opening these abscesses, in order to avoid the possible introduction of air into the abdominal cavity.

Unless there is a very decided fluctuation of the tumor along some portion of the vaginal wall or roof, or you are positive concerning the presence of pus therein — from having brought it away with the exploring needle — you will not be warranted in opening it per vaginam. For there is danger in such a case of wounding some of the pelvic viscera. But when there is a point of fluctuation, you may puncture very carefully and evacuate it as you would if it were a more accessible hæmatoma. It is safer, as in hæmatocele, to lance such an abscess through the vaginal septum, than from the rectal side of the tumor, because of the greater number of small vessels that are supplied to the latter. Whenever it is possible the sac should be entirely emptied, else a fistula may form and remain.

After-treatment.

After the abscess has been evacuated, it may be poulticed again for a short time, and then dressed with a lotion of calendula, or of a weak solution of carbolic acid in water. If fistulæ have formed, either of these mixtures may be injected into them.

Mrs. S. is now taking of apis mellifica 3, a dose every three hours. The camphorated oil is still being applied locally, and she has the best diet the hospital affords.

VAGINISMUS.

Case.—Mrs. N——, twenty-three years of age, married, has been out of health from the time her menses made their appearance, which was while she was at school, in her fourteenth year. She had all the usual symptoms of neuralgic or spasmodic dysmenorrhœa with each monthly return. The flow, after the first day, was quite free, and it usually continued about a week. She was married at eighteen, five years ago. Soon after this the dysmenorrhœa ceased, and the "period" has been quite easy and natural until now. She has never borne any children, nor ever had a miscarriage. She menstruated as usual last week. A slight and temporary leucorrhœa sometimes succeeds the catamenial flow.

She complains of great fatigue on slight exertion. This is

especially marked at intervals, which intervals have no known relation to the monthly cycle. At other times she is as active and vigorous, and can walk or ride as far as any one almost. There is a good deal of pain and soreness along the superior portion of the spinal column, extending from the upper cervical to the last dorsal vertebra. Sitting, standing, and writing increase this pain and aching, which do not appear to be influenced by exposure to changes of weather. Sometimes she says there is a burning sensation along this portion of the spine, and again the burning is referred to the region of the left ovary. Occasionally the pain leaves the back and goes to that ovary. While it remains there, the left iliac region becomes tender to the touch, and she involuntarily retracts, or flexes the thigh upon the abdomen.

Her chief complaint is of pain and extreme tenderness at the ostium vaginæ. This orifice is so sensitive, and the slightest contact is so very painful, as to render marital intercourse almost impossible. For more than four years she has consented to it only a very few times, and then has suffered an indescribable martyrdom.

Physical examination finds the parts quite normal, excepting that just within the vaginal orifice, there is great tenderness to the touch, and the moment that the finger comes into contact with the marginal remains of the hymen, there is an immediate spasm of the muscular coat of the vagina, which causes extreme narrowness of that canal, and prevents its admission without considerable force. The superior portion of the vagina is flaccid and capacious enough. The uterus is in its proper place, and does not appear to be changed in any respect. The bladder and the rectum are healthy.

This complaint is a very painful one, and one from which women sometimes suffer in silence for years together without the courage to consult a physician for its relief. I believe that, in its milder forms, it is more frequent than is generally supposed. It may occur in the virgin, or in the case of those who are married, but not in those who have ever had a child or children.

Symptoms.

The symptoms are similar to those which our patient has detailed. There is almost always spinal tenderness, soreness, and lameness, which are generally located between the shoulders and along the cervical portion of the spine. Sometimes, however, it is lower down the spinal column, and is described as a weakness of the back and hips. The soreness or weakness is paroxysmal, and is aggravated by exercise, but more especially by sexual excitement. In its recurrence it is very apt to alternate with ovarian pain, burning and irritation. A hysterical cough, aphonia, headache, or a tendency to general spasms, are not unfrequent accompaniments of this spinal irritation. Spasmodic dysmenorrhœa and strangury often complicate the case, and cause additional suffering. (*Exit the patient.*)

Local hyperæsthesia.

But the peculiar and distinctive symptom of vaginismus is the hyperæsthesia of the vulva and of the outer extremity of the vagina, which is so very sensitive that even the slightest touch causes a spasm of the sphincter vaginæ, and a closure of that canal. The closure may also extend to the sphincter ani. The location and extent of this sensitive surface varies in different subjects. In virgins, it may be limited to the outer face of the hymen, which membrane, in these cases, is thicker and more firmly organized than usual. In those married women in whom the hymen has been ruptured, the tenderness is frequently most marked somewhere along the marginal remains and attachments of this membrane. The carunculæ myrtiformes may be exquisitely sensitive. In many cases the most tender point is upon the side of, or near to the meatus urinarius. In others, it is about the orifice of the vulvo-vaginal gland, and sometimes at the fourchette.

In this condition the contact of the finger, or even of a camel's hair brush, or of a feather, may cause the greatest agony, and perhaps throw the patient into convulsions. Coitus is impossible, and you can not introduce the smallest speculum without almost killing her; indeed, in some cases that I have treated, the vaginal orifice was so closely and tightly constricted that I could not pass my little finger, or even a female catheter, into the vagina without exercising undue force. The sexual act being more or less completely performed, the suffering finally becomes so great that the parties are forced to desist, and most of these patients confess either that they have altogether relinquished the attempt and concluded to live apart, or, as they sometimes do, as brother and sister; or that it is undertaken only at long intervals. Usually such women remain childless. It has happened, however, that even under these embarrassing circumstances, conception has taken place, and gestation and parturition have cured the case spontaneously.

If these symptoms continue for years, and the patient is subjected to all the mental worry that is their indirect consequence, and to the contingent diseases which such a state of the nervous system is almost certain to induce, her general health will finally become impaired, and she will pass into a state of decline. She will become prematurely old, emaciated, dyspeptic, hypochondriacal, and a wretched "nervous wreck." The worst results may happen to her household and family. She is very apt to conclude, and may even be told by her physician, that she has an incurable disease of the womb. Her husband is likely to become estranged, and her married life to prove a disastrous failure.

Causes.

This disease is frequently complicated, either as cause or effect, with spasmodic dysmenorrhœa. Sometimes it arises from a pruritus of the vulva, which is due to vulvar eruptions. Or it may be caused by caruncles of the meatus urinarius, vulvar folliculitis, vesical, urethral or rectal tenesmus, hæmorrhoids, fissures of the anus, or of the vulva, vaginitis, uterine displacements, an irritable uterus, nodular neuromata of the vagina or vulva, or by the contact of acrid discharges in utero-vaginal leucorrhœa.

The most cultivated and gifted women, those of a high moral or emotional nature, are most subject to this affection. This is especially true of such of them as inherit the hysterical disposition, and who are liable to the different forms of spinal irritation. All this large class of women are exceedingly prone to be mismated, and to suffer from personal antagonisms which jar their sensibilities and derange the sexual sphere. Thus it may happen that a delicate, sensitive, impressible woman, who, if she were properly mated, would be exceedingly happy and contented, is tied to one whose brutal approaches become more and more loathsome and repulsive, until finally this morbid sensibility which ruins her health and happiness is developed. I have seen one case of the kind which really was more painful to witness than anything beside that has ever occurred in my professional experience. There are no toxical influences which are so difficult to antidote as those which arise from sexual incompatibility.

You need have no difficulty in establishing the diagnosis. First examine the patient by means of the "touch." If she is extremely nervous and apprehensive, shakes like one in a fit of ague, and is almost or quite convulsed the moment the vulva is touched; if there is a manifest spasm of the sphincter and the constrictor muscles of the vagina, so that the finger cannot pass into the canal without causing her more or less agony, you had better desist, and proceed to put her under the influence of an anæsthetic. A few whiffs of ether, or of chloroform, will quiet her apprehension, overcome her opposition, allay the super-sensitiveness of the vulvar mucous membrane, and more than all relax the spasm so that the finger, or speculum, will enter quite readily.

Diagnosis.

Dr. Sims has given us the differential points in vaginismus in one of his laconic sentences: "The supersensitiveness is diagnostic; the spasm pathognomonic."*

The prognosis is generally conceded to be favorable. If, however, the disease is the result of a profound lesion of the nervous centers, as sometimes, although very rarely, happens, it is not likely to be radically cured. Something depends also upon the duration of the disease and the serious inroads it has made upon the general health. But, in almost every case of vaginismus, you will expect to cure your patient, providing your instructions are carried out, and she has the patience to wait for the result.

Treatment.—The treatment is both medical and surgical. The remedies most frequently indicated are those which are suited to the relief and cure of the intercurrent disorders, more especially of menstruation, innervation, and digestion, and to the pain and suffering in the bladder, the urethra and the rectum. These should be carefully chosen and affiliated. I am not aware that any of them hold an especial curative relation to the vaginismus separately considered; nor is there on record a well authenticated cure of this disease by the use of internal remedies alone. Belladonna, atropine, thuja, macrotin, sepia, cocculus, conium, platina, nux vomica, pulsatilla, hyoscyamus, ignatia, and mercurius, include those which are more likely to be indicated than any others. If necessary, (and it often is,) either of them can be given in conjunction with the surgical treatment.

Medical treatment.

*Clinical Notes on Uterine Surgery, by J. Marion Sims, M.D., etc., etc. New York, 1866, p. 320.

As usual in gynæcological questions, authorities are divided on the question of employing the knife for the radical cure of vaginismus. My own opinion, based upon the successful treatment of numerous cases, is that, unless there is some especial reason why the cure should be speedy, it is best to try the milder means first. This is especially true of cases which are not very severe.

Surgical treatment.

One of the means designed to overcome this disposition to spasm of the vaginal muscular fibre is the dilatation of the canal, or rather of its constricted portion, by graduated bougies. An ordinary rectal bougie may be cut in two, and one half anointed with simple cerate, glycerine, olive oil, or with an ointment consisting of the extract of belladonna, one part, and lard or simple cerate, six parts. This may be very carefully introduced and allowed to remain, according to circumstances, for a period varying from a few minutes to an hour or more, when it should be withdrawn. Of course the patient should keep the horizontal posture meanwhile. You may be obliged to commence with a very small instrument of this kind, but gradually the larger ones can be used, and their presence will be tolerated so that they will no longer occasion pain. The patient can soon be taught to introduce and to remove them herself. After a time, with proper diet, remedies and regulation of the habits in every respect, you will find that it is possible to pass the largest size of the rectal bougie without suffering, and that the case is practically cured. The complete interdiction of coitus while this dilatation is being effected, is a condition of the cure.

Dilatation.

Case. — March, 1862, Mrs. —— consulted with me for the relief of an irritable and sensitive condition of the vagina which, during her three years of married life, had caused her untold suffering, and interfered most positively with sexual congress. She was a most intelligent person, frank and candid in her manner, and extremely anxious that something should be done for her relief, more especially lest her husband should become disaffected, and her family and friends continue to ridicule her for never having become a mother.

On physical examination there was nothing abnormal about the external generative organs, except the hyperæsthesia of the vulva and of the vaginal outlet. The slightest and most delicate touch with the finger caused the vaginal spasm immediately, and she was thrown into the same state of suffering which she said she had always experienced in the conjugal act. I placed her under the influence of sulphuric ether by inhalation, and these symptoms disappeared. The dilatation with bougies anointed with the belladonna and simple cerate, was begun and continued every two days for a fortnight, then every day for another week, and the barrier to intercourse was removed. She soon conceived, and now has a son, a beautiful boy, nine years old. I gave her no medicine.

In most cases to which this plan of dilatation is equally well adapted, the cure will not be so speedily effected. It generally requires about two months, sometimes a little more, and sometimes less, to accomplish the desired result. If you prefer, you can make use of a series of conical glass dilators, such as I hold in my hand, instead of the bougies. These were invented by Dr. Sims, and answer a very good purpose. The warm bath and electricity are useful auxiliaries to this treatment, in which I have great confidence. Scanzoni treated one hundred cases of vaginismus by a very similar plan and cured them all without recourse to the knife.

Excision of irritable tumors.

A very few cases are reported to have been cured by excision of the irritable tumor which is sometimes found at the mouth of the urethra. Others have been remedied by the removal of the vaginal neuromata, the cure of vaginitis, fissures of the parts, and such diseases as could be more easily reached and removed by local and general treatment.

Dr. Tilt's operation.

Dr. Tilt recommends to effect the forcible dilatation of the constrictor muscles of the vagina in the same manner as your professor of surgery, only a few days since, overcame a spasm of the sphincter ani in a patient which he had before you. Having anæsthetized the woman, he introduces both of his thumbs with their backs toward each other, into the vaginal orifice, and then stretches it firmly and forcibly for the space of five or six minutes. After this a plug, or dilator, is introduced and kept in position for several days by a T bandage. This mode of treatment, however, is not applicable, while there is any coincident or remaining uterine or vaginal disease.

Dr. Sims practices deep incisions on the right and left side of the mesial line of the vagina posteriorly. The patient should be placed upon the back, and brought thoroughly under the influence of ether or chloroform. With a pair of curved scissors remove the remains of the hymen. In order to separate the labia laterally, to open the canal as wide as possible, and to draw the fourchette very tense, the index and middle fingers of the left hand are to be passed into the vagina. Then with a common scalpel you make an incision through the vaginal tissue, a little to the right side, bringing it from above downwards, to the raphé of the perineum, thus making one side of a V; then insert the knife on the left side and cut obliquely toward the other incision, so as to join it at the raphé. Follow along through the raphé itself until the cut is Y shaped. Thus the incision will pass across the sphincter vagina for about half an inch, but not through it, and, in all will be nearly two inches in length, varying in different subjects according to the development of tissue in each.

Dr. Sims' operation

If there is considerable hæmorrhage, pressure, the local application of ice or of the per-sulphate of iron will arrest it. If the flow of blood is free, but not excessive, the dilator may be introduced immediately, and the pressure which it exerts will serve to arrest it. Usually the dilator is not applied until twenty-four hours after the operation, when it is kept *in situ* by an appropriate bandage, after which it is worn "for two hours in the morning and two or three hours in the evening, according to the tolerance of the patient." Dr. Sims says: "I have been often astonished at the rapidity with which the cuts heal, the process being seemingly facilitated by the pressure of the glass dilator, which is to be worn daily for two or three hours, or until the parts being entirely cured, and all sensitiveness removed, the patient may be pronounced competent to fulfil comfortably and pleasantly the duty of a wife."*

In brief, therefore, Sims' operation is preferred to that of Burns', which consisted in dividing the pudic nerve. Some very interesting cases cured by Sims' method have been reported by Drs. H. B. Clarke, T. G. Comstock, W. Tod Helmuth and others. You will find a suggestive report on this subject by one of our former pupils, Dr. W. A. Burr, of Nebraska, in the current issue of the United States Medical and Surgical Journal.†

*Bulletin of the N. Y. Academy of Medicine, vol. I, p. 434.
†Volume VII, page 367.

In some of my cases, where the remains of the hymen have constituted the focal point of the hyperæsthesia, I have removed them with a curved scissors and then finished the cure by means of dilatation and without any incision. This treatment will be followed in the case which you saw a few moments ago.

Another expedient.

Attacks of vaginismus that are incidental and transient in their duration may be relieved by a more simple but equally useful expedient. A mixture consisting of chloroform, one drachm, and olive oil and glycerine, each one ounce, may be applied by means of a cotton tampon, providing the spasm of the vagina does not prevent its introduction into that canal. In that case it may be thrown into the rectum, when the spasm will very soon cease. Afterwards the proper medical and hygienic treatment can be resorted to for the radical cure of the conditions, or diseases, upon which these paroxysms are contingent.

Local anæsthesia.

PHYSOMETRA.

Case.—May, 1864. Mrs. B——, aged twenty-four, of sanguineo-nervous temperament, has been married six years, and is the mother of two children. She was delivered of the youngest of these one year ago,—during the riots in the city of New York. She says she had a short and easy labor, after which she did well until the third day, when, the report having been circulated that the house in which she was living would be fired or destroyed, she was obliged to remove to another. The distance being only two squares, she insisted upon walking, and really accomplished the task, but under great mental excitement. The result was at first a partial, and, after the fifth day, a complete suppression of the lochia.

In a short time her present symptoms began to trouble her, and they have continued during the whole year. There is a circumscribed enlargement of the abdomen, situated in the mesian line, and extending from the pubis towards the umbilicus. This tumor increases in size so that at times she is quite as large, and looks as if she were seven months advanced in pregnancy. At other times, and especially after a good night's rest, its size is greatly reduced. Exercise and excitement increase its volume.

When she reclines the tumor gravitates or rolls toward the side upon which she is lying, but without any change in its form, and without borborygmus. It is still circumscribed, and always tympanitic. The neighboring parts yield their normal sounds on percussion. The only pain she has had is a species of soreness from outward pressure, or distension. She is at times sensible of having had a discharge of flatus per vaginam, but has never had eructations.

Sometimes, she says, this tumor or swelling feels as if it were rising into the stomach, and again into the throat. Occasionally she has headache and a flushed face, especially in the afternoon. She is a very intelligent woman, and is confident that she has never before had any uterine difficulties. The urinary function is normal, and in every other respect she is healthy. She was unable to nurse her child.

It may be a long time before you will see so good an illustration of this curious affection as we have here this morning. Indeed, owing to its rarity, many physicians of large experience have never seen a case of this kind. If you observe the physical characters of this phantom tumor, you will note that its outline is as well-defined as that of an ovarian cyst. It may be very hard, or it may yield to pressure, like a soft foot-ball, and is tympanitic on percussion. You hear this sound distinctly. The tumor changes its position when she turns upon either side, and rolls about to a limited degree, but there is no bulging in the lumbar region, and no flattening of the anterior surface of the tumor when she lies upon her back, as in ascites.

The tumor.

Physometra, or the collection of flatus in the womb, is almost always, directly or indirectly, related to gestation, or to the parturient state. Sometimes, however, it occurs during menstruation, and again in consequence of the presence of uterine hydatids, moles, polypi, and such intra-uterine growths as are liable to become decomposed, either before or after their detachment. Whether as cause or effect, hysterical symptoms are always present in these cases, as in other forms of tympanites to which women are more especially, but not exclusively liable. The lochia, the milk, and the menses, are suppressed. Sometimes, however, the breasts fill as they do in pregnancy. The nervous symptoms predominate.

The most commonly accepted cause of this singular infirmity is the retention and decomposition in utero of the fœtus, of some portion of the secundines after delivery; or similar changes in fragments of intra-uterine growths which have failed to be expelled by nature, or removed by the physician. The gas that is formed in consequence of the decomposition of organic matters is fetid, and is incarcerated in the cavity of the womb by the spasmodic closure of the cervical outlet.

Causes.

Decomposition of matter retained.

It is possible that similar changes may take place in the menstrual excretion, and also in the membrane (decidua menstrualis), which is sometimes exfoliated during that process, and which if it is retained by closure of the uterine neck, might also undergo chemical decomposition. Occasionally the arrest of the lochia results in the development of this form of uterine tumor. This cause is more powerful when conjoined, as in this case, with apprehension and anxiety, as well as with premature exposure and excess of fatigue almost immediately after the birth of the child.

Some writers ascribe the uterine enlargement in physometra to a collection of atmospheric air in the womb, which is either drawn into that organ by a species of suction, or passes into it when the os uteri is open and other matters have so escaped as to leave a vacuum, into which the air may rush until it is filled. Dr. Harley cites a case of alternate admission into, and expulsion of air from the vagina.* Something of this kind, it is thought, may, in very exceptional cases, take place in the womb.

Suction of air into the womb.

But there are instances in which, unless we ascribe it to mental excitement, it is quite impossible to detect any cause for this tumor. Acting upon a hysterical predisposition, there is no valid reason why an excess of flatus might not be as readily secreted or formed within the uterus, as it obviously may in the bowel or the stomach from a similar cause. And nothing is more common than hysterical tympanites from emotional causes in this class of patients. But I will not detain you with further remarks on this subject.

Mental causes.

The diagnosis is much easier than it was a few years ago. You have only to put the patient under the influence of chloroform or ether, and the differentiation of this species of tumor will declare itself. For if it is a case

Diagnosis.

*Transactions of the Obstetrical Society of London, Vol. IV., page 173.

of physometra, or indeed of a phantom tumor of any kind, the enlargement will disappear altogether. You can satisfy yourselves that the accumulation has been in the womb and not in the bowel, by passing a small canula, or a male catheter, through the os uteri. Then, by placing the outer extremity of the instrument under water you can evacuate the tumor through it, and be assured of the escape of gas therefrom. I tried this experiment on our patient yesterday, and, therefore, am confident in my diagnosis.

Treatment.

The treatment consists in removing any decayed substances that may have remained in utero; and in preventing their retention in the future. The cervix may be kept open for the free discharge of such matters, and of the gas also, by the use of the sponge-tent and the ordinary means of dilatation. If the case is a recent one, and the lochia have been suppressed, they should, if possible, be restored. If the patient is hysterical, this tendency should be counteracted by appropriate medical, moral and hygienic means. If the excessive size of the tumor worries her, it may be evacuated a few times for her comfort. Mrs. B. will take a dose of belladonna 3 every four hours during the day.*

*In four weeks this woman was well and menstruating normally.

LECTURE XXVIII.

AMENORRHŒA, WITH PROLAPSUS UTERI AND OBSTINATE VOMITING.

GENTLEMEN:

I doubt if it would be possible to occupy the first part of this hour more profitably than in the clinical review of a case from my private practice. It interested me greatly, and may contain something of value to you. It was a case of amenorrhœa, with prolapsus uteri and obstinate vomiting. The patient did me the favor to write out her symptoms in detail.

Case.—I am 22 years of age, and married; have been ill with an intractable gastric difficulty at intervals for six years. This affection first manifested itself after a severe attack of diarrhœa, which was followed by spitting up of the food while it was partially digested, or still unchanged. This symptom used especially to trouble me in the evening, after supper, but sometimes followed the other meals also. Coffee, pastry, and all rich food, new vegetables, and many kinds of fruit, were the first articles to be rejected by my stomach. Consequently, my diet was reduced to meat and bread. For a time all kinds of fresh meat were well borne, but finally beef-steak was the only one that would be tolerated.

The first attack of this indigestion came on late in the summer and continued for several months. It returned the next year at the same season, and lasted until the middle of the following winter, being accompanied by three months of suppressed menstruation. These combined troubles occasioned severe headache, and bloating of the stomach and the abdomen. However, I rapidly gained in flesh, which was soon lost when the menses returned. The next season I derived much benefit from a residence of nine months in Saratoga. After drinking its waters I returned home with my disease apparently cured. Two years of comparative health followed, with occasional symptoms of the old trouble, which were generally relieved by the regulation of my diet.

The third attack was preceded, accompanied and followed by

bilious fever and dysentery, with which diseases I was very ill for several weeks. The gastric difficulty did not leave as usual in the winter season. The symptoms continued for more than a year, the nausea and vomiting increased in frequency and violence, and were accompanied by great acridity of the matters ejected, distress and burning. I could compare the feeling which predominated to no sensation except to that which would be produced by many pieces of apple-core moving about in the stomach. Constipation and bloating of the abdomen were constant symptoms. Medicine seemed powerless; one article of diet after another was abandoned; my strength gradually decreased; I became nervous; my nights were wakeful, with unpleasant dreams, and a dumb ague at last set in. Meat and other solid food could not be tolerated by my stomach, and soon the entire system yielded to utter prostration and debility.

The region of the stomach now became very hard to the feel, but extremely sensitive to the touch. For seven months menstruation was entirely suspended. From September to the middle of December, I became weaker and weaker. I then began gradually to improve, but the vomiting continued nearly every day for about four months longer. For six months I had eaten no solid food whatever, but had subsisted on porridge and farina. For two months I lived exclusively on milk, and a weak strained broth.

The first discharge of matter or pus by vomiting took place in September, and from that time on I continued to raise it. In November this matter became more copious, and was thrown up as often as every hour in the day. The most abundant of these discharges of pus were preceded by sinking spells, with difficulty of breathing and numbness. Beside this matter there was also vomited a clear fluid which made the throat, mouth and lips burn and smart severely. But a thick froth resembling the beaten white of an egg, generally accompanied the pus.

Intense nervousness, wakeful and often sleepless nights, and severe pains in the head, and also in the back and hips, racked my delicate constitution terribly. For six months, with but a few exceptional days, the vomiting spells followed each other every one to six hours. I was entirely confined to my bed for four months.

This was the condition in which I found this patient on my first visit. She was a bride of a few months. Her husband and family were extremely solicitous concerning her, for, excepting that at times she had a rosy English complexion, she really appeared like one who could not live very long. Further examination of the case from time to time, as she could bear it and as opportunity offered, elicited the following additional symptoms:

A large portion of the time, during which she suffered from these attacks of vomiting, the appetite was craving and almost ravenous. This was accompanied by extreme depression of spirits. For several months after the vomiting came to be of almost daily occurrence, there was little or no loss of flesh, the cheeks were red and the eyes bright as in perfect health, but the complexion had a peculiar bluish hue, especially in the morning. The feet and hands, which at other times were almost as cold and colorless as marble, became hot and burning. The perspiration had a strong, disagreeable odor. This odor was especially bad when the vomiting of pus was most frequent and copious. For many weeks the stomach was so sensitive that she could tell the moment the food entered it, and in what part of the organ it was lying. A marked and peculiar feeling for months prior to her illness was that of a sharp distress (the "apple-core" sensation) just at the entrance to the stomach. This was accompanied by a feeling of faintness from lack of food, which eating only increased.

Each of these attacks was characterized by a more or less prolonged arrest of the menses. She also complained of weakness and lameness in the small of her back and hips, with dragging down sensations, occasional dysuria and obstinate constipation.

Prolapsus the exciting cause.

My first impression of the pathology of this case was, that it was one of perforating ulcer of the stomach, and, as you may suppose, my prognostications were very cautiously given. My second visit disclosed the menstrual complication, and the third interview decided me to request an examination per vaginam. It was accordingly made. I found the vulva in a state of hyperæsthesia, with considerable constriction of the vaginal orifice. The uterus was prolapsed upon the floor of the pelvis, and exquisitely tender to the touch. After a little delicate manipulation this organ was lifted as far toward the superior strait as possible, and the patient directed to lie for the most part upon the left side. I prescribed nux vomica[3], a dose to be taken every three hours.

Effect of replacing the womb.

The next morning her pelvic and sacral pains had vanished, the headache was relieved, the vomiting had been less frequent, and she was hopeful. In brief, she kept to her bed for about three weeks more, on account of the prolapsus, and also of the menstrual flow, which returned within a fortnight. Once in four or five days the womb was restored, in case it had fallen, with the index finger. Calcarea carbonica[3] was the only remedy that she took after the first few days, excepting caulophyllin and coffea, which were given incidentally to promote rest and sleep. Menstruation soon became regular and normal in every respect. The gastric difficulty lessened until almost any kind of food could be taken, relished and retained. Her "dumb ague" disappeared, and her old flow of spirits returned. In a few weeks her health was perfectly restored. In six months she became pregnant, and now she has a bright, healthy child, which is about a year old. She passed through gestation without any morning sickness or vomiting; and through labor and lactation with no untoward or unusual symptoms. Two years have elapsed and there has been no return of her disease.

Subsequent history.

My object in reporting this case is not to reflect upon either of the physicians who preceded me in its management, but to make a few practical points that will be available to you bye and bye as practitioners. The first of these is that your skill in diagnosis, and your success in treatment will depend upon the thoroughness with which you examine and analyze the case in hand. Much has been said of the importance of the "totality of the symptoms" as the basis of treatment. In a knotty, complicated case like this, the "totality of the symptoms" includes a great deal. It classifies and arranges the gastric, the alimentary and the nervous symptoms as the more prominent and suggestive; but it is found that those physicians who claim to prescribe in accordance therewith are very apt to overlook the menstrual and uterine complications, or, at least, they do not always give them their due prominence. And this fact explains some of their failures. For if we should place undue stress upon the character of the matters ejected, or the frequency and other peculiarities of the vomiting, as interpreting the nature of the disease, and as indicative of the remedy, which is characteristic and most appropriate for its relief—the result would be that our pathology would be at fault, and our therapeutical progress would take the wrong direction.

Practical points.

"Totality of the symptoms."

In a case of this kind it is sometimes very difficult, and even impossible to decide which class of symptoms is really the most significant. If our judgment concerning them is based upon their objective consequences, and

The cardinal symptoms.

not upon their subjective cause and relation, we shall be very apt to declare in favor of the former. Hence, it frequently happens that the most clamorous signs get the credit of being characteristic and sufficient when, in fact, they are not so.

Practical deductions.

This is a case in point. The uterus was badly prolapsed, and evidently had been each time that she had suffered from the gastric derangement. The cause of her illness was mechanical and, while it acted, was constant in its operation. The reflex functional disorder of the stomach was so severe and long-continued that it finally developed into an undoubted ulceration of that organ. But even when the symptoms connected with that ulceration were at their worst, there was nothing distinctive in them either as to the cause of the difficulty, or the best mode of curing it.

Must give due weight to proper symptoms.

The second proposition is that while we are careful not to exclude some of the symptoms arbitrarily, or through neglect, we should not exalt others to an unmerited prominence indiscriminately, and without good reason. The uterine deviation and the menstrual arrest were the cardinal peculiarities of the case under review. When they were relieved the more remote gastric symptoms disappeared. Now it would not be safe to conclude and to insist from this that pessaries and emmenagogues are the best means of cure in a case of ulceration of the stomach with similar vomiting; neither to declare that these symptoms are invariably due to the same, or to any remote cause, whether sexual or otherwise. It is the inference we deduce, and the lesson we learn from such an experience that interests the profession, and our patients also. It is the physician's tact in taking hold of the right thread that enables him to unravel the tangled skein of disease.

Also to proper clinical influences.

Key to success.

And whoever, in a case of utero-gastric disease, can tell which is the primary lesion, and which is the secondary one; which symptoms are first in importance, and which are not; will have a key to the choice of the treatment proper to these compound cases which he could not otherwise obtain. Starting from this point, he may select the remedy or remedies, surgical or medical, by a reference to his experience, to his library, to his materia medica, or through a species of "unconscious cerebration;" but he will gain his object more speedily, safely and surely than if he took a less comprehensive view of the case, and always persisted in beginning at the other end of the series.

You will readily understand how the extreme and persistent irritability of the stomach, in a case of this kind, might finally involve the most serious consequences. When all the food that is swallowed is rejected, and the vomiting is so nearly constant, it is impossible for the patient to be properly nourished thereby. Her assimilative functions are sure to be impaired. The digestion, the circulation, respiration and innervation cannot escape. And thus the general health will be undermined. Organic disease will be the indirect consequence, and prostration, debility and death may follow.

Ill effects of excessive vomiting.

Indeed the diseases of any portion of the gastro-alimentary mucous membrane are more serious when complicated with uterine and menstrual disorders than when they do not co-exist. For this reason, in women, the worst cases of intestinal derangement, and indigestion, constipation and diarrhœa are those which are complicated with intra-pelvic difficulties of various kinds, as for example, uterine displacements, ulceration, chronic cervicitis, ovaritis, menstrual retention, leucorrhœa, and menorrhagia. The remoteness of these several lesions, — which complicate even when they have not caused the alimentary disorder, and the absence of any very prominent signs of uterine or ovarian trouble, may lead to their being overlooked as prime factors in the case. If we add to this that a proper physical examination of the pelvic organs is usually the last thing to be thought of under these circumstances, you will see how it is possible for such complicated diseases to resist treatment, and finally terminate fatally.

Serious nature of utero-gastro-alimentary disorders.

These cases vary so much, and are so unlike, that one description will not answer for them all; nor will one kind of treatment cure them indiscriminately. Whatever the nature of the indirect cause, its effect should be counteracted by its removal. Possibly not one in a hundred cases of chronic and persistent vomiting may depend so directly as this upon uterine displacement. But the fact that it may happen should not be forgotten, for the very first case to which you are called may be one of this kind.

Nor need there be any clashing or mischievous interference on account of what may be termed the surgical and the medical indications sometimes presented by the same case. The uterus can be reposited, its cervix dilated, or the os uteri medicated topically, if needs be, while the constitutional treatment, based upon other and different indications, is still being pursued.

Surgery and medicine not antidotal.

IRRITABLE UTERUS. — HYSTERALGIA.

Case.— Mrs. J——, 27 years old, married, with three children, the youngest of which is two years of age, has been an invalid for nine years. She is naturally delicate and sensitive. She was married at eighteen, and left home directly for a wedding trip, which was to consist of an excursion to a distant city and a visit of a fortnight to her husband's relatives. When she reached home she felt as if her nervous system was very much shattered. She attributes this result to a want of entire sympathy and accord with her husband, who, she says, never understood her, and never took any especial pains to please or to gratify her. During her girlhood, after fourteen, she suffered a great deal at her monthly periods, more especially for the first ten or twelve hours. For this she usually took hot teas, and gin, and kept to the bed. Since the birth of her children this dysmenorrhœa has not returned, but she has not been well for a moment. Her chief complaints are of a fugitive character. She is wretched when she goes out, and when she comes in; in the morning and at night. The only pains that she has are shooting, shifting and transient, mostly in the lower part of the back and of the abdomen. At intervals she has spells of lying in bed with these pains for several days. Sometimes there is strangury, particularly after coitus, which always worries and unnerves her. Menstruation is regular, but less free than it should be. She is most happy when in general society. When she can forget herself, and be thoroughly diverted, she feels like another person. For this reason she likes to go away from home on a visit. Her nights are wakeful, and she dreams of every event, whether pleasant or painful, in her past life. Her feet are always cold.

Examination does not reveal any sign of organic disease about or within the pelvis. The uterus is very irritable and tender to the touch. It seems to be slightly enlarged, but is not displaced. When the finger comes into contact with it she says it produces the same painful tension and disagreeable feeling which she has always experienced during intercourse, and which is so intolerable to her.

There is a large class of diseases, of which this case is an example, in which the obvious organic lesion of the uterus and its appendages is the poorest possible criterion of the real nature of the complaint, of the suffering involved, and of the difficulty of curing it. The irritable uterus is not inflamed or ulcerated, congested or displaced. There is no lesion of structure connected with it necessarily. It yields no characteristic or critical discharge. Its measurements are normal, its regional anatomy is unchanged, and it offers no especial obstacle to menstruation, conception, or parturition.

Has no definite lesion.

So far, therefore, as its morbid anatomy is concerned, it resembles nitrogen in being negative in its character; for it consists essentially in an excitable or irritable condition of the womb, in which its nervous sympathies and relations are exaggerated and discordant. Inflammation of this or adjacent organs may exist as a sequel, or complication, but they are not a necessary part of the disease. So, also, in some cases there are incidental symptoms of spinal irritation, and of reflex disorders of every conceivable kind, which are contingent upon the morbid exaltation of uterine sensibility.

A species of hyperæsthesia.

This disease is limited for the most part to menstrual life. It occurs in the case of the married and the unmarried, but is more frequent among the former. Those who have been pregnant, whether they have gone to term or not, are believed to be more subject to it than such as have never conceived. There are, however, many exceptions to this rule. In general, those women who are weak, nervous, and impressible, and who have been subject to slight, spasmodic and painful irregularities of menstruation, are very prone to this disorder in after life. Unhappy marriage, the loss of property and of position in society, the lack of occupation, disappointment, solitude, the dread of having some "female weakness," inordinate use of tea and coffee, chagrin, jealousy, frequent abortion, too rapid child-bearing, erotic thoughts, and sexual excesses, belong also to this class

Limited to menstrual life.

Predisposing causes.

of causes. The rheumatic and neuralgic diatheses are powerful predisponents of this form of hysteralgia.

Exciting causes.

The exciting causes are also numerous. Whatever can directly or indirectly exalt the nervous susceptibilities and sympathies of the uterus (even if the stimulant be natural and harmless under different circumstances) is likely to work mischief if too frequently and carelessly applied. The emotions, which properly controlled are healthful and useful, may be in league with the passions to derange the uterine nervous system, and either or all of the functions connected therewith. Under their influence the womb may become so irritable that menstruation shall be suppressed, or become intermittent, scanty, profuse, or perhaps very painful. Or, through the uterine irritability that is induced, a fruitful intercourse may be impossible, and sterility will be the result.

Ungratified sexual desire is undoubtedly almost, if not quite, as injurious to the female in many instances as an excess of venery. For women are not only subject to sexual passions and propensities similar to those of men; but they are also under the dominion of a periodical crisis, that is attended by a peculiar exaltation and excitement of the generative system. These crises can not always be passed with impunity. They involve certain vicissitudes which derange the uterine innervation. And coming as they do so frequently, these nervous derangements are perpetuated. It is sometimes as difficult to tide a woman over "the month" as it is to carry a popular patient, who is very ill, over the Sabbath, or through a holiday, without a relapse, or an exacerbation of his disease. The contingent excitement and re-action are so mischievous that it is almost impossible to counteract them. The result is an irritable condition of the uterus and of the whole sexual system.

Other causes of this kind are the fitful, too frequent and incomplete performance of the sexual act, without regard to the menses, or to the emotional state and desire of the female; exercise, as in riding or walking while menstruating, or directly after the flow has ceased; getting up too soon after delivery, and especially after abortion; too prolonged lactation; frequent miscarriages; the use of harsh or cold injections with a view to prevent conception; constipation, from paralysis of the rectum; dancing, skating, horseback riding, blows and falls upon the spine; excessive or constrained muscular effort, as in running the sewing-machine, prolonged standing upon the feet, or sitting in a confined posture at a desk; prolapsus, retroversion or retroflexion of the uterus; pressure of the bladder, of the bowels, of the ovaries, or of some pelvic or abdominal tumor against the womb; spasmodic and mechanical obstructions of the cervix uteri; ulceration of the vagina or vulva; nymphomania; vaginismus, and ovarian irritation. The uterus is generally exempt from this form of irritation until after puberty.

From an early abortion.

Some of the most intractable and painful cases of irritable uterus that I have ever treated have occurred in those women who, having been married for several years, have had no children. In many of them conception took place almost immediately after marriage, but for reasons which seemed to them to be justifiable at the time, and without any adequate idea of the harm involved, measures were taken to force the flow, and, in short, to bring on an abortion. These measures were successful. The uterus was emptied of its contents. But the indirect consequences remained to torture them, and to impair their health and happiness for years to come. I could tell you the story of more than one beautiful woman who has suffered with this trying disease, whose health has been ruined, who has remained childless, and who would give the world if, when she was the bride of a few weeks, she had not swallowed somebody's "never-failing pills," or taken the wretched advice of a neighbor in this respect.

From escharotics.

Another fertile source of this uterine irritability is the reckless cauterization of the cervix of which I have already spoken so frequently. There are certain subjects upon whose delicate organisms this species of refined cruelty reacts with a most damaging effect. And it is a singular fact that those physicians who resort to it habitually become blinded to these results and indifferent of the consequences. Let me cite you a case to which I was called yesterday:

Case.—Mrs. ——, an intelligent, active woman of twenty-two, of nervous temperament, mother of one child two years old, has not been well for six months. Her household cares, and the worry with servants, the heat of the weather, and having to entertain an avalanche of friends, had worn her down, and she was reduced in strength and spirits. She had no positive symptoms to complain of, excepting that she suffered from more frequent and severe attacks of sick headache (to which she was accustomed) than usual.

For some weeks she tried to cure herself by means of domestic remedies from her own case, and finally by tonics of various kinds at the prescription of some of her friends. But her symptoms remained as before. She continued her household drudgery, did her own shopping and marketing, and, as usual, went to church and to Sabbath-school.

Finally, through the advice of a neighbor, she consulted a lady physician, who cauterized the neck of the womb, and continued to do so twice each week, excepting the menstrual week, for six weeks. From the first application, she felt herself very much injured, and made worse; but was advised to persevere, on the theory that, when she had once passed this purgatory, her feelings and experiences would be blissful enough. Each repetition of this cruelty unnerved her more and more. She could not sleep, but walked the floor at night, lost her little remaining appetite, had cold, fainting spells, in which she would be unconscious for a long time; she became discouraged and disheartened, melancholy, and, so her husband told me, practically insane for many hours after the caustic had been used. With this there developed a most tormenting strangury, and, after the second week, a corrosive, itching leucorrhœa, although she had never had the slightest sign of either of these complaints before.

At the end of the seventh week, after having had twelve of these "treatments," she deliberately came to the conclusion that her health would be utterly ruined should she persevere in this course. She therefore relinquished it, discharged her physician, and sent for me.

Symptoms.—It would be quite impossible to give you all the symptoms of this curious disease in detail. In general the pain that is experienced is disproportionate to the uterine lesion. It varies in its seat, and character also. Usually it is located somewhere in the lower part of the back, or within or near the pelvis; but very often it is situated in the head, the spine, the chest, or the abdomen. The pains are transient, paroxysmal and neuralgic, being for the most part, unaccompanied by any profound or peculiar constitutional disturbance. They are greatly influenced by emotional states, being either aggravated or relieved by certain conditions of the mind. Posture modifies the recurrence and severity of the paroxysms.

Location of the pain.

Most women who have an irritable uterus find it difficult to maintain an upright position for any considerable length of time. They can not stand or sit more than a few minutes without great suffering, and going up and down stairs is almost impossible for them. Often the reclining posture is the only one that can be tolerated. They may have a mortal dread of defecation and of urination, either of which is apt to be followed by extreme pain, exhaustion or faintness. Sometimes there is an irresistible desire to pass water, especially when she lies down; again the urging to stool is equally tormenting whenever she sits up. And still the urine may be unchanged in quality, and the bowels remain costive.

Effect of posture and of motion.

To these symptoms we must add those which simulate certain local disorders, as in the mimicry of Hysteria. The most common of these are dyspnœa, aphonia, palpitation of the heart, angina pectoris, pleurisy, neuralgic pains in, and swelling of the breasts, especially before or during menstruation, ovarian aching and irritation, headache, facial and orbital neuralgia, gastrodynia, dyspepsia, chronic vomiting, depression of spirits, monomania, numbness of the extremities, muscular paralysis, and stiffness and uselessness of the joints.

May simulate other diseases.

The nervous symptoms include insomnia, flatulent distention of the abdomen, dejection of spirits, emotional distress, great fluctuation of the feelings, sourness or suspiciousness of temper, loss of self-control, lassitude, indifference, hypochondria, extreme sensitiveness to ridicule or to reproach, fickleness, jactitation, unrest, local or general spasms, tremors, partial paralysis, and circumscribed alterations in the temperature of the part affected.

Nervous symptoms.

Of course these symptoms are not all present in every case of irritable uterus, but for every one of them that is lacking, you may find that ten or twenty others have been added. In brief, the symptoms are subject to the same variations, and are many of them as inexplicable as they are in hysteria, to which disease this affection is so closely allied. They are generally aggravated at the month, and are largely influenced by the state of the patient's emotions. She may be suffering severely, for example, with a pain which

Symptoms may be capricious.

alarms her family and makes her seriously ill. A friend calls to invite her to a drive, or a visit, and forthwith the symptoms vanish. The family are horrified at her going out so soon; and the doctor, who left her an hour before at home, may meet her miles away on a mission of mercy or of pleasure.

Contradictory nature of.

Such a patient, who can not sit upright in her chair for five minutes consecutively, will sometimes get into her carriage, and in a half-reclining posture, ride by the hour, or all the day long, without the least sign of fatigue or suffering. Or she will manage the affairs of her household, of the church, or of some charitable enterprise, with all the executive ability of one who is well and able to withstand any amount of fatigue. And yet, in so far as the mastery of her own movements is concerned, she may be as helpless as an infant.

Physical examination.

An examination per vaginam, as in the case of Mrs. J., reveals a more or less sensitive condition of the womb. The cervix is tender to the touch, and if you push the organ toward the superior strait it pains the patient exceedingly. In some cases the pain upon pressure is limited to a small spot. The most delicate manipulation with a view to introduce the sound or the speculum occasions more of suffering than usual. Sometimes the uterus feels swollen and slightly enlarged. Occasionally it is more or less prolapsed, and in very rare instances it is either retroflexed or retroverted.

From coccyodynia.

Diagnosis.—This disease is sometimes confounded with coccyodynia. But, in coccyodynia, whether from an injury sustained during labor, or from a fall or a blow, the patient can not sit down squarely, or rise again without immediate and most excruciating pain, which is always referred to the point of the coccyx. In irritable uterus the pain is not always so limited, and she can usually sit from five to fifteen minutes before the pain and the ill feeling come on. In the former the reclining posture is as painful as the upright one in sitting; but not so in the latter. In the former there is likely to be a great increase of the neuralgic pain while at stool, and pressure with the finger in any direction induces a local paroxysm; in the irritable uterus the suffering at stool is such as usually attends a constipated state of the bowels, and pressure upon the coccyx does not cause any very distinctive or extreme pain.

You would differentiate this affection from organic diseases of the womb by the absence of such discharges as are produced in uterine ulceration, and leucorrhœa. It need not be confounded with dysmenorrhœa, for in irritable uterus, although it is apt to be worse at the month, the pain recurs without any regard to menstruation, and often continues from one month to another.

From organic disease.—Dysmenorrhœa.

Treatment. — Whatever predisposition the patient may have inherited or acquired should, if possible, be removed, in order that the proper remedies may work more efficiently. So also of the avoidable causes, providing you can determine what they are, which in some cases is extremely difficult. To fulfil these indications may require much time and an infinite deal of tact, but, if you have the full confidence of your patient, and are sufficiently persevering, you will succeed in making life tolerable to her, if not in performing a radical cure.

Remove the cause.

In general you should remember that this class of patients are weak, debilitated, and badly nourished. If they take a sufficient quantity of food, it does not build them up as it should. Their vital force is low, and their strength is below par. They are too prone to depend for subsistence upon tea and toast, and crackers, and various little delicacies which can not sustain them properly. They are very apt to loathe meat of all kinds, milk and all varieties of animal food, and from their habits in this regard to develop a species of neuralgic dyscrasia, which frequently underlies and may even cause the worst form of hysteralgia.

Build up the general strength.

The first thing to be done for such patients is to fortify their general strength and vigor by stimulating their digestion, and supplying them with the proper aliment. Instead of mincing their meals and eating under protest in their rooms, apart from the family and alone, they should be brought to the table with others and tempted to eat more freely of good, substantial food. Let them "follow copy," as the printers say, and imitate those who have better appetites.

The mode and time of eating.

The fresh air and sunlight are indispensable; but the amount and variety of exercise to be taken must depend upon the patient's original strength, and the peculiar complications and history of the case. The more marked the hysterical tendency, the greater the need of will on her part, and determination to overcome the physical obstacles that lie in her path. Some of these patients need almost to be put out of doors before they will make the necessary effort to walk or ride, and thus learn for themselves that locomotion is among the possibilities.

Fresh air and exercise.

But it will not do to insist that all are alike in this respect. For, on the contrary, some of them will go too much and too far. They overdo in this direction, and need to be restrained. And others are absolutely too weak and too ill to take active exercise, regardless of its cost or consequences. The best rule with which I am acquainted is to observe carefully how each one is influenced by the effort of going to ride or to walk, and thus to learn what she can bear and take within the limits of actual fatigue. She may be able to ride three squares not only with impunity, but with decided benefit, when to add one more square to the length of the drive would do her a positive injury. Long journeys are more tolerable for this class of our patients than they were before the days of the sleeping-car, but notwithstanding this improvement, many are yet injured by travel on the railways. When it is possible, and convenient, it is best for them to journey by water.

Varying ability to take exercise.

You will have so much trouble in regulating the habits of some of these patients in many particulars, that I am tempted to let you into a little secret which may help you to carry your point, and to adapt your counsel to the end in view. First, make up your mind deliberately what practice, or habit, or influence it is that lies in the way of their recovery. Then set to work to reform or to remove that custom or influence, whatever it may be, by gaining the entire and willing assent of the patient herself. These indications cannot always, or perhaps frequently, be met in an off-hand or intuitive manner. They require the exercise of thought and of tact. And unless you can secure her confidence and co-operation, you certainly will not succeed. It may need a large measure of skill and of perseverance to bring it about, but you will learn that the art consists in having your own way, while she is under the impression that she has hers also.

A practical hint.

A very common error in the treatment of the irritable uterus is to suppose that uterine surgery, as it is technically styled, and ordinarily practiced, will help to cure it. For the truth is that, in this class of cases, it does more harm than good. There is not a single operation, or expedient of this kind, that is advisable in an uncomplicated case of hysteralgia. Caustics, the knife, the sponge-tent, the bistourie cachée, the sound, the probe, and pessaries of whatever variety, are so many instruments of torture. They invariably aggravate the disease. It is only when some of the incidental conditions that require such aid are superadded to the irritable condition of the uterus itself that the intelligent physician employs them in this disease at all.

Surgery contra-indicated.

For the relief of the spinal, sacral and pelvic pains various topical applications are permissible and useful, the same as in other forms of neuralgia. Bathing the back with salt-water, dry frictions along the spine from above downwards, hot or cold water locally, the shower bath, pediluvia, wearing a thick layer of cotton batting along the back, the wearing of silk undervests and wrappers to insulate and protect the person against sudden electrical changes, painting the painful part with the oleaginous collodion, dry cupping, porous plasters, arnica plasters, magnetism, electricity, galvanic belts and plates, and the use of bland and soothing injections per vaginam are the most common and useful of these expedients.

Topical expedients.

I once called an old physician in counsel in a case of diphtheria. We had agreed upon the internal remedies, when my friend suggested that something, and the simpler the better, should be prescribed for external use, chiefly in order to keep the nurse and watchers busy with that which would do no positive harm, even if it did but very little good; for, said he, you know that "Satan finds some mischief still for idle hands to do."

Why we should use them.

Acting upon this principle, and remembering the propensity of human nature to overdo in the matter of nursing especially, you had better advise some simple expedient that will "keep the nurse and watchers busy," rather than let them "fly to evils that they know not of."

It is unnecessary to repeat what I have already said of the

choice of remedies when speaking of the treatment of hysteria.*

No specific treatment.

There is no specific for the relief and cure of the irritable uterus. If the proper conditions are supplied and secured, medicines will achieve the most marked results. Otherwise they are powerless. The symptoms are so complicated, and oftentimes so contradictory, that you will find it very difficult to choose the most appropriate remedy.

The new remedies in.

It is very probable that among the newer remedies, which of late have attracted so much attention, we may yet find a more ready means of cure for the various nervous disorders which are symptomatic of uterine disease and irritation. For myself, I have come to place a deal of confidence in macrotin, gelseminum, caulophyllin, the lilium tigrinum, and senecin. Other members of this class are scutellaria, ambra grisea, cypripedium and veratrum viride. But the old polychrests should not be forgotten.

Prescription.

Mrs. J. will take a dose of macrotin three times daily, and have electricity applied along the spine twice per week—every Tuesday and Friday evening. I think it best in these cases that electricity should be used in the evening rather than in the morning or the early part of the day. She must also play the part of a good Christian philosopher, and not let her little domestic cares and trials fret and worry her too much.

* See page 315.

LECTURE XXIX.

THE UTERINE SOUND.

GENTLEMEN:

While we are waiting this morning for our first patient to be brought in, I will speak of the Uterine Sound. And in order to make my remarks as practical as possible, I will arrange them so as to consider (1) *why*, (2) *when*, and (3) *how* we should avail ourselves of this invaluable instrument.

1. *Why, or for what purpose do we employ the sound?*

You are doubtless aware that this instrument, of which you will find several varieties upon the table, has been in use for centuries. By the ancients it was regarded as a *curative* means. They scarcely used it for any other purpose than to replace the uterus when it had become dislocated. But, in the hands of modern gynæcologists, it is regarded almost exclusively as an aid to *diagnosis*. In this manner it enables us to diagnosticate:

In diagnosis.

(*a.*) *Certain Diseases of the Uterine Cervix.*—If we know what the proper dimensions and length of the neck of the womb are, or should be, by passing this instrument, we can decide if the case is one of hypertrophy, atrophy, or immobility of this part of the organ; if it is imperforate; if there is cervicitis, or a polypus, or uterine displacement. Atresia, obliteration and flexures of the cervix, as well as a more or less permanent closure of the internal os uteri, in mechanical and spasmodic dysmenorrhœa, are also recognizable by means of the sound.

In diseases of the cervix.

(*b.*) *In diseases affecting the cavity and body of the uterus.*—The very ease of introduction of the sound through the internal os uteri, during the inter-menstrual period, suggests that all is not right within the cavity of the womb. It is a sign of endometritis, or of the presence of some foreign growth, as, for example, either submucous or interstitial fibroids, polypi, hydatids, cauliflower excrescence, or of cancerous degeneration.

In diseases of the uterine cavity.

(*c.*) *To measure the size of the uterus.*—In health the unimpregnated womb measures about two and a half inches from the os to the fundus uteri. But this organ is so distensible, so given to development and to variations in its size and capacity from pathological, as well as from physiological causes, that we may sometimes learn much in a diagnostic way from its actual measurement. This, of course, is best accomplished by means of the uterine sound. Passing the instrument in the direction of the axis of the organ, through its whole length, and taking care to indicate the extent to which it has entered the uterus, we obtain the longitudinal measurement of that organ. If it is lengthened to four, six, or more inches, and the woman is not pregnant, or has not very recently been delivered, the information thus obtained makes us confident that something is wrong. By this means, therefore, we may be able to diagnosticate a longitudinal hypertrophy of the womb, a very interesting case of which I will take an early occasion to show you. By it, also, we may detect sub-involution and super-involution, as well as enlargements of the uterus due to the development of various kinds of tumors, as, for example, uterine fibroids, within its cavity. Thus, in the case of Mrs. H., you will remember, although she had a large ovarian cyst which was removed in presence of the class, the uterus measured six inches, and was found upon actual inspection to be very considerably enlarged.* In order to be accurate in this kind of measurement, it is well sometimes to use the graduated sound.

For measurement.

In uterine hypertrophy.

(*d.*) *To test the mobility of the Uterus.* — In not a few cases the non-susceptibility of the uterus to motion is a diagnostic test of great value. We apply this test by introducing the sound, and then observing whether, when we move it laterally and carefully, the womb moves along with it. If it does, the organ is free, and

* See page 363.

not bound down by adhesions or organic change; but if it does not, some pathological change has been going on which has resulted in its becoming glued or adherent to the neighboring parts.

In uterine carcinoma.

This sign is present in cancer of the inferior segment of the womb, and in certain confirmed cases of pelvic cellulitis, and more frequently in pelvic-peritonitis. We also meet with it, but more rarely, in old, chronic cases of retroversion and of retroflexion of the womb, in which the organ is anchored, so to speak, by strong adventitious bands attached to the rectum and the posterior pelvic tissues.

In uterine tumors.

This, as you know, is one of the means of differentiating between uterine and ovarian and other abdominal tumors. Placing the left hand over the abdomen, and moving the sound in utero with the other hand, as I have just indicated, if the motion of the womb is communicated to the tumor, or, in other words, if the womb and the tumor move simultaneously, in the same direction and to the same extent, we are assured that the tumor is uterine. But if the uterus can thus be moved independently of the tumor, there is no doubt of its being extra-uterine.

In deviations of uterus.

(*e.*) *In the diagnosis of Uterine Displacements.*—It will occur to you, without doubt, that any considerable disorder of place in the womb would necessarily include a deviation of its axis from the normal one. The direction of its long diameter, and therefore of its curve, would be changed. Now, in order to ascertain what direction the luxated organ has taken, and the extent of the displacement, more particularly in versions and flexions thereof, we must depend almost entirely upon the sound. If the womb is *in situ*, what might be termed the pelvic curve of the instrument (as we speak of the pelvic curve of the obstetric forceps), looks forward, toward the symphysis pubis, and the point thereof corresponds with the axis of the superior strait. But if the womb is bent forwards, or backwards, or laterally, the curve or concavity of the instrument will be found towards the bladder, the rectum, or the right or the left iliac fossa, as the case may be. Sims' uterine probe, which is a modified or attenuated sound, is sometimes very useful in this class of cases.

In prolapsus the sound enters more readily, and its point takes the direction of the axis of the inferior strait or of the vagina, and looks toward the hollow of the sacrum, or toward the sacro-vertebral eminence. In procidentia, the os being at the lowest part of the tumor, the sound may be readily introduced. By this means we differentiate between procidentia and inversion of the womb; for, in the latter, the os uteri can not be found before the organ is reposited, and therefore in inversion it is quite impossible to pass the sound until that operation is performed.

For the reposition of the womb.

Of late years, as I have already said, the ordinary sound is not often used as a means of replacing the uterus. In exceptional cases, however, it may still be used for this purpose. Drs. Elliott, Sims, and others, have brought out such improvements upon the old instrument as render it much more safe and valuable as a means of fulfilling this indication.

2. *When should the Sound be introduced?*

In the morning.

I have known physicians to fail to learn anything from a resort to the sound because they did not have tact enough to discover, and no one had told them, that there were certain times and seasons in which this instrument could be used to more advantage than in others. As a rule, I think you will find that the sound can be more readily passed in the early than in the later part of the day. If you can be permitted to make the operation early, before the patient is up, or has been upon her feet in the morning, it may be much more easily and thoroughly accomplished than if you wait until toward evening or bedtime.

In advance of the monthly flow.

Sometimes it is well to select a time which is a few hours, or perhaps a day in advance of the menstrual period. The preparatory dilatation having been effected in advance of the flow, the internal os uteri is lazily agape, and less irritable than usual, and the sound is made to enter with but little delay, pain or trouble.

When the patient is calm.

You would not attempt to pass it when the patient is very much alarmed or excited, agitated and apprehensive. Neither would it be advisable in case of menstrual retention with softening of the cervix, lest the woman might prove to be *enceinte*, and you might bring on a miscarriage. Nor would it do any good, but might possibly do harm, to introduce it too soon after menstruation, or directly after delivery.

3. *How shall it be passed?*

Unless the cervix uteri is closed by an atresia of its canal, which is comparatively rare, the chief difficulty in introducing the sound is met with at the internal os. This obstruction is caused either by a change in the course of the utero-cervical canal at that point, or by an irritable condition of the muscular fibres (which form a sort of sphincter about the orifice) which causes them to contract spasmodically on the approach of the instrument.

Difficulty at the os internum.

It is a very common error to suppose that the healthy uterus is nearly straight, when in fact it is not so. Cruveilhier, and other anatomists, have shown that, even in little girls, its fundus is thrown forward, as in anteversion, toward the bladder. Opposite the junction of the neck with the body of the organ, there is a curve which is in the form of an obtuse angle, as is shown most clearly in this beautiful model, and in the diagrams on the black-board.

Uterine axis not straight.

Now, in order to enter the uterine cavity, the instrument must follow this curve at the internal os uteri, otherwise its point can not reach to the fundus. If the curve, or flexion forward, were uniform and unvarying, in different women, there would be little trouble on this account. But it is not so. For we find that, even in healthy persons, there is the greatest possible difference, not only in the shape, size and position of the womb, but also in the course and direction of its canal. This explains the fact to which I have before alluded, that, having learned the individual peculiarity of a patient in this respect by the passage of the sound, it will be less difficult to perform the operation upon her in the future. There are many exceptions, however, to this rule.

Variation in uterine curve.

It is because of the varying course and curve of the uterine canal in different subjects, and in health and disease, that it is best to use a flexible sound, which is capable of adapting itself to the existing curvature, instead of a very stiff one, which would not yield,

Kind of sound that is preferable.

and which would require more of force to introduce it. For this reason, the copper sound, and in some instances the whalebone probe, is preferable to Simpson's old-fashioned sound. This copper sound will insinuate itself, whereas in a considerable proportion of cases, the old one can not be introduced without an unwarrantable degree of force. Where the uterine canal is bent acutely, forming an elbow, or the uterus is twisted upon itself spirally, we may sometimes pass a Sims' probe, such as I hold in my hand, and then withdraw it so carefully that it will retain its shape. The larger sound can then be bent into the same form, and afterwards passed more readily.

Position of the patient.

Concerning the best position for the patient to assume, something will depend upon the nature of the case which is to be examined. Usually, it is best for her to lie upon her left side, on the bed or couch, to have the thighs flexed on the abdomen, and the legs on the thighs. This will enable you to find the cervix most readily, and to give the proper direction to the point of the instrument, when it has passed into the cervical canal. If she lies upon the back, and the uterus is not prolapsed, more especially if the vagina is long and your index finger is short, you will experience considerable difficulty in reaching the neck of the womb at all. And when you have reached it, the finger will come against the anterior lip, and the organ will recede into the hollow of the sacrum, so that it may be next to impossible to pass the sound even through the external os uteri.

An exception.

There are exceptional cases in which the womb is displaced in an upward direction, in which, no matter what the position of the patient, it is very difficult to pass the sound. In these cases, it is recommended to let the patient stand upright, with her back against the wall, while the operation is being performed. But ordinarily this is not requisite.

In displacements backwards.

If there is retroversion or retroflexion, the woman may be placed on the bed, couch or table, as for the introduction of Sims' speculum, on the left side, far over upon the abdomen, with the right thigh flexed and the left one straight. Or, if this is not sufficient, with the aid of gravity, to bring the fundus forwards, so that the sound may pass readily, she may take the knee-elbow or prone position. In the latter case, before she gets upon the knees, you had better secure the cervix for fear it may recede and pass beyond your reach. This indication may be met by means of the uterine tenaculum, an ordinary vulsellum, or what answers equally well, and is less painful, by introducing the sound as far as may be before she turns over, then keeping it within the cervix while she is changing her position.

In anteversion and anteflexion you may take the precaution to recommend her to lie on the back for a number of hours before you pass the sound. She should also be instructed not to void her urine unless it is absolutely necessary, for about the same interval, in the hope that its accumulation in the bladder may help to restore the womb to its proper position. Indeed, you should not forget that the fullness or emptiness of the bladder and the rectum may greatly influence the facility with which it is possible to pass the uterine sound.

In displacements formed.

It is the habit of some physicians always to use the speculum as a means of facilitating the introduction of the sound. Since the invention of Sims' speculum especially, this practice has become quite popular. My own opinion is that, while in rare cases it may be necessary to use these instruments conjointly, in ordinary practice we can get on quite as well, or even better, without the speculum and the tenaculum. You can learn to pass the uterine sound without the help of vision quite as soon and as adroitly as you can learn to pass the female catheter by the sense of touch alone, and without any exposure of the patient's person. And I think you should try to do so.

Conjoined use of speculum and sound.

The chief things to be done in acquiring this species of tact are to place the patient in a proper position, to ascertain the direction of the uterine curve, to manipulate carefully rather than forcibly, to have the proper instrument,and not to be in too great a hurry. I have already spoken of the proper time and posture to be chosen. In order to learn the course of the uterine canal, the "touch" must precede the attempt to pass the sound. By passing the finger carefully on every side of the cervix, as high up as possible, you can get the direction of the cervical axis, and recognize any marked flexion of the

Points to be observed.

uterus, which is most apt to take place at a point opposite the internal os uteri, where the peritoneal coat is lacking in front. In case of the different versions the os and cervix must be located before the sound could be introduced.

Mode of introduction.

In ordinary cases, and with the tip of the right index finger at the external os, the sound can be passed along its palmar surface, while being guided by the left hand, and made to enter the canal of the cervix. When it has passed an inch or so within that canal, the handle of the instrument should be depressed toward the posterior commissure of the vulva, and its curve turned toward the symphysis pubis. A little delicate manipulation and tact will now cause it to pass through the internal os uteri and into the uterine cavity. Sometimes, however, it may be necessary to withdraw the sound and to change its shape somewhat. Or it may have failed to pass because its point was lodged in one of the lacunæ which are so numerous in the cervical canal.

Danger from too much force.

If you use too much force it is possible for the instrument to pass not into the uterine, but into the abdominal cavity. This is especially liable to occur in case the sound slips and passes into the Douglas' cul-de-sac ; and also where the tissues of the uterine cervix have been softened and somewhat disorganized as the result of chronic disease. Fatal peritonitis has sometimes resulted from this accident.

Explain.

If the patient is young and nervous, tell her precisely what it is that you propose to do ; that there will be no cutting, and but little pain ; that, in truth, this is only another means of extending the "touch" farther than the length of your finger will permit. Her attention should be diverted while the operation is going on.

Choice of a sound.

There is as much difference between two of these sounds which, to all appearance are precisely alike, as there is between two catheters. One will find its way like an intelligent agent, but the other almost invariably goes wrong. When you have selected a good one, let me counsel you to use it habitually and exclusively.

Above all things do not be in haste. This a delicate little operation upon the careful performance of which more may depend than you perhaps imagine. At any rate you will be more likely to fail than to succeed if you are rash and precipitate. It is better to take fifteen, twenty, thirty, or more minutes and do no harm, than to hurry the thing over without doing any good, or learning anything. If you fail altogether at one session, make another appointment with your patient, and try again. You may be more successful the next time.

"Festina lente."

The instrument should be anointed with oil, lard or glycerine, or better still with soap and water at the dressing table.

THE CLIMACTERIC — THE CHANGE OF LIFE.

Case. — Mrs. C. W——, is forty-two years of age; has eczema of the hands and forearms. This eruption commenced one year ago and has continued ever since, being worse at times and then better. It is not an hereditary disease. She never had it but once before, which was in her thirteenth year. At that time it remained out for about six months and finally disappeared without any bad symptoms. Her general health has always been good. She has not been subject to any cutaneous disorder. She has five children, the youngest of whom is thirteen years old. Her menstrual life has not been peculiar in any respect excepting that she had some trouble when the flow was first established. This was in her thirteenth year. She was in poor health at that time for about half a year, and did not recover entirely until the flow came on freely and regularly and the old eruption had altogether disappeared.

The life of woman is a succession of epochs, or crises. Puberty, matrimony, gestation, parturition, and lactation, bring their peculiar experiences and are beset by peculiar contingencies. But there is still another epoch which has its physiological and its clinical history. I allude to what is variously styled the "change of life," the "grand climacteric," the "critical age," the "cessation of the menses," the "turn of life," and the ménopause.

Crises in the life of women.

The age at which this period arrives in women varies as much in different individuals as does that which dates the advent of puberty. Indeed it bears such a general relation to the early or late establishment of the menstrual function that we ordinarily estimate from puberty to

Varying age.

determine when the catamenia should naturally cease. Thus, the usual duration of menstrual life is thirty years. If our patient was "unwell" for the first time when she was but thirteen years old, and we add thirty to that number, we shall have forty-three years as the most natural limit for the return of the monthly cycle. If, instead of beginning at thirteen the function had failed until she was fifteen, then she would most naturally continue to menstruate until she had reached the age of forty-five years.

Duration of menstrual life.

But this calculation is approximative, and not exact. We must make allowance for modifying circumstances of various kinds, among which hereditary peculiarities are, perhaps, the most marked. There are families in which all the women cease to menstruate prematurely at as early an age as thirty, others at thirty-five, and still others in whom the ménopause is adjourned until fifty, or even to the 60th year, when it degenerates into a species of sexual hæmorrhage. In these cases the advent of the change of life bears no particular relation to the age of the individual at the time that puberty was established. It not unfrequently happens that those who begin to menstruate the earliest continue to do so for a longer period than those who began later in life.

Exceptions.

Physiologically considered, the "change" which closes and terminates a most important function of the female economy, is truly an eventful and a marvelous one. It must work such a complete revolution as to invest this crisis with numerous contingencies. For this function, which represents the maternal instinct and relation, which made it possible for the woman to become a mother, which was suspended while the child was being developed in utero, and while she nourished it at the breast; and which was restored again in due season, is not one that can be begun, continued for so many years, and then stopped, without great expense and risk to the general organism.

Importance of the change.

Hence we find that the approach of the climacteric predisposes women to various diseases which are of a more or less serious nature. And, what is very strange, it not unfrequently happens that the disease from which they may have suffered at puberty re-

Predisposition incident to this period.

turns. It is so in the case before us. The class of affections which are most likely to recur in this manner are eruptive and nervous disorders, and hæmorrhages from certain mucous membranes. In cases of this kind, it may happen that many years have elapsed without any sign of the difficulty, but when this change begins to take place the first symptom noticed is the reappearance of the old enemy. Very nervous and plethoric women are more likely to suffer in this manner, and indeed to be ill, at the change of life, than those who are of a lymphatic temperament.

Diseases incident to puberty may return.

But in this respect the ménopause is not absolutely or always in relation with puberty. Very often the experiences that have intervened since the woman first began to menstruate have so changed her nature that she has acquired a predisposition to other and different diseases. Pregnancy, labor, and lactation, leave their impress upon her organization, and it is as impossible for her youthful susceptibilities always to return, as it would be for her to become the same in feeling after the change of life that she was in her girlhood.

New disorders induced.

Another peculiarity worthy of note is that many diseases are cured, or disappear in consequence of the climacteric. The ovarian atrophy and paralysis removes a constantly recurring source of disease. The monthly cycle and its attendant excitement of the nervous, vascular, and glandular systems is withdrawn. A season of continued quiet, and comparative tranquillity supplies a favorable condition for the restoration of health. And when the critical period has passed it is found to have been the scape-goat of a thousand ills. Slender women may become corpulent and even obese, bed-ridden invalids get up and walk, and an entire and radical change of physical condition is the consequence in those who escape the perils of this period. They enter upon a new phase of life, with new hopes and relations towards the present and the future.

Old diseases cured by.

Symptoms.— The manner of approach of the critical period varies in different individuals. With some women the change is abrupt, but with the majority it is more prolonged and gradual. Not infrequently the flow becomes intermittent, or, rather, the periods become irregular. One, two, three, or perhaps six months, and sometimes a year or more, may elapse between them.

In many cases they are too frequent, as well as too profuse, for a season, and afterwards are more tardy and abnormal in this respect.

Hæmorrhage.

In a considerable proportion of cases the amount of the flow lessens gradually, so that it may finally come away drop by drop, or until there is nothing of it left. But as the change approaches, many women find themselves flowing more freely than ever before. Indeed, the tendency of the catamenial discharge to develop into a hæmorrhage is often observed. Out of 500 women at the change of life, Tilt observed that 208 had hæmorrhages of various kinds. Of these, 138 had either a single terminal flooding, or successive floodings.*

Other forms of hæmorrhage, which are in a sense vicarious of the monthly flow at the climacteric, are hæmorrhoids, entorrhagia, epistaxis, hæmoptysis, cerebral hæmorrhage and apoplexy, hæmatemesis, hæmaturia, bursting of varicose veins, bleeding from the ear, and cutaneous ecchymosis. In plethoric women these losses of blood are in a sense critical, and although they are often dangerous in themselves, yet as a kind of safety-valve, they are sometimes salutary.

Simulates pregnancy.

The sudden arrest of the accustomed flow, when the change comes on abruptly, and more especially in those who are in good health, is often the occasion of alarm with such persons lest they be pregnant. This suspicion finds apparent confirmation in the coincident gastric derangements that not unfrequently ensue. There is something resembling morning sickness, caprices of appetite, a sense of fullness and discomfort, and pelvic bearing-down and aching which women recognize as very similar to, if not identical with the symptoms of early pregnancy. You will certainly be consulted in cases of this kind, and in making a diagnosis should not forget that some women cease to menstruate as early as the twenty-fifth year.

Alimentary symptoms.

Sometimes the most violent, and again the most persistent and intractable indigestion, colic, diarrhœa, hæmorrhoids, dysentery or constipation, come with the first symptom of the menstrual decline. In many cases, these

* The Change of Life in Health and Disease. By Edward John Tilt, M.D., etc., London, 1867, page 65.

attacks are self-limited, and subside of themselves when the crisis has finally passed. In a few they supplement the catamenial flow, and may pass into the chronic form.

Disorders of the circulation.

The circulation is very irregular, as is shown by flushes of heat in the face and elsewhere, local congestions to the head, giddiness, blushing and discoloration of the skin, coldness, tingling and numbness of the extremities, sudden outbreaks of perspiration, chilliness, rigors, and active hæmorrhages.

Nervous symptoms.

The nervous symptoms and sequelæ of the climacteric are marked and sometimes very troublesome. In degree they vary from the slight mental perturbations, vulgarly styled "the fidgets," to the most profound convulsions and paralysis. Headache, vertigo, nervous irritability, pseudo-narcotism, self-absorption, insomnia, jactitation, palpitation, dyspnœa, horrible dreams, fainting, erethism, depression, debility, twitchings, spasms, mania, and full-fledged hysteria are by no means uncommon at this period. Either of these affections may precede, accompany or follow the cessation of the menses. In many cases the disorder is ephemeral; but in others it becomes seated and confirmed. Spasmodic affections are very apt to continue, and to take on a regular periodical type, which is most difficult of cure. The ganglionic nervous system is always implicated.

Epilepsy.

There is a form of epilepsy which is not unusual at this period. I have seen several cases of the kind that were in no way connected with the hereditary form of this disease. Only yesterday I was consulted by my friend, Dr. W. R. McLaren, for the relief of the following

Case.—Mrs. ——, aged forty-five, is now passing through the grand climacteric. The menses recur every four to six months. They are quite profuse. About every seven weeks she has the epileptic seizure. There is no very strong muscular contraction or rigidity. The face is pale, and during the paroxysm there is stertorous breathing, with foaming at the mouth. The fit, during which she is quite oblivious to everything external, lasts about four minutes. After it she sleeps for three-fourths of an hour. The change of life commenced with her one year ago, at which time she first began to have the epileptic paroxysms. Epilepsy is not hereditary in her family, although her mother also had fits at the change of life.

Disorders of the special senses.

Disorders of the nerves of special sense are not infrequent. Deafness, blindness, aphonia, loss of the sense of taste or of smell, and of tactile sensibility in various portions of the skin, are among the more common of these affections. These complications are most apt to occur in weakly, nervous, debilitated women in whom, for some reason, the climacteric is very much prolonged or exhaustive.

Diseases of the respiratory system.

The respiratory system comes in for its share of the contingent ailments. Those women especially who are predisposed to pectoral complaints, who inherit this bias, and who have suffered some of the consequences of incipient organic disease of the lungs at or before puberty, are most likely to have something of the kind at the climacteric change. Perhaps the first thing noticed is a more or less copious spitting of blood, or a nervous, irritating cough, which by and by settles into a confirmed habit, and is accompanied by free expectoration. In some cases these symptoms develop into a rapid decline, and the patient may not live more than a very few weeks. In others they subside of themselves when the first cause is removed, and the menstrual crisis is safely over. In not a few instances the boasted cures of phthisis pulmonalis are really to be ascribed to the fact that such cases as these are self-limited, and frequently get well of themselves.

Disorders of the generative system.

But, as you would suppose, it is the generative function and the sexual organs which are most seriously disordered in consequence of the final cessation of the menses. Thus Dr. Tilt* found that of 500 women at the change of life, 463 suffered from uterine affections. Among these contingent disorders are uterine cancer and catarrh, cervical inflammation and hypertrophy, uterine ulceration, hæmorrhage, hysteralgia, leucorrhœa, displacements, tumors, hydatids, polypi, and fibroids. Either or all of these diseases are more serious if the patient has already suffered from them.

Other complications are ovaritis, ovarian induration, atrophy and paralysis, the development of cystic tumors, and of ovarian

* Op. citat., p. 82.

abscess, and hæmatocele. And still another disease of the generative system, properly speaking, is cancer of the breast, the development of which appears in many cases to be hastened by the permanent arrest of the menstrual secretion.

Incidental diseases.

Women sometimes suffer from a species of rheumatism and others from neuralgia which worries them exceedingly, and may perhaps wear away their remaining strength very rapidly. Again these affections are combined, and either or both of them may be located within the pelvis. The arrival of the critical period may act as an exciting cause, and really occasion an attack of rheumatism in one who not only has never had it before, but who was thought to be free from any predisposition to it. I could cite you many cases of this kind, but it must suffice merely to call your attention to the fact itself.

Rheumatism and neuralgia.

Prognosis.—Where serious diseases occur at the climacteric, or follow it almost immediately, you will be puzzled in your prognosis. Eminent authorities are of opinion that the ovarian activity is commensurate with the constitutional vigor; and that, as a rule, life is longest in those women in whom puberty is retarded and the menstrual function most prolonged. Therefore, it will be a safe criterion upon which to base an opinion if we say that the patient's previous health (especially in so far as ovulation is concerned) has been good or ill, habitually. If she has been weakly and sickly, and suffered from menstrual derangements, such as dysmenorrhœa, menorrhagia, and amenorrhœa, or her nutritive resources have been sapped and drained by a chronic leucorrhœa, or diarrhœa, or mal-medication, or starvation, whether mental, moral or physical, the case is not of the most hopeful kind. The same is true of the bad effects of scrofulosis, and of too rapid child-bearing, as tending to undermine the general health and vigor, and to leave the patient a more easy prey to the contingencies that beset the ménopause.

The general health the best criterion.

We are therefore compelled to make due allowance for previous ill health, and to qualify our prognosis; for it is a crisis through which the woman must pass, and whether she will survive it or not, will depend very largely upon the stock of strength that she has in reserve to begin with.

Critical catamenial hæmorrhages are dangerous, not because, as the ancients believed, that certain poisonous matters from the menses are retained in the blood-current, and need to be eliminated, but because of an overwhelming afflux of blood to a delicate tissue or organ, which may soon result in disorganization and death.

Cause of the danger.

If the cessation of the periodical flow shall re-act upon the lungs, and light up the tuberculous diathesis, it will not be safe to promise to cure the patient. And so, also, of the alimentary disorders, of which I have spoken; for, although some of these utero-intestinal affections subside of themselves, when the menses are entirely disposed of, still in many other cases they only run a more rapid and fatal course.

The tuberculous diathesis.

Treatment.—The critical period, therefore, is beset with so many dangers that its treatment becomes a very important matter. The first thing to be done is so to regulate the habits and surroundings of the patient as to protect her against these dangers. The state of her mind, the amount and variety of her physical exercise, and her food, must be prescribed and regulated according to the rules of hygiene and of good, sound common sense. Nothing wears upon a woman who has reached the turn of life like a want of sleep, of rest, and of freedom from the petty cares and annoyances which she could once overcome by her own strength of will.

Hygienic rules.

She should be encouraged and stimulated by cheerful society, and pleasant intercourse with a few friends. Her thoughts should not be introverted. She should not be permitted to brood over such reflections as will make her nervous and wretched, but should become interested in the welfare and happiness of others; for this is the line of thought that henceforth must engage her attention.

Diversion.

Especially should you guard against the development of any disease to which she is predisposed. If she is liable to hæmorrhagic attacks from plethora, let her diet be plain and unstimulating, her habits as active as possible within the limits of prudence, and give her such remedies (according to their specific indications) as aconite, belladonna, veratrum vir., gelseminum, bryonia, or ipecacu-

Guard against hereditary predispositions.

anha. If, however, the hæmorrhage is passive, and the result of an anæmic or vitiated habit, you may consult the merits of nitric acid, china, arsenicum alb., secale cor., sabina, crocus, trillium, erechthites, pulsatilla, ferrum met., and carbo vegetabilis. Cool acidulated drinks ought always to be preferred in this class of cases. Tea and coffee should be interdicted, and so, also, should very active or violent exercise.

For the hæmorrhage.

Next to this tendency to hæmorrhage, which is always alarming and frequently dangerous, especially at this time of life, the possibility that the patient may pass almost insidiously into a decline from tuberculosis in some of its forms, renders it necessary to antidote this predisposition whenever it exists. For this purpose certain precautionary measures are requisite. A limited amount of exposure is not necessarily harmful, but care should be taken that these patients incur no risks in this regard. They should not be suffered to take cold, to get the feet wet, to go out in a storm, to wear insufficient clothing, no matter how fashionable, or to talk or to sing too much and too long at one time. They should keep in from the night air especially, and not be permitted to sit in the open air, as many women are in the habit of doing. Such a patient should not be removed from her old home into a new house, for example, in which the walls are not dry. In brief, without being fussy, she should take unusual care of her health at this period, for a slight indiscretion, or an otherwise trifling cold might act as an exciting cause for the development of a latent disease that would soon carry her off.

For the tendency to phthisis.

The remedies to be thought of in this connection are calcarea carb., calcarea phos., sanguinaria, phosphorus, stannum, mercurius jod., kali jod., kali brom., kali carb., hepar sulph., lachesis, sepia, lycopodium, nitric acid, ignatia, bryonia and silicea. The greatest possible care should be taken to recognize and to remedy the first symptoms of tuberculosis in a woman who is passing the critical period; for if this is done there is little doubt that much trouble and suffering may be spared, and her life prolonged.

The symptoms of coincident digestive disorders may be treated upon specific indications, always giving preference, however, when possible, to those remedies that have a curative relation to the generative, as well as

For the digestive disorders.

to the alimentary function. Nux vomica, colocynth, arsenicum alb., mercurius, pulsatilla, natrum mur., bryonia, calcarea carb., cocculus, veratrum alb. and veratrum vir., chamomilla, sulphur and belladonna belong to this class. The diet should be regulated with the greatest care.

For the disorders of the circulation.

The wonderful influence of aconite over most of the derangements of the circulation at the climacteric, has long been known. It is an invaluable and almost indispensable remedy. Other available remedies of this sort are veratrum viride, gelseminum, and belladonna. They are not only indicated physiologically and pathogenetically in many cases, but the indication includes their special relation to disorders of the sexual system, more particularly to such as depend upon certain crises in the uterine and ovarian circulation. For the "flushes" and flashes of sudden heat, which constitute the most troublesome symptoms in milder cases, Dr. Madden recommends lachesis, either in the sixth or twelfth dilution; Dr. John F. Gray, sanguinaria; and Dr. Trinks, sulphuric acid. You will find the indications for these and other remedies in Dr. Richard Hughes' excellent work on Therapeutics.*

For the nervous symptoms.

The nervous epiphenomena demand such remedies under almost the same identical indications, as would be prescribed for them if they were incident to the more common menstrual disorders, as for example, dysmenorrhœa, amenorrhœa or menorrhagia. Belladonna, ignatia, hyoscyamus, coffea, chamomilla, moschus, pulsatilla, caulophyllin, macrotin and senecin, are most freely indicated.

For the disorders of the generative system.

And so likewise of diseases of the generative organs that are incident to the critical period. The rules which I have so frequently repeated with reference to their medical and surgical management should be carried out in practice with even more than ordinary care and skill. Whatever can possibly interfere with the structural changes which result in the atrophy of the ovaries and the uterus, as a part of the critical process, should be removed. For these structural changes, brought about through fatty metamorphosis, really pertain to the period through which the patient

* A Manual of Therapeutics, by Richard Hughes, L.R.C.P. Ed., etc., etc., N. Y. 1869, page 455.

is passing, quite as decidedly as the cessation of the flow itself. Since it might therefore interrupt this retrograde metamorphosis of the tissues if inflammation were established in them, you should see to it that such a contingency is averted; or if it has already begun, to cure it and remove its consequences as speedily as possible.

For rheumatism and neuralgia.

For the rheumatic and neuralgic complications, macrotin, rhus tox., atropine, the valerianate of zinc, mercurius, and similar remedies will be required.

LECTURE XXX.

SPINAL IRRITATION—NOTALGIA—"BACK-ACHE."

GENTLEMEN:

Some of the more advanced members of the class have frequently consulted me with regard to the treatment of spinal irritation. This woman has suffered from that disease for many years, and her clinical history will doubtless interest you.

Case.—Mrs. M., aged fifty, enjoyed excellent health until her eleventh year. At that time, while running at play, she fell and struck the back of her neck against the corner of a table. The blow was upon the most prominent of the lower cervical vertebræ, (*vertebra prominens*). In consequence of this injury she was for six weeks very ill in bed, and so extremely weak and sensitive that they had to move her on a sheet. Several months elapsed before she could wear a dress. She finally got around again, but for several years her physicians did her but little good, and none of them referred her poor health to the injury that she had received. Finally, another physician, Dr. ——, while visiting her mother one day, touched the spot where the blow was received upon the neck, and she suddenly fainted away. Then followed a thorough course of blisters, with tartar emetic dressings, cups, leeches, and four years of barbarous treatment, which to think of, makes her "shudder to this day." With this treatment, there was much sloughing of flesh from the back, which is all scarred up now. It was a regular field-day when these sores were dressed. She cried, her mother cried, and all hands cried, but they could do no better, and she facetiously says, "it was equally impossible to do anything worse." In consequence of this injury, the left foot and limb were changed, the heel being drawn up as in a form of club-foot (*pes equinus*), in which position it remains.

She did not menstruate until she had reached her eighteenth year, and then only once. She "never saw anything again" until after she was nineteen years old. From the time that menstruation was really established, she began to improve, and kept tolerably well. At twenty-two she was married, and for eighteen months more her health remained pretty good. Then she skipped one month, and was supposed to be pregnant. At the eighth week she began to flow excessively. The hæmorrhage continued, better and then very much worse, without interruption for two months more. Despite this flooding, her size increased until she measured one and one-quarter yards (forty-five inches) around the body over the abdomen. She was said by the physicians to be four months advanced in pregnancy.

The flooding reduced her to death's door, and was not relieved until labor pains came on and continued severely enough to expel an enormous mass, which proved to be hydatids. With this mass many gallons of water were also discharged. The mass consisted of small bodies, which "varied from the size of a pea to that of a walnut, and which were strung together like grapes upon a stem."

Two months elapsed before she could sit up. The lower limbs became powerless, and remained as if paralyzed for many weeks. In a little while the most severe and agonizing headaches commenced. These recurred frequently, and kept her ill the whole summer. They were excruciating, and so severe that "it seemed as if she would go crazy with them."

In eighteen months more her first child, a son, was born. In two years from his birth she had another child, which did not live but a year; and in five years her third and last child, a daughter, was born. In every instance pregnancy and labor were normal in all respects. The labor was very severe, averaging about twenty-four hours, and the children were large. Her first and third children are still living.

When she had been married thirteen years, she received a second injury. While on her way to church, and walking on an icy place down hill, her feet slipped from under her and she fell. She thought of her back and neck, and "tried to save them." For this reason she struck upon her right elbow and her head was twisted backwards. She was lifted upright, and, with a woman's courage, walked home again. When she got up her head was fixed backwards, the muscles of the neck were rigid and spasmodically contracted, so that she could not turn the head or straighten it without taking hold, as she did, with her hands upon either side, and forcibly bringing it into position. When it turned, "something cracked as if a bone had suddenly gone into place." To this day she can not look up to the ceiling without supporting her head from behind with her hands.

In consequence of this second accident she was kept in bed for about three months. The head could not be moved except by others, or rather excepting by her husband and one lady friend. This had to be done most carefully else it brought on paroxsysms of screaming, and agony that was almost unbearable. The headache returned, but in a different form. The first symptom of an attack was a feeling "as hot as fire almost," in a spot on the top of the head. If the husband began early and promptly when this burning commenced, to rub first over the spot and then to follow along down the body and extremities, the pain in the head would vanish.

From that time until now, the region of the spine, for the space of nearly an inch on either side, and running from the base of the skull to the last dorsal vertebra, has been so exquisitely tender that the weight of a feather brush would excite the keenest suffering. Even if one should point the finger towards the back it would make her "scringe."

The lower part of the spine has remained perfectly well. In no sickness that she has ever had, so her husband says, has her mind seemed to be affected in the least. She has frequently been unconscious and oblivious to passing events, but never in the least delirious or "out of her head."

Before the birth of her last child, and for a short time only, she had some pain with menstruation. With this exception, she has never had dysmenorrhœa, or indeed any "female weakness" of any kind. The spine is not as straight as it should be, but is curved posteriorly at a point midway between the shoulders. She can lie best upon her back, and could do so during all her sickness; but, on account of pulling sensations in the opposite direction, cannot lie upon either side. At times the head has felt very heavy, as if the shoulders could not sustain it, and as if it pushed directly downwards toward the body. It is impossible for her to sit upright without something to lean her head against. She can use her hands from the wrists automatically, providing her head and body are snugly fixed and padded, and there is no necessity for moving them.

Beside the experiences in falling she has incurred other risks, among which was the swallowing of a tea-spoonful of the strong tincture of iodine, which a druggist's clerk had put up for Indian hemp! Opium throws her into violent, frightful spasms, which last for days. She once suffered severely in this manner from taking a small quantity of this drug contained in a cough mixture. She cannot bear either very cold or very warm weather. Her worst attacks of prostration always occur in the winter and spring, generally in the months of February and March.

The menstruation is becoming scantier, the flow is very debilitating and very irregular. As she approaches the climacteric her general health is somewhat improved.

Here is a case that would puzzle a clairvoyant. A spinal injury of a very serious nature is received at the impressible age of eleven years. Its effect is to delay the establishment of the menstrual function. While the system is suffering, not only from the traumatic lesion of the spinal nerves and muscles, but also from retarded puberty, she is placed under such treatment as would undermine and ruin the health of the strongest person. This voluntary martyrdom was continued for four long years. And yet she lived. At eighteen, when she had discontinued these barbarities, Nature renewed the attempt to establish the catamenia. The flow came once, but was not repeated for more than a year. After her marriage she became pregnant as she supposed, and the doctors insisted. Then after two months of flooding on her part, and of blundering on theirs, she is finally rid of a hydatid mass. Months elapsed and she barely survived. Then followed the birth of her three children.

Résumé.

After thirteen years of married life she sustained the second injury, while on her way to church. (Perhaps it has never occurred to you that the *men* are almost never injured on their way to church.) Then the fearful suffering with the crampings in the muscles of the neck, the hyperæsthesia of the superior spinal region, the headache, and the confinement in bed for several months. And, finally, the incidental vicissitudes and experiences so common to the female portion of humanity. This is but an outline sketch of thirty-nine years' experience on the part of this good woman.

Causes.—Spinal irritation, as it is styled for the lack of a better name, most frequently arises from a traumatic injury, as, for instance, from a direct blow, or a fall upon some portion of the spinal column, or from a railway jar, or contusion. Of course men and women are alike subject to such accidents. But in women, who are more delicately organized, whose spinal muscles and nerves are softer and more susceptible of injury, the first shock is more severe, and its secondary effects are more lasting and permanent. Add to this the peculiar impressibility of her general nervous system, in many cases amounting to a decided hysterical predisposition; and the perturbing influences of the crises through which she is always passing, or is about to pass, and we find there are especial reasons why she should

Traumatic causes.

Peculiar organization a predisponent.

suffer more severely, and why such mishaps are more difficult of cure in her case than in men.

The full significance of this idea is not apparent at first. Not only does it concern the fact that women are especially prone to this kind of martyrdom, but that a large measure of their consequent suffering and mal-treatment is due to ignorance thereof. What a woman wants more than anything else when she is ill, is sympathy. And if her disease is largely nervous, there is still greater need for this kind of universal emollient. But her family and friends are usually the last to realize how a slight fall, blow or shock, can so completely unhinge and demoralize her physically. They talk about resolution and will on her part, and insist that she shall get up and go around, make some effort to throw off this incubus, and develop strength by the use of it. As a rule, the stronger they are, and the more muscular, the less their sympathy with this class of patients. This, of course, reacts upon the victim, and she can not accomplish what might be possible under different circumstances.

Practical inference.

A similar misjudgment on the part of the physician may lead him to adopt such a means of treatment and of exercise as shall only add fuel to the flame. This happened in the case of Mrs. M. While her nervous sympathies and susceptibilities were at their utmost tension, she was put upon the rack and tortured afresh. Her physician made no allowance for sexual impressibility and excitability, and hence the means employed were fitted to increase her suffering rather than to alleviate it.

A common error.

There can be no doubt that the doctor did the best that he could "with the light he had;" but it was the dark lantern of empiricism that he carried. He evidently mistook the case for one of spinal meningitis with effusion. But in this he was in error; for whatever direct injury of the meninges may have followed the first fall, received some years before, the symptoms showed clearly enough that dropsy of the cord was not the real cause of her illness at the time she fainted from pressure upon the spinous process of the cervical vertebra. If any considerable effusion had existed and continued for so long a time, there must have been chronic and complete paralysis.

The very fact that puberty was arrested, without any intra-pelvic lesion, and that menstruation came on spontaneously when the treatment was suspended, shows that the disorder was mainly, if not altogether, of a nervous character. And whatever had a tendency more and more to derange her nervous system could only produce further irritation, perturbation and unrest. The marvel is that she survived such unskillful and harmful treatment at all.

Of nervous origin.

Other causes of spinal irritation are strains, as from lifting, or jumping, lying, sitting or standing habitually in such a posture as to keep the spinal muscles on the stretch, and thus to weaken and paralyze them. Rheumatism and neuralgia being predisponents of this disease, persons who have either of them are more or less decidedly susceptible to changes in the weather. For this reason, among others, as with our patient, extremes of heat and cold, and more especially of dryness and moisture, influence it greatly. The jar of travel by rail, in a rough carriage, or upon horseback, may induce it. And so, also, of tight lacing, the wearing of high-heeled shoes, and of articles of dress which are fastened at the waist and not hung upon the shoulders.

Exciting causes.

Symptoms.—The symptoms are almost endless in their variety. If the disease has been caused by direct traumatic injury of the spine, the most severe pain will be located there, and we may accordingly find the suffering referred either to the lumbo-sacral, the dorsal, or the cervical region.

If it is in the sacral region the pain will be less acute than when it is higher up along the vertebral column. It will be dull, aching and heavy in character, with complaint of great weariness, exhaustion, and perhaps of numbness also. The patient wishes something to be pressed "into the hollow of her back," or to have her hips rest firmly upon something for support. She often stuffs a pillow or her shawl, or something of that kind, beneath her, or behind her, to rest her back and to give her ease. These pains are often accompanied by intra-pelvic pains, bearing down and distress, as if the womb were displaced. Indeed, they are often wrongly attributed to some slight and temporary deviation of the womb, and the attempt is made to cure them by pessaries, injections, etc.

From injury in the sacral region.

When the results of the injury, or the lesion, if there is one, are located in the dorsal region, the pain is more acute, with super-sensitiveness of the skin over the spinous processes of the dorsal vertebræ. Sometimes these processes are exquisitely tender to the touch. Direct pressure upon them, although it may be slight, may cause her to fall, to faint, to vomit, or to shriek as if she had been shot. I have seen two cases in which the pain produced in this way was compared to that from stabbing with a very sharp knife. The dorsal vertebræ are most frequently affected.

From injury in the dorsal region.

If the blow has been received, or the injury done to the spine, in the cervical region, the pain and soreness will vary according to circumstances. The suffering is apt to be very severe. Sometimes the arms become powerless from injury of the nerves which constitute the brachial plexus. Other branches of the cervical nerves being injured by the blow or the shock, the muscles of the back part of the neck are more or less implicated. These muscles, which you know are very numerous, including the splenius colli, splenius capitis, cervicalis ascendens, transversalis colli, the trachelo- and sterno-mastoid, complexus, spinalis cervicis, trapezius and the obliquus superioris, are those which were spasmodically affected in the case of our patient, It was the painful cramp or contraction of these muscles that caused her head to be almost as immovably fixed as it is in torticollis, or wry-neck. Pressure upon the tender cervical vertebra may even stop the pulse at the wrist.

From injury in the cervical region.

When the symptoms are produced by other than mechanical causes, they are usually less intense but more erratic in their nature. The spinal tenderness is more diffuse. It may be located in any portion of the back from the occiput to the point of the coccyx. Light pressure on the spinous processes of the tender vertebræ produces considerable pain, while firm pressure may be borne without flinching. This shows its neuralgic character.

From incidental causes.

Now, from what I have said you will infer that the causes of spinal irritation act either centrically or eccentrically. In the former case a mechanical injury is done to some portion of the vertebral column. The shock is felt by the spinal nerves, and the muscles

Their centric and eccentric action.

participate more or less in the painful result. In the eccentric variety, however, the cause is more remotely applied. The irritant is at work at the incident nerves in their distribution to some muscle or organ, and, in a reflex way, the spinal center may become implicated even to the extent of producing absolute organic disease of the medulla, or of its enveloping membranes. The pain and trouble may become localized, but the irritation caused in these nerves is more apt to be reflected from the cord again to some particular organ or apparatus, as, for example, to the stomach or the bowels, to the bronchi and the lungs, to the heart, the head, or the liver.

Spinal irritation and uterine disease.

It is in this manner that utero-meningeal disorders originate and are perpetuated. There are undoubtedly many cases of spinal irritation that are in no way connected with uterine disease. And there are other cases in which, for sexual reasons, and on account of the perturbing influence of the menstrual molimen, or of maternal contingencies, the womb becomes indirectly and secondarily implicated. But there are other cases also in which the uterus has been the prime factor in this morbid process; cases in which the spinal nerves and the medulla itself have become deranged and diseased in consequence of some pre-existing uterine lesion. For this reason there are few confirmed examples of "irritable uterus," in which these two affections do not co-exist.

Reflex symptoms.

Moreover, most of the fugitive, peculiar, inexplicable local pains, burning and suffering that are incident to confirmed diseases and deviations of the womb, arise from uterine irritation which is conveyed by the sensitive nerve filaments to the cord and then reflected to these different points. It is thus that the infra-mammary pain is produced. You remember that Dr. Simpson said this pain was as characteristic of uterine disease as the pain in the point of the shoulder is of hepatic disorder. We may refer the occipital headache of menstruation to a similar cause. The point which I wish to make is this, that the continued application of this irritant, brought from the suffering part to the sentient center, in the person of delicate, nervous women, is almost certain to cause a greater or less degree of spinal irritation.

And what is true of the uterus is also true of the ovaries. The most troublesome cases of spinal irritation that I have ever treated originated in ovarialgia. The contingencies that beset ovulation even when the periods are regular; that may derange the innervation of these organs at puberty and the climacteric; that may result from intemperate coitus and similar causes, are indirectly responsible for a large proportion of cases of what are termed spinal irritation. There may be cases in which the converse is true, and wherein the ovarian disease is secondary upon the spinal lesion. Indeed, it is sometimes extremely difficult to decide between the cause and its effect, and to say positively whether the ovarian lesion is idiopathic, or *vice versa*.

From ovarian implication.

As a rule, however, I think you will find that the other coincident disorders which sometimes attend upon spinal irritation are almost always secondary. Such are the diseases of the respiratory system. It is seldom that aphonia, spasm of the glottis, dyspnœa, or a violent nervous cough, in these cases is not directly referable to the spinal lesion. So also of functional troubles of the heart, and of the digestive system. We look to the spinal center for their cause, and hope to relieve them by its cure or removal.

Secondary diseases.

Diagnosis—Providing it has been caused by direct injury, and is therefore traumatic, the diagnosis of spinal irritation is not very difficult. This is true, no matter how long a period may have elapsed since the injury was sustained. It holds in Mrs. M.'s case, for example, although thirty-nine years have passed since the date of the accident. For this reason you should take especial pains to enquire whether such a patient has ever fallen, or received a blow upon any part of her back. It is possible that so long a time has elapsed since the accident occurred, or that the mischief itself was attended by so little pain and immediate illness, that it may have been forgotten. She may have tumbled down stairs, fallen upon the ice, from her horse while riding, or from a chair upon which she was about to sit, and hurt her back long ago, but because she thought it a trivial affair at the time, may forget to mention the circumstance unless you enquire for it.

In post-traumatic cases.

Or it may happen that on account of mechanical injury to the coccyx during labor, a similar train of symptoms may have been induced. In a word, whenever you can refer the lesion to a traumatic injury, however complicated the attendant symptoms, or trivial and remote the date of the accident, the original idiopathic disease will not be difficult of recognition.

May arise from coccyodynia.

But, under different circumstances, the case is very different. When neither the patient nor her friends can recall such a misfortune, and there is no reason to believe that any portion of the vertebral column has ever been directly injured, it will not be so easy to decide the question. The tenderness of some portion of the spine upon contact and pressure, more particularly if it is constant, or habitual in certain positions of the body, is quite characteristic. If this tenderness is aggravated by the return or interruption of the menses, by coitus, by emotional states, or by sudden displacements of the womb, there is manifest spinal irritation of a reflex nature. Sometimes this exacerbation of pain and super-sensitiveness in the spine alternates with the sexual infirmity or excitement, and this fact will help you to differentiate it properly. In very rare cases there is a cutaneous anæsthesia, which is allied to the pseudo-narcotism of hysteria, and which is almost invariably due to uterine or ovarian disease.

Difficulties in the way of diagnosis.

Spinal irritation should not, and need not be confounded with inflammation of the spinal cord or of its membranes. Its advent is not characterized by a chill, rigors or fever. The pain is circumscribed in extent, erratic in character, and, in general, is worse upon slight, than upon steady or firm pressure. There is less dread of motion, and, unless in case of traumatic myalgia, more ability to move about than in real meningitis and myelitis. In the adult, meningitis is almost always either traumatic or epidemic. If paralysis occurs in spinal irritation, it is self-limited and not permanent, as it is apt to be in consequence of inflammation with serous effusion into the spinal canal.

Diagnosis from inflammation of the cord, etc.

This disease may be distinguished from true neuralgia by the diffuseness of the pain which does not follow the track of any nerve or nerves, but is characterized, so far as it extends, by a general cutaneous tenderness. The reflex irritability is exaggerated, and sometimes intensely so. Spinal irritation bears a pretty close resemblance to neuralgia, however, in such cases as we have had under review this morning. For where the cervical vertebræ are injured, it presents many of the symptoms of cervico-brachial neuralgia. This is especially true in highly neurotic patients.

Prognosis.—The prognosis will depend upon the location, nature, extent, severity, and duration of the spinal lesion, the age of the patient, her peculiar nervous impressibility, and the more or less serious derangement of the menstrual function. The danger is not usually proportionate to the degree of suffering. Coincident disorders of respiration may be more grave in character than such as implicate digestion. The nervous symptoms are usually more alarming than serious, although it is possible that permanent paralysis of some of the voluntary muscles may follow. In some cases there is a form of hysterical mania that is quite unmanageable by the ordinary means, which is, however, likely to terminate of itself, providing too much is not done in the way of treatment.

In case the irritation has been caused and maintained by a lesion of the generative organs, the possibility of cure will depend upon one of two things ; (1), the curability of the uterine or of the ovarian disease, whatever it may be, and (2), our ability to remove such sequelæ as may remain when the antecedent affection has been remedied. Patients with spinal irritation frequently recover when the climacteric has passed.

Treatment.—These are the patients who travel from one physician to another. By the time you have them fairly in hand you will find that they are experienced itinerants. They have run the whole gamut of the professional possibilities, and, at last, are persuaded that, if you can not benefit them, nobody can. But, in a short time, unless you are very skillful in treating them, or successful in satisfying them that you do really understand the case and expect to cure them, they will be adrift again.

Itinerant patients.

If from any cause the symptoms of spinal irritation are developed, as they were in this case, at a time when the menstrual function is about to be established, or when the changes that are incident to puberty have already begun, you should take the greatest possible care to do nothing that can interrupt this process, or pre-

Guard the menstrual function.

vent its accomplishment. Your aim should be to remove all obstacles thereto, and so to regulate the operations of the nervous system as to favor and assist Nature in her critical effort. For it is manifest that if puberty is not delayed, and the catamenia appear as they should, the nervous and other functions can not be in a very bad condition.

If the symptoms of spinal irritation appear when the menses have been suppressed, as after pregnancy, lying-in and lactation, or from amenorrhœa, a similar indication will exist. And if they come on with the climacteric period, you will bear in mind what I said in my last lecture concerning their treatment under these circumstances.

In amenorrhœa and at the climacteric.

Incidentally, whatever disease may drain the patient's strength or exhaust her energies, should be remedied as speedily as possible. A quarter of a century ago, when this poor woman suffered for two consecutive months with uterine hæmorrhage that was due to the presence of a hydatid mass in utero, there may have been some excuse for a lack of promptness in emptying the womb and stopping the flow. For the sponge-tent was unknown, and physicians had almost as great a dread of manipulating or operating upon the uterine cervix as surgeons had of opening the cavity of the peritoneum. But now such a hæmorrhage should not be permitted. The neck of the womb could be readily dilated and the foreign body removed.

Remove any dangerous condition.

In order to counteract the peculiar impressibility of your female patients, and thereby to put them in a condition that is favorable to the cure of spinal irritation, you will need to exercise a great deal of tact and a large measure of sympathy and discretion. Rough treatment may sometimes be tolerated in other cases (although it is inexcusable), but in this disease it will not be borne. The patient's perceptions are too acute, and she is too susceptible and sensitive to be treated in such a way. Your manner should be kindly, your words fitly chosen, your tone sympathizing, and your faith in her desire to get well, and not to deceive you, unbounded. If you are fully impressed with the tenderness and delicacy of her organization on the one hand, and with the irritable, excitable and wretched state

Tact and sympathy.

of her nervous system on the other, you will never be guilty of adopting such a mode of treatment as must necessarily make her worse instead of better.

For the effects of the spinal injury.

If the attack originated in a strain, shock, blow, or fall, although years may have passed since the injury was sustained, arnica, rhus tox., calendula, or the hypericum perf., will be indicated. I have great confidence in the latter remedy given internally and applied locally at the same time for traumatic injuries of the spine and its membranes. The other medicines named may also be used both constitutionally and externally.

For rheumatic and neuralgic symptoms.

For rheumatic and neuralgic complications the most prominent remedy in many cases is macrotin, after which there are rhus tox., bryonia, spigelia, belladonna, atropine, aconite, veratrum alb., veratrum vir., colocynth, lachesis, caulophyllum, nux vomica, colchicum, and gelseminum, with the leading indications for which you are already familiar.

For the uterine and ovarian symptoms.

Whatever uterine or ovarian diseases have been sufficient to cause or to complicate the spinal lesion, should first be treated as if they existed separately and idiopathically. But when these are removed or cured, such spinal and nervous sequelæ as remain may be treated more directly and specifically. Uterine deviations, cervicitis, hypertrophy, and ulceration of the cervix uteri and hysteralgia are the more frequent of these affections, which have the first claim on our professional attention. To these may be added subacute and chronic ovaritis, and ovarian neuralgia.

For contingent disorders.

The respiratory, digestive, hepatic and general nervous derangements which are secondary upon the spinal trouble, will usually yield to treatment that is addressed to the cure of the lesion upon which they are dependent for a cause. The symptoms must be carefully studied and the remedy affiliated properly, else there will be but a poor prospect of success.

Local treatment.

Local adjuvants are sometimes of the greatest possible service in the treatment of this troublesome complaint. They are not only grateful and useful on account of the relief which they afford, but do really assist in the cure. I suppose that their *modus operandi* is by excluding the presence and pressure of the atmosphere upon the tender surface along the spine. My own preference for these local expedients has been based upon the following indications:

If the muscles of the back or of the neck are cramped and very painful, I direct that the surface shall be thoroughly anointed with camphorated oil. This may be gently rubbed over the painful part, or applied by means of flannel compresses. The oil soothes and softens, and the camphor relaxes the muscular spasm. Bathing with spirits of camphor is less efficacious, because both the camphor and the alcohol evaporate so quickly.

For painful cramping, etc.

Where there is less pain and more diffuse tenderness, it gives great relief to coat the surface with the oleaginous collodion.

If the disease has resulted from a mechanical cause, you will not forget the local use of arnica, hypericum, calendula and hamamelis. I believe these topical applications have the best effect, in this disease especially, when they are diluted in and applied by means of hot, instead of cool or cold water. In mild cases, a porous plaster will sometimes afford relief. Dry cupping, and the exhaustion of the air by means of cups to which the air-pump is attached, affords a useful expedient in some cases. But sinapisms, blisters, pustulation by croton oil or tartar emetic, and issues and setons of all kinds are harmful and unnecessary.

Topical expedients.

The spine should bo insulated as it were, by a layer of cotton batting, or of oiled silk, worn next the skin. The cotton may be sewed into the clothing and kept constantly applied, day and night. It should extend from the neck throughout the whole length of the back. In many cases, more particularly in those who are predisposed to rheumatism, the patient should wear a silk vest, or under-wrapper, to protect her from sudden vicissitudes of the weather, and from electrical changes.

Domestic expedients.

Sponging the back from above downwards with warm, or hot water, may help to remove the extreme sensitiveness of the integument. It should be done very carefully however, and, if possible, by a person who is in sympathy with the patient, and towards whom she has no feeling

Available expedients.

of antagonism. In chronic cases, with marked debility, salt-water spongings along the spine are sometimes very beneficial. In certain cases, the shower-bath, electricity, and animal magnetism may also be useful. They should, however, be administered with care and discrimination, else they may only serve to increase the difficulty. The electrical bath answers as an available tonic, when the general strength is very much reduced, and the patient's nervous system needs a ready means of support of some kind.

Faradization.

An ancient writer says: "There is one special phase, however, of spinal irritation which is very amenable to a direct treatment, viz.: cutaneous and mucous tenderness. Whenever the 'hyperæsthetic' part is within reach, so that we can apply Faradization, we can almost certainly eradicate the morbid sensibility very quickly. The secondary current of an electro-magnetic or volta-electric induction apparatus is to be employed; the conductors should be of dry metal, and the negative one, which is to be applied to the painful surface, should be in the form of the wire-brush. The positive pole is to be placed on some indifferent spot, and the negative is to be stroked briskly backward or forward over the sensitive skin, a pretty strong current being employed. The process is painful, so much so that it will often be advisable, with delicate patients, either to administer chloroform or to inject morphia subcutaneously before the Faradization. A very few daily sittings of four or five minutes length, will generally remove the morbid tenderness completely. When the tender part is within one of the cavities, as the rectum, bladder, vagina, or pharynx, we must of course use a solid negative conductor of appropriate form, and must content ourselves with applying it to one point after another of the sensitive surface." *

HYSTERICAL HEMIPLEGIA.

Case.—Mary J——, aged 29, seamstress, unmarried, had been in poor health for more than a month, complaining of headache, fatigue, debility, drowsiness, loss of memory, and disinclination to work. Two weeks ago she was suddenly seized during the night with a violent fit of hysteria. The spasms of the voluntary muscles were very severe. She talked foolishly of her little

* Neuralgia and the Diseases that Resemble it. By Francis E. Anstie, M.D., etc., New York. D. Appleton & Co., 1872, p. 299.

love affairs, of church matters, and upon all kinds of topics. In about half an hour the paroxysm passed off with alternate laughing and crying, and finally with the escape of a large quantity of colorless urine. The next morning her right arm and leg were paralyzed. The muscles were relaxed. She could move the leg a little, but only with the greatest effort. The arm was quite powerless. Her consciousness was complete, and had been from the subsidence of the fit. The face was not paralyzed, nor did the tongue turn to the right angle of the mouth when she protruded it; her speech was unimpaired, but it was sometimes difficult for her to swallow. She complained of frontal headache and inability to sleep. The right pupil was considerably enlarged, but the left one remained unaltered. The bowels were obstinately constipated.

The menstrual flow, which had begun only a few hours before the hysterical attack set in, was arrested, and did not return. She has been subject to amenorrhœa, and sometimes passes several months without any "show." She has frequently had hysteria in a mild form, but these paralytic symptoms are new, and have alarmed both herself and family very much.

Hysterical mimicry.

This case is *apropos* to the preceding one. It furnishes another illustration of the hysterical mimicry of which I have already spoken. One would say, at first thought, that it would be quite impossible for this or any other affection to imitate so grave a disease as hemiplegia. But here you see a case in which the right half of the body is powerless. This poor girl had to be carried into the amphitheatre, for she cannot stand alone. When she attempts to walk, the right limb, which seems a little stronger than it was at first, swings with a pendulum-like motion, directly forwards and backwards, but its abduction and adduction are impossible. You will observe that the arm hangs helpless by her side.

A practical test.

There is an evident paralysis of the nerves of motion. Let us see if the nerves of sensation are in the same state. For these two forms of palsy have no necessary relation to each other. Observe that when I stuck the pin into her arm, to test this question, it was done without her knowledge. If I had told you in her hearing what I intended to do, and she had seen the point of the pin coming towards her, she would have imagined that she felt it, whether she really did so or not. We must be cautious in these little matters. I once introduced a sound into the female bladder, and on turning it about observed a clicking noise, which exactly resembled that caused by the striking of a metallic instrument against a calculus, which disease she was supposed to have. Having withdrawn the instrument, I was about to declare that my patient had stone in the bladder, when, upon turning its handle, I discovered that it had become loosened and gave forth precisely the same click that I had heard before. This shows the importance of being always on our guard, lest we arrive at wrong conclusions in diagnosis.

Caution.

Naturally enough you would like to know what variety of unilateral paralysis it is from which this patient is suffering. I have no doubt but that it is hysterical, and my judgment is based upon the following reasons.

Diagnosis.

1. She is of the hysterical temperament. This peculiar constitution is as different from the apoplectic habit as the scrofulous cachexia is from the sanguineous temperament. The fact that she has been subject to hysteria before precludes the probability that her paralysis is due to effusion, either of blood or of serum, within the cerebro-spinal cavity.

Points.

2. Hysterical attacks commence abruptly, and are not accompanied by marked signs of congestion, fever, coma or constitutional disturbance. There are no lesions of the perceptive centers in hysteria, as there are in apoplexy, whether it be nervous, serous, or sanguineous.

3. The relation of the menstrual arrest to the initiatory paroxysm. A mere suppression of the menses in one of her slender form and delicate organization would not be likely to induce such a determination of blood to the head as to result in apoplexy, or such a disorder of the cerebral nutrition as, in the short space of a fortnight (more especially in one so young), to cause softening of the brain. In such subjects as this the menses are very apt to be scanty and irregular. Hysterical paralysis is more frequent at puberty and the change of life, when these particular crises influence the general nervous system so decidedly, than at other times.

4. The sweeping motion of the leg, and the absence of paralysis of the face and tongue, enable us to exclude the more ordinary forms of hemiplegia, and to identify the hysterical variety.

Other signs are classed as diagnostic of this singular affection.

Among them are the ability to move the palsied extremity under sudden and powerful emotional impulse. Such a patient may sometimes be so shocked or startled as to use the limb automatically, and without thinking of what she is doing. One of my neighbors, who had not walked a square for months, left her bed suddenly, the night of the great fire in this city, in October last, and marched three miles in order to save her life.

Other differential signs.

If the patient feigns paralysis of the arm especially, you will observe that when she stoops forward she keeps it close to her side. In absolute paralysis of that member it would be impossible for her to do so, for, having no voluntary control over it, it would fall forward when she stoops towards the floor.

Position of the arm.

Another distinguishing peculiarity of the hysterical paralysis is that there is very little atrophy of the muscles of the affected part. If the arm or the leg, or both, are helpless and useless for months, their size is not so apt to be diminished as in ordinary palsy. The limb does not become shrunken and attenuated, but remains as plump and fleshy as the sound one.

Absence of atrophy.

In many cases, the hyterical fits recur from time to time, with or without choreic movements of the other voluntary muscles. Sometimes there is an incidental aphonia, and globus hystericus is the rule and not the exception.

Hysterical hemiplegia is not a very common form of paralysis. Hysterical paraplegia is more frequently seen. In the former it is said that the left side is more apt to be affected than the right one. Being largely the result of emotional causes, there is no doubt that it may occur in men as well as in women. Indeed it is very probable that a large proportion of the cases of paralysis that are cured by itinerant pretenders through the "laying on of hands," animal magnetism, and every species of mummery, are hysterical, functional, emotional, circumstantial, self-limited, and not dependent upon any structural lesion whatever.

May occur in measles.

Unless the disease is complicated with some serious lesion, either of the brain or spinal cord, the prognosis is generally favorable. It may require a long time to effect a cure, but the patient and persistent use of the proper means will ultimately succeed.

Prognosis.

In many cases the affection leaves as abruptly as the hysterical aphonia or meteorism are apt to do. If the paralysis comes on during the climacteric, the more or less serious nature of the incidental disorders, and the condition of the general health will modify your judgment of its severity.

Treatment.—The auxiliary treatment of this affection is very important. It includes the proper employment of friction, elec-

Adjuvants.

tricity, animal magnetism, the movement cure, the health-lift, Faradization, bathing, and exercise, both physical and mental. It prescribes fresh air, sunlight, change of scene, travel, pleasant and agreeable society, good, healthy, and nourishing food, and the careful use of stimulants. It orders the removal of whatever may cause her to become impatient and irritable, or that can in any way disturb her mental equilibrium.

Internal remedies.

Ignatia, gelseminum, belladonna, secale cornutum, cuprum, plumbum, rhus tox., cocculus, causticum, baryta carb., caulophyllin, phosphorus, and zincum metallicum, are the remedies most frequently indicated.

LECTURE XXXI.

FIBROID TUMORS OF THE UTERUS.

GENTLEMEN:

A course of lectures on our specialty would be very incomplete without some remarks upon the clinical history and treatment of uterine fibroids. This is true not only because of the interest which attaches to neoplastic growths in general, but especially because those which are uterine are more readily diagnosticated and cured than they were a few years ago.

Relative frequency.

These tumors which, according to various authors are found in from 20 to 40 per cent. of those women who are ill with uterine disease after their thirty-fifth year, are benign and not malignant. Nor do they ever degenerate into cancer, or any other form of malignant growth. This fact is interesting in a prognostic point of view, and also with respect to their cause and mode of development.

Pathological anatomy.

I need not remind you that the fibrous and cellular structures of the uterine wall exist in a rudimentary state until they are especially developed in consequence of conception, or of the growth within the uterine cavity of a foreign body of some kind. The possibility of this extraordinary increase necessitates such changes in the circulation to and through the organ as will supply sufficient nutritive material therefor. It is because the depth and dimensions of the uterus may be so much increased, in consequence of a physiological stimulus, that these fibroids are formed. In all essential particulars, their growth and development is identical with that which takes place in the muscular coat of the womb during pregnancy. The only difference is that in fibroids the actual increase in the substance of the uterus is circumscribed, instead of being general; and that it is pathological and more or less permanent, instead of being physiological and of limited duration, as it is in pregnancy.

Unless they have undergone some form of benign degeneration, fibroids are therefore homologous and not heterologous. There is indeed a new growth of tissue, but it is of the nature of a local hypertrophy, and, excepting in a mechanical way, is not foreign to the part affected. Sometimes these tumors consist exclusively of a prematurely developed muscular fibre, constituting veritable myomata, but in most cases the connective tissue is also involved, and hence it has been customary to style them myo-fibromata. Microscopically considered, there is nothing distinctive in these growths, excepting perhaps, that the arrangement of their fibres is more irregular, wavy and tortuous than in the proper uterine tissue.

Homologous growths.

These tumors are either single or multiple. There may be but one of them; there have been as many as forty within and upon the same womb. They generally assume a rounded form at first, and afterwards change their shape, according to circumstances. They may remain sessile, but are more apt to become pedunculated. Their size varies from that of a marble to a man's head, or even larger. They may weigh an ounce, or as much as twenty, thirty, fifty, or even a hundred pounds. Their solidity varies with their location and vascularity, the rapidity of their growth, and their tendency to undergo cystic, carneous, calcareous, or fatty degeneration. The more strictly fibrous the tumor, the more succulent it is.

Number, weight and texture.

There are three varieties of uterine fibroids which are named from their location with reference to the cavities of the womb and of the abdomen, and also to the uterine wall. I will speak of them separately.

Varieties.

I.—SUB-MUCOUS FIBROIDS.

As their name implies, these tumors are situated directly beneath the endometrium, or lining membrane of the womb. They are really contained within the uterine cavity, and hence are frequently styled intra-uterine. Their mode of development appears to be as follows: From some cause, which may be known or unknown, the fibro-cellular tissue

Sessile or pedunculated.

of the uterus becomes thickened, and of increased vascularity at a particular point. This growth, nodule, or hypertrophy, continues to increase in size, perhaps for months, or even for years, without any untoward symptoms. Being located in closer proximity with the mucous than with the peritoneal coat of the organ, it pushes in that direction, and finally invades the uterine cavity. Here it may continue to grow in all directions as a round tumor, with a broad base, which gradually fills the womb; or it may become pear-shaped, and finally develop into a fibrous polyp, with a neck or stalk which is sufficiently long and slender to allow it to drop into the os internum, or even into the vagina. As in ovarian tumors and polypi, the pedicle is the means of keeping up the vascular connection with the uterus.

Symptoms.—The symptoms indicative of the presence of such a tumor are objective and subjective. The patient complains of a sense of weight and dragging down, intra-pelvic pains and distress, lumbo-abdominal aching, vesical or rectal tenesmus, inability to walk without great dread of procidentia of the pelvic organs, uterine colic, pains in lying upon one side or the other, sick headache, nausea, morning sickness as in pregnancy, copious and sometimes very painful menstruation; the catamenia are too frequent as well as menorrhagic; weakness, prostration, constipation and unrest. Of course these symptoms vary in different cases, and also with the size and shape of the tumor or tumors. The larger the tumor the greater the coincident suffering. Pediculated fibroids are, in general, more likely to excite strong uterine contractions than those which are sessile. Indeed, there is a theory that, in some cases, the force of the peristaltic contractions of the womb, or the uterine tenesmus, is the cause of this particular form of the tumor, and that these bear a constant relation to each other. My own observations confirm the truth of this theory. There are, however, some exceptions to the rule.

The hæmorrhage.

The most alarming and constant of these symptoms is the hæmorrhage which, however, is a menstrual flux. Seventy per cent. of intra-uterine fibroids are accompanied by hæmorrhage. The flow, which is very free, is usually, but not always painful, and very debilitating. If it has continued long, the patient becomes anæmic, bloodless, and perhaps dropsical also. It returns every fortnight, or three weeks; she does not recover from one attack before another is upon her. It is astonishing how small a fibroid may serve to perpetuate such a hæmorrhage. For it may happen that a little body of this sort, which is not larger than a grape, may cause as great a loss of blood as sometimes does the fragment of placenta which is left in the womb after an abortion. Leucorrhœa, serous discharges and obstructive dysmenorrhœa are often due to the presence of uterine fibroids. More rarely the tumor blocks up the outlet, and there is complete retention of the menses.

Uterine displacements.

Incidental symptoms of uterine deviation are always present. The larger the tumor the greater the displacement. Being attached more frequently to the posterior wall of the womb, retroversion and retroflexion are very common. If, however, as sometimes happens, the point of attachment is to the fundus, and the tumor is a very large one, the organ may be inverted. Anteversion, anteflexion and prolapsus are not infrequent. Latero-version, a state of things in which the body of the womb is forced towards one side of the pelvic basin, is sometimes caused by the presence of an intra-uterine fibroid.

Changes in the cervix.

Beside the morning sickness, anorexia and caprices of appetite, the development of the mammary glands, of the areolæ, and of the abdomen, there are other signs simulating those of pregnancy, that are caused by the growth of a fibroid in utero. The cervix is shortened, and may become flaccid and patulous. More frequently, however, after some months, it forms a ring which is resistant and sometimes very sensitive to the touch. Auscultation through the abdominal parietes (providing the tumor has passed above the pelvic brim) reveals the uterine *souffle*, which you remember was once regarded as a positive sign of pregnancy.

The uterine souffle.

Tolerance of the tumor.

In exceptional cases there is a singular tolerance of the presence of these tumors. Some women carry them for years and become so accustomed to them that they make very little if any complaint of them. It is only in consequence of the hæmorrhage, or the pressure they occasion, that they are led to take measures for their removal. They do not always interfere with pregnancy, although they grow more rapidly in the gravid than in the non-gravid uterus. They sometimes cause abortion.

These tumors, as they grow, lead to an enlargement of the uterus and an increased size of its cavity. Hence, if the organ is not quite filled with the fibroid, the sound will pass quite readily, and perhaps farther than you would have supposed. For the depth of the uterus may be as great as it is at term. In order to get the best idea of the size, and the point and mode of attachment of the growth, you should select a flexible sound, which will adapt itself to the contour of the tumor without force, and, therefore, without inducing pain or hæmorrhage.

Increased size of the uterus.

As felt through the abdominal parietes, the outline of the tumor can usually be very well recognized. There is dullness on percussion over the whole anterior surface of the womb. It is not unusual for the patient to complain that one particular spot is and has always been painful and tender to the touch; but there is no diffuse soreness. The uterus is hard and resistant to external palpation.

Physical signs.

These tumors, being invariably attached to the body and fundus of the womb, a vaginal examination by the touch is of little use unless the growth is large enough to be felt, or so to displace the uterus that it can be reached. In case the tumor is very large, the whole organ may be displaced upwards, above the brim of the pelvis and the "touch" reveal nothing. In some cases the "touch" may be conjoined with pressure with the tips of the fingers of the free hand over the uterus and just above the pubes, as in Sims' bi-manual exploration.

The "touch."

Bi-manual examination.

Causes.—The causes are not well known. That the growth of these tumors bears a certain relation to the menstrual function, and to that of procreation also, is evident from the fact that they are most frequently developed at a period when these functions are most active. But precisely what that relation is has not been determined. In a certain class of cases it is probable that the fibroid is a sequel, or a consequence, of the incomplete involution, or folding upon itself, of the uterus after delivery. It has happened that a clot has been found to form the nucleus of a uterine fibroid.

Menstruation and child-bearing.

Diagnosis.—The diagnosis is difficult. I have already told you how to diagnosticate a case of intra-uterine fibroids from one of ovarian dropsy.* The hardness and mobility of the tumor; the absence of fluctuation; the depth of the womb, as shown by the distance to which the sound will enter; the co-existence of hæmorrhage, which may be menstrual, but is often inter-periodic; the pain and uterine tenesmus; the uterine souffle in either groin; the uterine displacement and leucorrhœa; and the comparatively slow rate of the growth of these fibroids, are sufficiently characteristic. The occurrence of uterine fibroids and of ovarian dropsy are not very frequent in those who have never been pregnant.

From an ovarian cyst.

The incidental hæmorrhage, with its tendency in most cases to return at or near the month with tolerable regularity; the tardy and protracted growth of the tumor; the absence of quickening and of the fœtal heart sounds; the rounded outline and hardness of the tumor as felt through the abdominal walls; the patulous state of the os uteri; and the persistent displacement of the womb, are so many signs which will help you to differentiate this variety of uterine fibroids from pregnancy. The altered and peculiar shape and consistence of the cervix in case of placenta prævia, would be as different from that which is proper to uterine fibroids, as it is from that of ordinary pregnancy. You should not forget that it is possible for a woman with any variety of uterine fibroid to become pregnant, although, in case of the intra-uterine variety especially, they seldom reach term without aborting. It is therefore best not to pass the sound in all cases indiscriminately, and without thought of the possible consequences. Perhaps, in a majority of cases the large fibroid becomes impacted in the pelvis and does not rise into the abdominal cavity, as the gravid uterus does, at or about the fourth month.

From pregnancy.

In the case of uterine hydatids the abdominal tumor is larger, grows more rapidly, is characterized by smoothness, fluctuation and decided distention, which subsides somewhat with occasional discharges of serum and blood. Sometimes small portions of the mass are detached and extruded, from which specimens it is possible to recognize the nature of the growth. When there is copious or continued hæm-

From hydatids.

*See page 369.

orrhage, the diagnosis from a uterine fibroid is more difficult. In this case a decision can be reached by dilatation of the cervix and an exploration of the uterine cavity by means of the finger or the uterine sound.

From fibrous polypi.

It is quite impossible, in most cases, to distinguish an intra-uterine fibroid from a fibrous polypus, without artificial dilatation of the cervix and careful exploration, unless the polypus is large enough, and its pedicle sufficiently long to enable it to drop into the canal of the cervix, or into the vagina. Their differential diagnosis is, however, not a matter of very great importance. The only real difference between them is that the fibroid is enclosed in a proper capsule, which really disconnects it from the surrounding tissue; while the polypus is a true out-growth, which is continuous with the substance of the uterus and covered only by its lining membrane. These differences are not observable, however, until the growth has been removed.

From inversion of the womb.

These fibroids have sometimes been confounded with the tumor formed by inversion of the womb. They have many symptoms in common. But inversion follows the evacuation of the uterus. Either the woman has recently been delivered, in abortus or at term, or the organ has first been distended and developed by a contained tumor, and finally turned inside out during or in consequence of its delivery. The best test between these tumors, however, is a very simple one. In inversion the tumor is sensitive, and if you stick a pin into it the patient feels it; but not so in case of the fibroid.

From retroversion and retroflexion.

By means of the uterine sound or probe alone you can diagnosticate retroversion and retroflexion of the uterus from a sub-mucous fibroid.

May die suddenly.

Prognosis.—There are several sources of danger in this disease. The hæmorrhage may drain away the strength, and so undermine the health as finally to destroy life. Sometimes such patients die very suddenly from excessive loss of blood. In consequence of the mechanical pressure of the tumor upon the pelvic viscera, or upon the ureters, serious disease may be caused in the bladder, the bowels, or the kidneys. The reflex disorders occasioned by the same cause are harassing and exhausting. The impairment of digestion, respiration, and especially of the circulation are sometimes very serious.

In some cases the symptoms are very deceptive, and give no reliable criterion of the gravity of the disease. Women who have carried these tumors about with them for years with almost no complaint, and at last find themselves ill, are apt to drop off very suddenly; while those who complain most bitterly are often in a less dangerous condition.

Symptoms deceptive.

The risk of operative interference is less than in either of the other varieties of uterine fibroids. There are two reasons for this fact: (1) because the tumor is more readily reached and removed, and (2) because the danger of consequent inflammation is in proportion with the liability of wounding or cutting into the peritoneal surface of the womb.

The risk of an operation.

Treatment. — The treatment is medical and surgical, or palliative and radical. Whatever contingencies beset the case must first be removed. The hæmorrhage is the source of danger and must be controlled. For this purpose such remedies as ipecacuanha, china, arsenicum alb., hamamelis, erechthites, crocus sat., cinnamonum, trillium, secale cor., sabina, belladonna, nitric acid, or ferrum met., may be given each under its appropriate indications. The suitable remedy will generally suffice to relieve the pain as well as the excessive flow.

Medical.

If the hæmorrhage is copious and continuous, and it becomes necessary to stop it at once, in order to husband the patient's strength and to save her life, and internal remedies act slowly or fail altogether, recourse must be had to such local treatment as was recommended in my lecture on uterine hæmorrhage.* You doubtless remember what I then said of such available expedients as cold water locally and by injection, ice, ice-water, pouring cold water from a height upon the abdomen, colpeurysis, and the tampon. In some cases the sponge tent makes an excellent tampon for the cervix ; and Palfrey† recommends to introduce the speculum, to draw down the anterior lip of the cervix, and then, with the uterine sound to pack its canal with a long and narrow strip of lint. The lint, which may have been soaked in carbolized water, should be

Palliative.

* See page 80.

† Medical Press and Circular, Vol. VII, p. 516.

allowed to remain for about twenty-four to thirty hours before it is removed.

Among the improved methods of hæmostasis, which also include a more or less permanent exemption from the flow, there is no simple expedient that is more valuable than the introduction of the sponge tent. I have known it alone to prevent the return of the menorrhagia, and to secure a natural flow for months in succession.

The sponge tent as a hæmostatic.

In obstinate cases nicking, slitting or incising the os uteri with a curved, blunt-pointed bistoury, a pair of scissors, or the hysterotome, has also been practiced with marked success. Whether these latter means are efficacious because they unload the engorged vessels, or because by dilating the os uteri, they empty the womb of its more fluid and distensible contents, and thus remedy the difficulty, I am not prepared to say. But that they certainly present a valuable means of relief, which is always available, and which, until quite recently, was unknown, I am well assured.

Incision of the cervix.

If this treatment fails to bring the desired relief, Dr. Atlee* recommends to follow up the section of the os uteri with a free division of the capsule of the fibroid in utero. This he accomplished by means of a long-handled, curved and probe-pointed bistoury, which is to be passed into the uterus as far as the guiding finger will reach, and then drawn firmly down over the tumor so as to cut through its capsule and into its substance to the depth of half an inch. This operation not only lessens the hæmorrhage, but so impairs the nutritive vitality of the fibroid that its destructive metamorphosis is soon established, and it will be either enucleated spontaneously, or thrown off with a kind of leucorrhœal discharge. This practice seems to me to be especially adapted to tumors with a broad base and margin of attachment.

Dr. Atlee's operation.

But unless Dr. Atlee's operation shall result in the extrusion of the fibroid, either as a whole or in fragments ; or it shall be spontaneously detached and expelled, as it sometimes is, by strong uterine contractions; or unless it shall undergo some form of degeneration, and there-

Excision of the tumor.

* Transactions of the American Med. Association, 1858, page 558.

by escape or cease to be troublesome; a radical cure will only be possible by its excision and removal. This is to be effected by a ligation of the tumor. And two obstacles are in the way of its accomplishment. The first of these is the narrow state of the cervix uteri. To overcome it we must resort to free dilatation. If the tumor is quite large, and the cervix is shortened and softened, as in the later months of pregnancy, two or three sponge tents of various sizes may be introduced successively. These will expand the neck so that the fingers can be passed within the womb, the exact site of the tumor ascertained, its mode of attachment also, and the instrument adjusted. For this must be done by the sense of touch, and not by sight.

First obstacle.

In the more rigid and unyielding states of the cervix, the sea-tangle tents are preferable. Of these quite a number are to be passed through the internal os uteri one after another, until it contains from three to seven or eight of them. The longer these tents the better. They should be allowed to remain for from twelve to twenty-four hours. On their removal, if the dilatation is not sufficient, one of Barnes' rubber dilators may be inserted through the cervical canal, inflated, and left in situ for some hours longer. These expedients will provide a mode of entrance that will make the further steps of the operation possible. To secure a free expansion of the cervix, it may perhaps be necessary to incise it at the same time that you dilate it.

Dilatation the first step.

The second obstacle in the way of operating in some of these cases is the difficulty of adjusting the ligature, or rather, the chain or wire of the écraseur. If the tumor is in the vagina, and is not very large, there will be no trouble in this respect; but if it is in the uterus, and more than all if it is attached to the fundus, and has a broad base, instead of a pedicle, you will find that it is not so easily done as you might have supposed. Indeed, it may require repeated trials before you succeed in carrying the loop of the ligature over and beyond the tumor. A few authors insist that, to facilitate this object, the uterus should be dragged down to the vulva. But, unless in very exceptional cases, this proceeding is barbarous and unnecessary.

The second obstacle.

The ligation of the tumor.

To obviate the difficulty of which I have just spoken, Dr. Sims added a porte-chain to the uterine écraseur, which so stiffened the instrument that its flexible part could be more readily and certainly adjusted. As thus improved, the chain écraseur is more useful than it was formerly; but the majority of gynæcologists prefer that the ligature shall be made of wire instead of the chain. This can be worked in the frame of, and upon the same principle as the ordinary écraseur. Dr. Braxton Hicks' instrument, which I hold in my hand, is a wire-rope écraseur.

A practical hint.

In order to ensnare the tumor most readily, let me give you a hint which I have found of great service. First ascertain as accurately as possible the precise site of the tumor, and its point of attachment to the uterine wall. Then place the patient in such a position that it will drop away from its pedicle, or base, towards the opposite side of the womb. If it happens to be centrally located the position of the patient is less important. Fortunately a majority of these intra-uterine fibroids, and fibrous polypi also, grow from the posterior wall of the womb; and therefore the patient is usually placed in what is now known as the left lateral position.

Caution.

When the instrument is finally adjusted, all that remains is to tighten it slowly and steadily until the tumor is cut off. This should be done very gradually, lest the wire break. Iron wire will not stand the strain; but the wire-rope or steel wire are more trustworthy. If the tumor is a very large one; it may need to be delivered with the obstetric or other forceps, or perhaps to be cut into pieces before it can be brought away through the os uteri. Fortunately, in écrasement, there is an exemption both from immediate hæmorrhage and from the danger of subsequent inflammation.

An exceptional case.

In rare cases, where the tumor is very large and pedunculated, and occupies the vagina, it is so difficult to excise it in the ordinary way, that it has been recommended first to seize it with the obstetric forceps, and then to draw it out at the vulva, after which the écraseur may be applied. This operation causes a temporary inversion of the womb; but the os having been stretched so widely by the tumor, and paralyzed by pressure upon it, is not likely to contract so firmly as to interfere with the reposition of the organ afterwards. If there is much hæmorrhage, the stump, or pedicle, may be seared with an iron at a white heat, or painted with the per-chloride of iron, before the uterus is replaced.

II.—SUB-PERITONEAL FIBROIDS.

These growths, which are located on the exterior surface of the womb, and beneath the peritoneum, are also known as sub-serous, extra-mural and extra-uterine fibroids. They are less frequent than either of the other varieties, but when they do exist, are almost always multiple. They grow more rapidly, are of various sizes, and may be very numerous. Not unfrequently the abdomen will be filled with one which is very large, while the exterior of the uterus is studded with a number of smaller ones that are undeveloped. Sometimes, however, two or more of these tumors may grow together and not differ materially in their size and form.

Frequency, number, size, etc.

Symptoms.—Since they have no necessary connection with the cavity of the uterus, neither with its mucous membrane, nor indeed with the generative intestine in any way, the disorders of menstruation which are almost invariably present in the case of sub-mucous fibroids, are lacking in the sub-peritoneal variety. There is no especial liability to hæmorrhage, or to serous discharges from the uterine cavity.

The symptoms are therefore chiefly mechanical. Small tumors of this kind occasion very little inconvenience, and may exist for years without symptoms. Larger ones drop into the retro-uterine space, against the bladder anteriorly, or press laterally in such a way as to cause pain within the pelvis or in the corresponding hip and thigh. If it becomes pedunculated, as it frequently does, the length of the pedicle may permit the tumor to float, as it were, and to change its position with reference to the pelvic organs, so as not permanently to displace the uterus. But, when there is no pedicle, and the growth has a broad base, the womb is almost certain to be dislocated and more or less fixed in an unnatural position.

Chiefly mechanical.

"Pressure on the bladder, even without co-existing anteflexion, may become so considerable as to compress it between the symphysis and the tumor, giving rise, in consequence, to secondary phenomena in the uro-poietic system. The hyperæmia of the pelvic blood vessels, occasioned by fibroid tumors, is frequently manifested in the mucous membrane of the bladder as a varicose distention of its veins, especially of those situated at the neck of the bladder; and Rokitansky even observed a case of rupture of a submucous cystic vein, with hæmorrhage into the bladder. Thomson relates a case in which a perforation occurred in the wall of the above organ from pressure of a large fibroid tumor, with adhesion of half of the periphery of the tumor to the borders of said perforation.

Effects of pressure.

"On the other side pressure affects the rectum, and defecation may be completely prevented by fibroids impacted in Douglas' space. They may also cause varicose distention of the hæmorrhoidal veins, and hyperæmia of the rectal mucous membrane in the same way as in that of the bladder."*

Hypostatic hyperæmia, or engorgement, of the utero-vaginal mucous membrane is a very common result of the pressure from these tumors. And hence they are likely to be attended, not only with uterine deviations, but with a coincident cervicitis, endo-cervicitis, endo-metritis, and vaginitis. Such local derangements of the circulation sometimes find vent in a critical hæmorrhage which is inter-periodic, and sometimes (though rarely in this form of fibroid) in copious or prolonged menstruation.

Coincident disorders.

In these extra-mural fibroids there is a marked and characteristic tendency to peritoneal inflammation. In many cases this lesion is latent and circumscribed, and as a consequence adhesions are formed which glue the tumor more or less firmly and generally to the neighboring parts or organs. At other times patients suffer from acute lancinating pains, are sick a few days, with a sharp attack of peritonitis, and then recover. All the suffering and all the sequelæ, however, are usually, but improperly, referred to the tumor itself. These are the adhesions which are encountered on section in gastrotomy.

Liability to peritonitis.

Diagnosis.—The frequency with which this class of fibroids is

* Pathological Anatomy of the Female Sexual Organs, by Julius M. Klob, M.D., etc. N. Y. 1868. p. 175.

located at the posterior cul-de-sac increases the liability of their being mistaken for retroversion or retroflexion of the womb. But the physical signs will enable you to distinguish them. Perhaps the "touch" reveals a tumor which lies in the hollow of the sacrum, but it alone is insufficient as a means of diagnosis. The bi-manual examination will help you to decide whether the upper and anterior portions of the uterus are enlarged or the seat of an abnormal growth. But it will not serve to differentiate between a fibroid tumor in the posterior part of the pelvis and a retroverted or retroflexed uterus. To settle this question, therefore, we must pass the uterine sound. If the point of the instrument looks towards the superior strait, as it should, when it has reached the fundus, the tumor is a fibroid, and the uterus is not displaced backwards. I should not forget to remind you, however, that, in certain cases, these two disorders co-exist.

From retroversion and retroflexion.

Having already detailed the signs by which you would diagnosticate an extra-uterine fibroid from an ovarian tumor or cyst, it is unnecessary to repeat my remarks upon that subject.*

From ovarian dropsy.

So much depends upon the length and size of the pedicle in these cases that it is difficult to establish a rule of diagnosis between this form of fibroids and pregnancy. The uterus will be increased in its dimensions if the pedicle is short, and if the womb should grow and develop, the presumptive signs of pregnancy will be all the more prominent. There is, however, some considerable difference in the form and general character of the abdominal tumor in the two cases. In fibroids, if there is more than one, the outline of each can be recognized through the abdominal parietes. If these walls are thin, and not inordinately developed, the fibroid is felt to be a hard, firm, resistant mass, which imparts an entirely different sensation to the fingers from that of the elastic fluctuating sensation of the gravid uterus. Sometimes it is possible to feel the rounded, knob-like masses caused by smaller fibroids which are attached to the exterior of the uterus.

From pregnancy.

The uterine souffle will be very similar in both; but the possibility of hearing the fœtal heart-sounds will sometimes enable

* See pages 371–72.

you to decide between them. In fibroids the tumor develops very slowly, while in pregnancy the relative rapidity of its growth is much more marked. By withholding an opinion for a few weeks you may sometimes be able to settle the question of diagnosis very positively, on account of the size of the tumor having very much increased meanwhile, providing she is pregnant. Unmistakable quickening would also be diagnostic, but it must be real and not imaginary.

In the later months, the condition of the os and cervix uteri, the more or less regular return of the menstrual flow, the inability to feel the movements of the fœtus, the depth of the uterus as disclosed by the sound (which should not be passed if the signs of pregnancy are at all prominent, or unless in very extreme cases), will generally enable you to determine the diagnosis correctly. Time is, however, an important element in this respect. It may require that you make several examinations before your final decision is given. If so, and the patient is not *in extremis*, it will be well to allow the intervals between these several examinations to be somewhat prolonged.

When pregnancy occurs in the case of a woman who already has one of these sub-serous fibroids, it is more likely to extend to term without accident than in case of the sub-mucous tumors of which I have spoken, probably for the reason that in the former the uterine cavity and its mucous membrane are nearly or quite normal.

Relative immunity from abortion.

In these fibroids the previous history of the case; the absence of grave constitutional symptoms, chill, fever, and a tendency to suppuration; the fact that the tumor has been growing for months or years, and has no necessary connection with parturition, whether premature or not; neither with any traumatic or surgical injury; would serve to distinguish this affection from pelvic cellulitis. Add to this that in cellulitis the uterus is almost always fixed and immovable, while in fibroids it is not so, and you can have no difficulty.

From pelvic cellulitis.

The tumor that is sometimes formed by impaction of the fæces is in no manner connected with the uterus, is posterior to it, does not move with it, is doughy to the feel and can be indented on pressure, is accompanied by symptoms of paralysis of the rectum, obstinate constipation, rectal tenesmus, and more or less of intestinal irritation.

From impaction of the fæces.

Course and Termination.—Having free space, within the pelvis at first, and then within the abdomen, in which to grow, these tumors may reach a considerable size, and exist in a dormant state for years before they are observed or detected. And being, in most cases, unaccompanied by alarming or dangerous symptoms, harmless in themselves, and benign in their tendencies, their presence may be tolerated for many years more.

Toleration of.

Extra-uterine fibroids tend to develop into fibro-cysts, such as you saw in the case of Mrs. C. D——, in this clinic, some weeks ago.* This cystic degeneration is one in which the tumor becomes composite, and instead of being made up exclusively of fibro-cellular tissue, as it was originally, is composed of compartments, or cysts, which contain a quantity of serum, blood, or pus, or of all these commingled. It is only in case of the larger fibroids that this particular degeneration takes place; and you should remember that, although it is by no means very frequent in the sub-peritoneal fibroids, yet it is much more rarely met with in either of the other varieties of this disease.

Cystic degeneration.

Prognosis.—Concerning ultimate recovery from this kind of a fibroid you had better promise nothing. Nature may extemporise a means of palliation and relief, through an arrest of the development of the tumor, or even amputate it spontaneously by attenuation or rupture of its pedicle, so that it shall float around like a loose cartilage in the knee-joint, causing little pain or inconvenience; but it is not probable that she will remove it entirely. Pregnancy is not so serious a complication in extra- as it is in intra-uterine fibroids.

Nature's attempts to cure.

Although such a tumor may possibly co-exist with carcinoma uteri, yet it is a settled fact that uterine fibroids have no malignant tendencies, and do not, therefore, develop into cancer.

No risk of cancer.

Treatment.—Physicians are agreed that, more especially in the early stages of these growths, internal medication *should* suffice for their removal and cure. But to say that it ever *has* cured them is to claim too much for our skill. In the present state of our knowledge, the

Short-comings of internal treatment.

* See page 426.

most that we can expect to accomplish with our remedies is the relief of contingent disorders and complications. And whether we shall ever improve upon this is largely a matter of "faith and works." If these tumors result from a simple hypertrophy of tissue, the resolvent powers of our medicines, locally and internally used, should be sufficient to arrest their development, if not indeed to cure them radically. Perhaps in the future we may be more successful with these means than we have been in the past.

Reasons therefor.

One grand difficulty in the way of this result, however, is the impossibility of placing such patients under proper treatment in the early stage of the disease, when the tumor or tumors are in their incipiency, and when specific means would act more promptly and perhaps successfully. Another is that the differential diagnosis is so difficult; and a third, that few women with these adventitious growths, or with uterine tumors of any kind (especially in these days of prize-surgery), are willing to take sufficient time to test the merits of internal treatment.

Surgical treatment.

Gastrotomy.

The only surgical resource in case of the extra-uterine fibroid is gastrotomy. If the tumor has a well-defined pedicle, and its attachments are not very extensive or vascular, it may be removed, and the pedicle ligated, as in ovariotomy. A similar operation may suffice in case its stem or stalk is broken, and it is floating in the abdominal cavity. But, even after the abdominal incision has been made, if it is found that the growth is glued on all sides, and thoroughly amalgamated with the uterus and the neighboring parts, it is thought to be best to relinquish the operation, to close up the wound and allow the tumor to remain. This course is deemed proper because of the danger that would almost necessarily follow from the final extirpation of the growth under such adverse circumstances. These dangers include the possibility of the shock or collapse, hæmorrhage, fatal peritonitis and septicæmia.

Extirpation of the uterus and ovaries.

Notwithstanding these dangers, however, surgeons have pushed forward, and not only removed the fibrous growth, but the uterus and ovaries also. The proportionate loss of these patients has been very large, but no larger, it is claimed, than was the relative number of deaths from ovariotomy in the early history of that operation. Out of 35 cases of uterine fibroids, in which the uterus and ovaries were extirpated, 7, or 1 in 5, recovered.

"No operator should undertake gastrotomy for uterine neoplasms without being prepared, if necessary, to remove the uterus with the tumor, for sometimes the connection is so intimate that an exact localization of the tumor is out of the power of the most skillful diagnostician. Indeed, even after the removal of the mass from the body, its relations to the uterus are often discovered only after patient and intelligent search. Dr. Farre tells of a specimen preserved in one of the London museums as a solid ovarian tumor which, upon careful examination, he proved to be uterine by tracing the Fallopian tubes into it. It was also in this way that the nature of the tumor removed by Dr. Storer was identified, Prof. Ellis, after a very minute examination, distinctly discovering the entrance of the tubes into the cavity of the body, and thus settling the matter."*

*A Practical Treatise on the Diseases of Women, by T. Gaillard Thomas, M.D., etc. 3d edition, 1872. p. 501.

LECTURE XXXII.

FIBROID TUMORS OF THE UTERUS.—(*Continued.*)

GENTLEMEN:

Having discussed the special pathology and treatment of those fibroids which are denominated intra-uterine and extra-uterine, we now come to speak of such as are located within the wall of the womb, midway between its mucous and serous coats. These tumors, which are not in the uterine, nor yet in the abdominal cavity, are commonly known as

3.—INTERSTITIAL FIBROIDS.

They also have various synonyms such as intra-mural, intra-stromal, parietal, and intermediate. These are the round tumors proper, for no matter what their size, unless they are forced into the uterine or the abdominal cavity, and thereby become oval or perhaps pedunculated, their shape is unchanged. They are always enclosed within a proper capsule, and, like the other varieties, are most frequently located posteriorly with reference to the womb. In very rare cases they are met with at the lower segment of the uterus, and even in the cervix. But, wherever they are found, the neighboring portion of the womb is hypertrophied, and all of its tissues are preternaturally developed.

Symptoms.—The symptoms are more or less grave and troublesome according to the size of the tumor and the tendency to inflammation within or about the womb. If the growth is large, and fixed in the posterior wall of the uterus, that organ will necessarily be displaced posteriorly. For this reason retroversion and retroflexion are almost invariably present in these cases. But if the tumor is attached to the side of the womb, the latter will, of course, be dragged, or made to incline laterally.

Uterine deviations.

In a considerable proportion of cases there is dysmenorrhœa. The difficulty of menstruation is due either to the partial closure or the tortuosity of the cervico-uterine canal, which is caused by the flexion of the uterus and the presence of the tumor; or to the fact that this foreign body almost necessarily excites painful contractions of the womb whenever anything is to be extruded.

Dysmenorrhœa.

In other cases, I think there can be no question that the obstruction to the ready exit of the flow in dysmenorrhœa may indirectly cause such a tumor to be developed. It is reasonable to suppose that such a derangement in the uterine circulation as almost necessarily accompanies very painful and tardy menstruation, would beget a vice of nutrition that might result in local hypertrophy. And thus, in exceptional cases, it might be very difficult, and perhaps impossible, to determine whether the dysmenorrhœa was the cause or the consequence of the interstitial deposit.

On account of their nearness to and intimate relations with the uterine mucous membrane, there is almost as great a liability to menorrhagia in the interstitial as in the submucous fibroid. The menstrual discharge is always too free, and the return of the periods is apt to be more frequent than natural. In many cases the flow is prolonged and continuous, the blood oozing away constantly. Or the hæmorrhage may be sudden and alarming, accompanied by violent pains and contractions like those of labor. Not unfrequently this condition of things is mistaken for abortion, more especially if shreds of membrane and coagula are expelled.

Menorrhagia.

The tendency to abortion is somewhat less marked than it is in the case of intra-uterine fibroids, but this accident occurs more frequently in this than in the extra-uterine variety. We can account for this clinical fact upon the theory that this adventitious growth diverts the nutritive supplies which are needed by the developing embryo. Perhaps a better explanation is that the tumor, or fibroid, excites such peristaltic contractions as are likely to empty the womb of its contents. The unequal development of the uterine wall is not without its influence also.

Abortion.

I have now under treatment two cases of sterility, which are due to the presence of parietal fibroids. In both of them the growths are so situated as to cause violent dysmenorrhœa, and so decided a retro-flexion of the womb as absolutely to prevent the ingress of the semen masculinum. Under these circumstances insemination is impossible. In order to cure these women it will be necessary to remedy the displacement. But if conception were attained, they would almost certainly abort afterwards, unless the fibroid had been disposed of.

Sterility.

Other incidental disorders are endometritis, cervicitis, leucorrhœa, cystitis, proctitis, rectal ulceration and paralysis, inveterate constipation, hæmorrhoids, pelvic cellulitis, and pelvi-peritonitis.

Diagnosis. — In separating these from other foreign growths we are obliged to depend mainly upon physical signs. Examination is to be made with the finger per vaginam, and per rectum, and with instruments also, of the cervical and uterine cavities. The tumor must first be located, and afterwards identified. These steps are less difficult, perhaps, than in other fibroids, because in most cases the tumor is pelvic and not abdominal, and because it is so located in the hollow of the sacrum as to be more accessible.

The bi-manual method facilitates the examination by the "touch." The patient should be placed upon her back, the limbs flexed, and the abdominal parietes relaxed. The left hand is then to be placed upon the hypogastrium and pressure made upon the uterus over the pubes, so as to cause it to descend as far as possible into the excavation, toward the ostium vaginæ; the index finger of the right hand being at the same time within the vagina, or the rectum, is made to explore the lateral and posterior surfaces of the womb in such a manner as to recognize any increased or abnormal development of its wall.

The bi-manual examination.

Depressing the uterus.

Or, if the woman is corpulent, it may be necessary to draw down the uterus with a Sims' or Nott's tenaculum, in order to examine it more thoroughly through the retro-uterine space.

The uterine tenaculum.

The probe may suffice to indicate the presence of a tumor which presses towards the uterine cavity; but in general it will not diagnosticate an intra-mural fibroid, excepting upon the principle of exclusion. Thus, if the

The sound.

sound is passed without difficulty or obstruction, and takes the direction of the proper uterine axis, the inference is that, if there is a fibroid in the wall of the womb, it cannot be of any considerable size. For one of these tumors must almost necessarily displace the organ. A sub-peritoneal growth with a pedicle might fill the hollow of the sacrum without changing the axis of the womb, but not so with an interstitial fibroid.

Dilatation.

However, if you can not satisfy yourselves of the existence of an intra-mural tumor, by the conjoined methods of which I have spoken, it will be necessary to proceed to dilatation, in order to be able to explore the cavity of the womb with the finger or other instrument. This may be done in the manner indicated in my last lecture. It should be done cautiously, however, lest you induce a severe hæmorrhage.

The differential signs between an interstitial fibroid and pelvic cellulitis, pelvi-peritonitis, and kindred affections, with which it is sometimes complicated, and for which it has been mistaken, are the same as those by which you would distinguish these diseases and other sequelæ from sub-mucous and sub-serous fibroids.

Relative curability.

Prognosis.—My own experience leads me to conclude that this variety of the myo-fibromata is more amenable to treatment than either of the others. Unless it be excessively developed, or attended by unusual hæmorrhage, or other dangerous complications, from which this class of fibroids is not exempted, you should not despair of curing your patient.

Influence of the change of life.

A favorable change is likely to follow the ménopause. This crisis once passed, the chances are that with the subsequent atrophy, or senile involution of the uterus and the ovaries, such a growth may also undergo a retrograde metamorphosis, and never occasion any more trouble. Sometimes, however, these fibroids cause the climacteric to be delayed, and the menstrual flux to be substituted by prolonged and dangerous hæmorrhages, which have a fatal tendency.

The condition of the cervix.

In bad cases, where the cervix is long and narrow, as well as dense and undilatable, occurring in women who have never been pregnant, the prognosis is generally unfavorable. Indeed, the texture, consistency and other physical characters of the neck of the womb, have more to do than almost anything else with the possibility and probability of cure, whether by surgical or medical means. Other things equal, multiparæ are more likely to recover than nulliparæ.

While the fatty, calcareous, cartilaginous, and even the osseous degenerations which these fibroids sometimes undergo, are to be considered as salutary in their tendencies, other varieties of textural change may imply increased danger. Suppuration, sloughing, œdema, and interstitial hæmorrhage are critical processes that will cause you the greatest anxiety, and which you will learn are beset with extreme peril. The spontaneous enucleation of the tumor is altogether favorable. An evident inclination in the fibroid to develop in the direction of the uterine cavity, and especially to become pedunculated, is not of necessity a bad sign, for it may facilitate its removal by surgical means, or otherwise.

Various forms of degeneration.

When complicated with other diseases, the danger varies with the grade and character of the contingent disorder. In women of a hæmorrhagic diathesis the chances of recovery are not the most promising.

Treatment.—I am aware that there is a sort of histological difference between a simple hypertrophy of the uterine wall and an interstitial fibroid ensconced in its capsule. But this difference is more apparent than real. The early clinical history of these fibroids is so closely related and allied to those changes which take place within the same tissues during utero-gestation, and their post-partum involution, as to convey a therapeutical hint which promises to be of especial service. And I am persuaded, as the result of experience, that, in their early stages, these tumors are often curable by the use of internal remedies conjoined with very simple local means.

Curable in their incipiency.

It is therefore a most fortunate circumstance that these parietal fibroids are more likely to be recognized, and to come under our care at an earlier period of their existence than either of the other varieties of this affection. It is for this as well as for diagnostic reasons, that I have chosen to treat of them separately.

Manifestly, the first duty of the practitioner is, if possible, to prevent their recurrence. This may sometimes be accomplished through the adoption of means that are calculated to ensure the complete and uniform involution of the uterus after delivery; the free and ready exit of the menstrual flow; to prevent such habitual or permanent deviations of the womb, particularly retroversion and retroflexion, as would result in its disproportionate development; the prevention of abortion, and its consequent arrest of the organic changes proper to pregnancy; the interdiction of intemperate and fraudulent intercourse; and of the wearing of pessaries, stays, abdominal supporters, and of whatever might interfere with a free and uninterrupted distribution of blood through the pelvic and abdominal viscera. This preventive treatment is very important.

Prophylaxis.

And so likewise is the medicinal treatment. The hæmorrhage and the serous discharges, as well as the symptoms which are attendant upon the local inflammation and the menstrual disorder, afford a series of definite indications for our remedies. We make requisition upon the materia medica for secale cornutum, sabina, sepia, belladonna, lachesis, crocus, calcarea carb., staphisagria, arsenicum alb., silicea, phosphorus, lycopodium, china, thuja, carbo vegetabilis, sulphur, or nitric acid. One of these is given upon specific indications—which should be as definite and accurate as possible—and its use is persisted in until the symptoms for which it was prescribed have disappeared. Then another may be chosen.

Medicinal treatment.

I could detail a number of cases in which the careful and persistent employment of belladonna has removed a limited hypertrophy of the womb which, but for it, would undoubtedly have developed into a fibroid. It was given in the third decimal attenuation.

Belladonna.

Lachesis is equally efficacious in certain cases. It seems possessed of remarkable virtues as a resolvent, particularly where there is a defective involution of the womb. I am not aware that any author has mentioned this fact, and you will therefore take my individual estimate of its value for no more than it is worth. No class of facts needs such abundant confirmation as those which are clinical. In my hands the best effects have been derived from lachesis in the sixth and the twelfth attenuations.

Lachesis.

In claiming that these tumors are curable in their incipiency by means that are so mild and available, I do not forget that there are many sources of fallacy which might lead to a wrong inference respecting the efficacy of this or any other plan of treatment. It is not unusual for these growths to increase or to decrease in size very rapidly, and sometimes to disappear spontaneously. A retrograde metamorphosis may take them out of the way. The climacteric may arrest their development; and other changes may cut off their nutrition and cause them to wither. These cures by limitation are often placed to the credit of such agencies as animal magnetism, spiritualism, electricity, and other imponderables, and even of medical treatment. But, making due allowance for all these exceptional cases, I apprehend, it remains that very great good of a positive kind may be done by means of fitly-chosen internal remedies.

Sources of fallacy.

Together with these remedies, as already indicated, I am in the habit of employing the cotton tampon saturated with pure glycerine, or with glycerine containing a few drops of the strong tincture of calendula, of hamamelis, hydrastis, or of the same medicine that is being taken internally. This is an excellent adjuvant to the cure, and has the effect in many cases to avert the recurrence of frequent and dangerous hæmorrhages.

Local means.

The surgical treatment contemplates the removal of the tumor either by excision or enucleation. Excision by the ligature or the écraseur, not being available in non-pedunculated growths, as a rule, and these fibroids being interstitial, the main dependence is upon some form of enucleation. This operation consists in making one or more free incisions into the tumor and through its capsule, from the interior surface of the uterus. The fibroid is then turned out of its bed and, if possible, detached and removed at once. In many cases it is only partially separated, and then allowed to slough away, care being taken meanwhile to avoid pyæmia and similar contingencies by frequent injections of carbolized or calendulated water, and appropriate internal medication.

Surgical treatment.

Enucleation.

Although the risks of this expedient are sometimes very great, still it is growing in favor. It is sometimes resorted to for the removal of the sub-mucous fibroids also, particularly in case of such of them as are attached to the uterus by a broad base.

Drs. Atlee's and Brown's operations.

Dr. Atlee's operation is a modification of this. And so also is Dr. I. Baker Brown's plan of coring or "gouging" out a piece from the middle of the tumor and filling the cavity with lint that has been dipped in olive oil. The idea in both of these operations is to impair its nutrition, and to facilitate the sloughing and separation of the adventitious growth.

Danger in dilatation.

In some of these cases there is such an exceptional intolerance of artificial dilatation of the cervix uteri, both on account of the hæmorrhage that may follow, and of directly fatal results, that the greatest possible care is requisite in the preparation of the patient for the removal of the tumor. Dr. Thomas reports two cases of sudden death from the use of the sponge-tent preparatory to enucleation, and sums up the dangers of this whole operation in the following forcible language: "If the cervical canal be well dilated, and the uterus susceptible of depression to the ostium vaginæ, or the vagina be so dilatable as to admit the hand, the case should be regarded as favorable to the procedure. If the opposite state of affairs exists, the case is not only an unfavorable one, but the procedure will in all probability fail. The prospect of success is, for these reasons, much better in multiparous than in nulliparous women."*

ALBUMINURIA IN PREGNANCY.

Case.—L. W. C——, 19 years of age, primipara, weighing 180 pounds, was admitted to the hospital at the eighth month of pregnancy. She is of full habit and is troubled with headache and "flushes." On being tested by heat and nitric acid, the urine was found to be highly albuminous. She had previously taken apocynum can., and arsenicum alb., without any benefit. The feet and legs were enormously swollen, so that she could not walk or stand with any degree of comfort. She felt wretched, nervous and apprehensive.

She took mercurius corrosivus in the 3rd decimal trituration once in three hours. The proportion of albumen in the urine

* The American Journal of Obstetrics and the Diseases of Women and Children. 1872. Vol. V, page 108.

lessened almost immediately, and continued to decrease, so that there was a mere trace of it the day before her delivery. Although we had anticipated convulsions, her labor came on naturally, and was completed without a single untoward symptom. Her child is now three weeks old, and all the dropsical and urinary symptoms have entirely disappeared.

I do not know where you will find a case of disease which is the cause of greater mental strain and anxiety than such a one as this has been. To feel and realize that in all probability a woman who is approaching term will have puerperal eclampsia, and that her life and that of her offspring depend almost entirely upon your skill, is a great load to carry. It should interest you to know how such a calamity may sometimes be averted.

A pregnant woman at the eighth month may have dropsical symptoms which do not forbode any ill of this kind. But if she has decided albuminuria, with dropsy of the face and extremities, with or without amaurosis, the probabilities are that unless this is relieved, her delivery will be accompanied by convulsions. How to remedy this single symptom may therefore be a very important question for you to decide.

Signs of convulsibility.

Experience has led me to place great confidence in the mercurius corrosivus. I have prescribed it very frequently to fulfil this precise indication, and it has seldom disappointed me. Dr. Adams has furnished me notes of another case which occurred in the hospital some weeks ago, in which the effect of this remedy was equally satisfactory.

Mercurius corrosivus.

Case.—Nancy J., aged 29, primipara, was eight and a half months advanced in her second pregnancy when she was admitted to the hospital. She reported that she had had dropsical symptoms for two weeks already. The legs and ankles were very much swollen, the ankles being so puffy that the infiltrated integument hung over her slippers. The face and eyelids were œdematous, and she complained of much headache. On examination the urine was found to be albuminous. She also had a partial amaurosis, which began and subsided with the dropsical symptoms.

She took the murcurius corrosivus 3, a dose every three hours. The albumen disappeared from the urine, so that the day before her delivery no trace of it could be discovered. She passed through parturition and lying-in without any convulsions.

In presenting these cases the idea which I design to convey is not that this, or any other remedy, is an absolute specific for ante-partum convulsibility. There is no real prophylactic of puerperal eclampsia. But if in one case in ten, you can recognise the incipient symptoms of this dreadful disease and avert it, you should know how to do it. Therefore, I recommend you not to fail to apply the tests for albuminuria whenever any of its symptoms are present in the later months of pregnancy, and not to forget that the mercurius corrosivus is in many cases an invaluable remedy for it. When Nature "flags the train" we should always take the hint.

There is no infallible prophylactic for convulsibility.

OVARIAN IRRITATION.

Case.— Mrs. K——, English, 54 years old, the mother of eight children, has been in poor health ever since her "change," which occurred seven years ago. Prior to that she had always enjoyed good health, although she confesses that she "was always very nervous." Once, however, she has had a pretty severe attack of gout in her right foot, and occasionally rheumatic lameness in her right arm. It was her habit, while she continued to menstruate to flow more freely than most women, and after the birth of some of her children she had severe hæmorrhages. But, notwithstanding this, the climacteric passed without any flooding, or any dangerous symptoms whatever. The only complaint for some months after the flow had ceased was of a congestive headache, which alternated with a severe aching, sickening, burning pain in the left hypogastric and iliac regions. Finally the headache left, but the ovarian sufferings continued.

For some weeks past she has been subject to occasional outbreaks of diarrhœa, which alternate with constipation, with scybalous stools and cutting colicky pains in the abdomen. She is extremely nervous and excitable, has globus hystericus and very copious urination now and then, and finds herself "very uncertain."

On inspection the abdomen is uniformly distended. There is evident meteorism, which is general. Palpation does not disclose the presence of any tumor or enlargement. The left ovarian region is tender to the touch and to moderate pressure, but not especially so to firm pressure with the tips of the fingers. The os uteri is not abnormal. The uterus is *in situ* and mobile. The sound passes readily to the depth of two inches by actual measurement. Bi-manual examination does not reveal anything abnormal.

Ovarian irritation is not an infrequent sequel to the climateric.

It is often the cause of ill health among those who, like this woman, have ceased to menstruate. But there is a combination of circumstances which constitutes a strong predisponent to this affection in such persons, and which is well illustrated in the case before us. Her habit of menstruating very freely, while that function was intact, and of flooding in childbed; her rheumatic diathesis; and her hysteric constititution, render it almost impossible for her to have escaped the disorder from which she is at this moment suffering.

At the climacteric.

Complications.

Fortunately, she did not experience any severe or alarming hæmorrhage at the ménopause. In this respect the menstrual function ceased without any untoward symptoms. In so far, her case was an exception to the rule that the hæmorrhagic diathesis predisposes to critical floodings, which may damage the general health, and endanger life. But this very exemption may have acted as an exciting cause, and prompted the development of the rheumatic and hysterical tendencies. As a matter of course, under these peculiar circumstances, the ovary (and the left ovary especially) would be more liable to implication than any other organ.

Analysis of the case.

Hence a train of symptoms that are compounded of hysteria and rheumatism. If, instead of being predisposed to these affections, she had had a constitutional bias toward cancer, dropsy, or tuberculosis, the result would have been very different, and the case would probably have developed into one of cancer of the womb, or of the mammary gland, or she would most likely have had an ovarian cyst, or some form of phthisis.

Clinical inference.

You can scarcely err in ascribing a sickening, burning pain, with aching in either of the iliac regions, to irritation or inflammation of the ovary. No matter what other symptoms are superadded, if this is frequent or constant, the primary lesion is in that organ. The patient may have any of the manifold signs of hysteria, or she may have indigestion and diarrhœa, or constipation, or all these in alternation, and yet the focal point of the disorder will be either in one or in both the ovaries.

A pathognomonic sign.

Among the exciting causes of ovarian irritation which we have not already enumerated, are the indulgence of such habits, and the subjection to such emotional influences as tend to derange the circulation and innervation of the generative organs. One of my patients had this disorder in a most intractable form in consequence of taking vaginal injections of cold water, and sometimes of ice-water, several times daily for more than two years. In another it was caused by horseback riding. It frequently originates in the sudden arrest of a leucorrhœal discharge by astringent injections. A fertile source of this affection is the habit of staying at home, and of going very little into the open air; for, contrary to what you would suppose, nothing allays a sur-excitation of the female sexual system like exercise or exposure out of doors.

Exciting causes.

In order to show you how these simple causes operate, and how complicated the resulting affections sometimes are, I will read you the notes of a case in which I was recently consulted by my friend and former pupil, Dr. A. W. Woodward, of this city, who has reported its history for me:

Case. — Mrs. B——, a middle-aged, slender, and somewhat delicate woman, with three children, has usually enjoyed good health. During the last few months she has been too closely confined with family cares, and spent too many hours at the sewing machine. In consequence, she began to be troubled with a more or less severe pain, sometimes acute in character, located in the left hypogastrium. This pain is aggravated by standing upon the feet for any considerable time, and is much more severe and continuous just before the menses. It extends through the whole length of the left limb. The flow had always been normal until within the last two months, since which time it has been both protracted and profuse.

A lady practitioner diagnosticated "retroversion and prolapsus," and treated her by a severe and prolonged application of galvano-electricity. As a consequence the patient was completely prostrated, the pain was greatly increased, and instead of being merely indisposed, she became quite ill. At this stage I was called in, and finding no signs either of retroversion or of prolapsus, or of anything to contra-indicate the use of stimulants, they were given, with good effect. Hot fomentations relieved the pain, and as this subsided it was followed by a copious diuresis, for which I gave ignatia.

This remedy was continued until the next day, when I found her with heat and slight swelling in the region of the left ovary, a rapid pulse, thirst and headache. The pain still continued, but was throbbing and not of the "sickening" kind that she had had before. I prescribed atropine and mercurius sol., and although she had a marked chill followed by heat during the afternoon, these remedies were given until the next morning. Arsenicum caused the strength to return, the pain to be lessened, and there was no sign of a chill for several days.

But as the ovarian difficulty subsided, the stomach began to be deranged. At different times anorexia, cramps, acid eructations and vomiting were present. The symptoms would yield very readily to nux vomica, and then be followed either by a return of the ovarian irritation, by diarrhœa, or by a chill, after which these different affections would terminate with a profuse flow of urine. Then the same series of gastric, intestinal, ovarian and febrile symptoms would recur and run through their course as before. There was, however, no apparent order in their coming, excepting that the diuresis came last.

The remedies that we prescribed jointly did this patient but very little permanent good. It was not until the cause of her suffering was discovered, or rather until it disclosed itself, and was removed, that she got well again. This cause proved to be the presence of a pestilent old female relative, who gave the poor woman no peace, upset her domestic affairs, and finally proposed to carry off her valuables in the wrong trunk!

A peculiar "thorn in the flesh."

Having already detailed the proper means of preventing this form of sexual irritation, and of its general management,* it only remains to speak of the remedies that may be indicated. Among these the most prominent is macrotin. In many cases it is an invaluable, and indeed an indispensable remedy. Belladonna, atropine, ignatia, rhus tox., zincum val., platina, colocynth, china, chamomilla, hamamelis, and the lilium tigrinum are equally useful under their appropriate indications.

Remedies.

The symptoms, in the case of Mrs. K., call for ignatia. She will therefore take this remedy once in three hours, and report. I have no doubt that it will relieve much of her suffering, but this does not justify me in claiming that it alone will effect a radical cure.

* See pages 165-6-7.

LECTURE XXXIII.

AMENORRHŒA. — MENORRHAGIA. — CONVULSIONS.

GENTLEMEN:

I have had frequent occasion to extol the virtues of Nitric Acid in a certain form of menorrhagia. Here are the notes of a case for which I am indebted to Dr. W. H. Parsons, of the Class of 1870-71:

Case. — Miss ——, twenty years of age, of nervo-bilious temperament, with dark hair and complexion, black eyes, and small in stature, had been ill for nearly four years. For the first eight years of her life she was puny and small, and, though never very ill, the skin was always of a yellowish hue, and the flesh very soft and flabby. At the eighth year she began to grow in height and breadth, and finally became very fat. She continued so until her fifteenth year, when her menses appeared. At the second month she began to have a peculiar discoloration of the skin in various parts of the body. There were dark circles about the eyes, with languor, a morbid appetite and a general chlorotic condition, and the catamenia did not return.

The doctor under whose care she was placed succeeded in bringing on the menses, but the flow did not cease at the proper time. The discharge was muco-sanguinolent, dark and offensive, and lasted at first about a fortnight. After this it became continuous, and she lost the record of the month. This state of things was unchanged for several months more when the mother besought the doctor to *stop* the flow. Some unknown medicine was given which had the desired effect, but she went into convulsions, and the doctor, having decided it as hopeless, relinquished the case. As soon as the effect of the drug passed off, the flow returned and the convulsions ceased.

This was followed, however, by twitching of the voluntary muscles. For about six months these symptoms continued and increased in severity, and her parents abandoned all hope of her recovery. Another physician was called, who diagnosticated the case as one of menorrhagia. He proceeded to suppress the discharge and re-produced the convulsions. He then declared them epileptic, and treated her for epilepsy. But the girl grew weaker and more nervous, and finally he also abandoned the case, saying that "she would either outgrow it, or would ultimately die of it."

At the beginning of the third year Dr. —— was called. He declared it to be a passive menorrhagia, and prescribed hamamelis, creasote, secale cor., pulsatilla, etc. With these remedies the flow was arrested without bringing on the convulsions, and for a time the patient seemed to improve. After this she had amenorrhœa (*suppressio mensium*), for several weeks, and then for six months more alternations of suppression and continuous flow. She was finally reduced to a mere shadow, passed sleepless nights, her right side was constantly in motion, and she was anxious to die for the sake of relief.

Another physician was called, the patient improved, under senecin, gelseminum, and secale cor., and the parents soon thought they could "get her along" without the doctor. So far as the discharge was concerned, she was in a somewhat improved condition. But generally she was no better. In a few months the old difficulty returned with renewed violence.

I found the patient in the following condition. She is very much emaciated, and hardly able to walk; flesh flabby, skin soft, discolored in spots, very sallow and dirty looking, hectic flush, sensitive, alternate chilliness and flushes of heat, eyes brilliant, with dark circles about them, and constantly moving from one object to another. Sometimes she sits and stares like an idiot, and acts in a very silly manner. She also complains of pains in the top and back part of her head. The pulse is quick, small and irregular; respiration hurried; her body is in almost constant motion, her right foot and hand are very restless, particularly at night; starts in her sleep as from fright. She rises at six A.M., but soon returns to bed, and almost immediately falls into a deep sleep which lasts about two hours, after which she feels weary and languid. She dislikes society, is fond of seclusion, and is very despondent. Complains of pain in the dorsal region of the spine. The stomach is very irritable, with a constant feeling of "goneness," eats little, food irritates and causes pain in the stomach. Craves acids, can not eat either pastry or hearty food. Tongue is coated and of a bluish white color. The bowels are bound, the urine high colored. No pain in the uterine region.

The vaginal discharge is of a muco-sanguineous nature, very dark and fœtid, darker than the proper flow, with occasional clots.

I stipulated that she should eat what I directed, and nothing else, that her room should be changed from a dark and curtained dungeon to an airy, pleasant one, exposed to the sunlight, and that she should continue under treatment until I pronounced her cured, whether it took a month or a year. She was to take all the apples and oranges that she could eat, to exercise lightly in the open air, and to forego her exhausting sleep in the morning. The remedy prescribed was nitric acid[3] (centesimal), four pellets three times each day.

April 17, two days later, no change excepting that her stomach is less irritable, and bears food a little better. Continue the medicine.

April 19, improved; thinks the flow less; appetite better; but is very nervous and wakeful. Coffea[6] one dose at bed-time, and nitric acid as before.

April 23. Continues to improve; rested much better; the discharge is very much lessened; appetite improved; pulse less frequent and more regular. Continue.

April 26. Improving. Repeat the acid only twice per day.

April 29. Flow completely stopped. Is very restless, can not lie or sit still; starts at the least noise, seems afraid of every one, must get out of bed, looks wildly about, can not sleep. Hyoscyamus[6] two doses at night. Nitric acid discontinued.

April 30. Slept well, feels refreshed; had the best night's rest that she has had for months. Hyoscyamus as before.

May 3. Better, sleeps well, is more inclined to talk, and less nervous; eyes less brilliant, appetite better, very little pain in the head. A slight discharge from the vagina. Nitric acid again, two doses to be taken each week.

May 15. Found my patient much improved. She has passed through her menstrual period, which lasted four days and ceased spontaneously two days ago. She feels like a new creature, sleeps like a child, appetite good, stomach bears food well, no head symptoms, is cheerful and hopeful, glad to see her family and friends, her skin is almost natural, and, in brief, she appears well.

Three months later (Aug. 10th), I called upon my patient and learned that she had quite recovered, and was in every respect the opposite of what she had been. The nervous symptoms had vanished, the menstrual irregularity had disappeared, and her health was entirely restored.

This case illustrates the ill effects of "forcing the flow" at puberty. Here is a young lady of fifteen years. Nature is making an effort to establish the menstrual function. She is passing through the preliminary stage of the crisis, has been sick once, and in due time all will be well.

Emmenagogues at puberty.

But her incidental ill-health alarms the parents. A doctor is called, and he decides that the "change" is not progressing as it should, and that all her difficulties are due to the delay in menstruation. Thus far his opinion is well enough. But, forgetting, if he ever knew, how delicate the function of ovulation necessarily is, with what contingencies it is beset, and how easily its proper performance may be deranged, he prescribes something that is designed, not to prompt, but to compel the flow.

The consequence is that a train of ills, which might have been avoided, is fastened upon her. The flow appears, but it is not physiological and healthy. Instead of being followed by a spontaneous return in four weeks, it does not come at all. A little more medicine, and more of tinkering with the most marvelous of all the wonderful processes of the living animal body, and, as if to revenge itself, the discharge commences and continues indefinitely, or until it is checked again by powerful astringents.

Bad practice.

Now, gentlemen, you know the mischief of the artificial induction of abortion. I have shown you how ruinous it is to the health of a woman to forcibly interrupt the attachments and growth of the germ. In this clinic your attention has been called to some of the sequelæ of this abominable practice. But, let me tell you that, leaving the fœticide out of the question, the consequences to the woman are no more serious and lasting than those which frequently follow the taking of emmenagogues by young girls who are but just beginning to menstruate.

Remote consequences.

The fact that with this patient the menses had already appeared should have been a sufficient guaranty that, if she were well in other respects, the flow would be regularly established. And besides, as every experienced practitioner will attest, nothing is more common than for the "periods," after having come once or twice at puberty, to be irregular. Sometimes they skip one month, or two or three, or perhaps even a year, before they return again. And this without any material damage to the general health. By and by, unless the doctor or the nurse is impertinent, ignorant or mischievous, they are resumed with very little risk, and afterwards become quite regu-

Menstrual intermissions common.

Let them alone.

lar. But, if you will observe carefully, I think you will find that in a very large proportion of cases of intermittent and irregular menstruation, amenorrhœa and menorrhagia, the difficulty is traceable to mal-treatment of this kind, at or about the period of puberty. In this manner it is quite possible for a single doctor, who has a passion for what he calls "demonstrative treatment," to sow the seeds of evils that fifty better men can not remedy.

The nervous and the menstrual functions.

The relation between the nervous system and the menstrual function is also shown in this bit of clinical history. When the hæmorrhage was suddenly checked the patient had a convulsion, and when the flow returned the convulsions ceased. Each time the discharge was lessened, the nervous twitchings and choreic movements became more manifest. And even when the convulsions were not induced by an arrest of the menses, these jerkings and twitchings were very troublesome and persistent. It really seemed as if the patient was "decreed" to have either the menstrual disorder or the convulsive affection. The problem in the treatment was how to cure the one without causing the other.

Illustration.

You are aware that the liability to hysterical convulsions, spasms and paralysis, is limited to menstrual life. In girls, chorea, or St. Vitus' dance, subsides as puberty approaches, and finally disappears when the catamenial function is established. There is a form of menstrual mania that may accompany amenorrhœa, or menorrhagia, which, in many respects, resembles puerperal mania. All of which illustrates the intimate and profound relation between the menstrual function and the function of innervation.

"Stopping" the flow.

Another item that we should consider in this connection is the folly of supposing that, in certain cases of uterine hæmorrhage, the disease is cured if we only stop the flow. There are cases of flooding in which if we fulfil this indication it is all that we can expect to accomplish, for in so doing we shall necessarily remove the cause of the trouble. Such cases are those in which the loss of blood depends upon the presence of polypi, fibroids, hydatids, or of the placenta in utero, upon cauliflower excrescence, or the more ordinary form of uterine cancer. These can

A practical distinction.

frequently, and indeed generally be relieved most speedily and certainly by surgical together with medical means.

But in such cases as this, where the hæmorrhage depends upon a pathological condition of the uterine mucous membrane, and a morbid state of the whole menstrual function, it will not suffice to check the discharge. For, even if the patient escapes having more alarming symptoms in consequence, the disease which has caused the flow is not cured thereby. The remedy must be possessed of an intimate, curative relation to the lesion that underlies and has occasioned this particular symptom, else it will do no permanent good.

The digestive derangement was a very natural and almost necessary consequence of the menstrual disorder. And so also was the chloro-anæmia. Nothing could be better adapted for their relief than the careful attention to the diet and to the surroundings of the patient. Fresh air and sunlight, acid fruits, a cheerful room, and pleasant society, were useful auxiliaries toward the cure. Indeed, as the result proved, nothing could have been more appropriate than the treatment adopted. The nitric acid was perhaps the only remedy capable of correcting the menstrual irregularity without aggravating the nervous disorder, of intercepting the convulsive paroxysms, and of curing the alimentary derangement. But alone, it was not sufficient to effect a radical cure. For, as an intercurrent remedy, the hyoscyamus did the best possible service. I hope you will remember this case.

The gastric and chlorotic symptoms.

NITRIC ACID IN UTERINE HÆMORRHAGE.

Every practitioner of considerable experience has encountered cases of metrorrhagia supervening abortion, or that were incident to the climacteric, that have resisted all the ordinary means of arrest. The hæmorrhage has continued for weeks, perhaps, in a passive and irregular manner. As a consequence, the patient has been greatly reduced and discouraged. There is a loss of appetite, headache, malaise, and a series of symptoms that are chargeable to the continued drain upon her physical resources. She cannot sit upright, or stand erect, but the difficulty is increased.

Metrorrhagia after abortion.

These cases are very annoying, perplexing, and tedious, and sometimes tax our skill to the utmost. Perhaps the various astringents have already been tried, but without avail. Or, the more usual and familiar remedies, such as ipecacuanha, china, secale cor., sabina, crocus, hamamelis, trillin or the erechthites, may have failed in your hands. In such cases, the nitric acid will sometimes answer an excellent purpose. My habit is to give it in the second or third decimal attenuation, the dose to be repeated every one to three or four hours, according to the urgency of the symptoms.

Nitric acid as a dernier ressort.

Case.—In consequence of a rough ride in a sleigh, Mrs. ——, aged 28, aborted at the second month. For the first few hours she had considerable pain. But the uterine contractions came on regularly, and the embryo was soon expelled. Of course, there was no well-formed placenta at this early period of pregnancy. The post-partum hæmorrhage was profuse and long-continued. When the pains had ceased the secale which she had been taking ceased to have any more influence over the flow. The flow then became passive, and the discharge dark-colored and shreddy.

As the result of keeping her in the horizontal posture, and upon the use of an appropriate diet and drinks, she grew better, but soon relapsed again. This was twice repeated. The usual remedies would cause the flow to cease for a little, but upon the least change of posture, the discharge commenced again. Matters went on thus for nearly four weeks, in all of which time she really had gained nothing, but lost much in strength, color and spirits. At 6 P.M. of Tuesday I prescribed nitric acid in the second decimal attenuation, twenty drops in half a glass of water, two teaspoonfuls to be taken each hour. On Wednesday she had had no flow since midnight. The same medicine was directed to be repeated once in three hours. On Friday there was no return of the discharge, and she sat up a little. The remedy was discontinued. On Sunday she came into the parlor, and afterwards recovered rapidly.

I am aware that there is little in the provings of this remedy that is suggestive of its superior efficacy in this variety of hæmorrhage; and also that I am not calling your attention to anything especially new or strange. In general terms, the nitric acid appears to be indicated in those hæmorrhages from the mucous surfaces which depend upon the destruction and desquamation of their investing epithelium.

Clinical deductions.

Hence we find it useful in passive hæmorrhages from the nose, the throat, and the respiratory, alimentary and urinary passages. The escape of blood by transudation in consequence of the removal of the protecting envelope, would occasion very different symptoms from those proper to an active and alarming hæmorrhage, while in the end the result might be equally serious.

Post-menstrual hæmorrhage.

The opinion that the decidua, or outer envelope of the embryo, is formed of the mucous membrane that lined the uterus before conception, is now very generally received. When abortion occurs prior to the third month, this lining is stripped off, and the cavity of the organ is left as destitute of its proper covering as is the spot where the placenta was attached, when that structure is cast off in labor at full term. If it is not exfoliated entire, the decidua may come away in shreds, in which case the attendant hæmorrhage persists for a much longer period, and is passive in character. The blood escapes slowly, and is for some time exposed to the action of the air before it is expelled from the uterus and vagina. The discharges resemble those of melæna. Occasionally they are quite profuse. In these symptoms, I apprehend, we have the most trustworthy and practical indications for this remedy.

Special indications for nitric acid.

In the case just cited the other remedies failed to give entire relief, because the first stage, and the active symptoms to which they were appropriate, had already passed. Then it was that the nitric acid could be used with the best results.

Post-dysmenorrhœal hæmorrhage.

Many cases of dysmenorrhœa, more especially of the congestive and membranous varieties, merge into menorrhagia. The patient suffers extremely in the first stage of the menstrual period. The flow is started with great difficulty and prolonged suffering, which is similar to the first stage of labor. But when the obstacle to its egress is overcome, the pain subsides and the discharge is correspondingly free and copious. The delay and retention of the blood in utero, and the violent efforts to force open the internal os uteri, have resulted in the partial or complete exfoliation of the endometrium, and therefore, whenever she menstruates, it is as if the woman had had a veritable abortion. In one sense the hæmorrhage is post-partum. In all important pathological respects, it is identical with that which supervenes upon a miscarriage, in the early months of gestation. The detachment and disorganization of the uterine mucous membrane develops the case into one of passive hæmorrhage, to the relief of which the nitric acid is frequently, but not invariably, adapted.

Hæmorrhage at the climacteric.

You are already aware that, at the climacteric, many women are liable to protracted hæmorrhage, which is apt to be of a passive kind, not profuse, but lingering, exhaustive and debilitating. This flow is sometimes intractable. It may or may not contain strips or shreds of what are falsely called "pseudo-membranes," but its existence often depends upon the morbid condition of the uterine mucous membrane of which I have spoken. In some of these cases the nitric acid is invaluable.

Case.—Mrs. ——, aged 46, had been ill for five weeks with a passive hæmorrhage, which dated from her last menstrual period. She was much reduced in strength, the pulse was weak and irritable, the lips, tongue and alæ nasi were very pale. She complained of occasional faintness, and disgust of food and drinks. The feet were cold, and she had almost complete insomnia. Her friends thought her going into a rapid decline. Motion aggravated the flow. Prior to the last period she had a similar attack, which continued about four weeks before the flow was arrested.

I prescribed nitric acid in the second decimal attenuation, to be taken as directed in the former case. In two hours the hæmorrhage ceased. She made a rapid and complete recovery without taking any other remedy.

Practical conclusions.

In these cases the state of the uterine mucous membrane is very analagous to that which we meet with in aphthous conditions and incipient ulceration of the alimentary mucous surfaces, as in stomatitis, typhoid fever, and in some forms of diarrhœa and dysentery. Here we have a similarity of texture, and there can be little doubt that these membranes are susceptible to disease-producing and disease-curing agents of a similar character. Possibly the sulphuric, phosphoric and muriatic acids might also be useful in some cases of uterine hæmorrhage. The great benefit derived, in the treatment of hæmorrhages, from citric acid in the form of lemonade and oranges, and of tartaric acid in grapes, may not be attributable alone to their being grateful to the taste. It is not improbable that they are of service in a medicinal as well as in a dietetic way.

CHRONIC CORPOREAL CERVICITIS.—CHRONIC CERVICAL METRITIS.

Case.—Mrs. Emma H. ——, aged 26, Irish, is of sanguine temperament, has had three children and two miscarriages, the last of which she induced herself six months ago. The menses have always been profuse, and accompanied with great pain. At present she complains of pain in the left hypogastric region which, at times, extends to the pit of the stomach. She also says she has pains through the womb. The bowels are habitually costive. The appetite is poor. Micturition is difficult, and the urine carries a heavy deposit of urates. She also has leucorrhœa, which is both cervical and vaginal.

Physical examination shows the uterus to be three and a half inches in length. The cervix is engorged, thickened and swollen in the direction of its circumference. Its diameter measures nearly two inches. It is smooth and firm to the touch. The introduction of the sound, although not at all difficult, occasioned great pain. There is nothing discoverable about the neck of the bladder or the urethra to account for the painful micturition.

She was first placed on belladonna[3] once in two hours. The cotton tampon saturated with pure glycerine, was to be introduced every evening and worn through the night. This treatment, local and general, promptly relieved the engorgement and tumefaction of the uterine cervix, and her general condition was very much improved. Since that time, however, she has treated herself and our clinical assistants, to a series of hysterical manifestations, of which the following is a list:

1st. Gastralgia, which continued at intervals for three days.

2d. Retention of urine—which she passed easily enough when left to herself—lasted one week.

3d. Paralysis of the right arm for three days, and

4th. Pseudo-pleuritic pains that continued for twenty-four hours.

Our patient was brought into this institution from a neighboring hospital where, she says, her case was decided by the physician to be one of uterine cancer. I do not credit her story, and yet it may be a true one. For excepting what the doctors sometimes say of each other, no kind of testimony is so unworthy of trust as that which patients bring us concerning the views of other physicians, and the treatment to which they have already been subjected.

Symptoms — This is a case of chronic cervicitis, or of cervical hyperplasia. For some reason, most probably on account of the abortions which she has suffered, such interstitial changes have taken place within the uterine neck as to result in its enlargement and hypertrophy. Its measurements are very much increased, so that, within the pelvis it acts like a foreign body, or a tumor, causing suffering in other organs, and making the patient wretched. It presses against the urethra in such a manner as to give great pain on passing water; upon the rectum so as to cause the bowels to be obstinately bound; and is sufficient to maintain a constant leucorrhœal flow.

Mechanical symptoms.

Other symptoms which usually attend upon this affection are pelvic and sacral pains; prolapse of the womb, which is dragged toward the vulva by the increased weight of its lower segment; dyspeptic troubles, as vomiting, loss of appetite, gastralgia, loathing of food and caprices of appetite; and inability to walk without great effort, pain and fatigue. The incidental nervous disorders are more prominent than characteristic. Hysterical symptoms are an almost certain outgrowth of this particular lesion. Reflex ovarian irritation is also very common, and pains in the left hypogastrium, such as this woman complains of, are almost always present.

Direct and reflex symptoms.

Menstrual disorders are frequent. Some of these patients have amenorrhœa. In many cases there is unusual pain and difficulty in the commencement of the "period," which is occasioned by a partial closure of the cervico-uterine canal. But when that obstacle is overcome, the cervix being so very much engorged, the flow becomes excessive and perhaps long-continued. It often arises from excessive or improper exercise or travel at the month.

Menstrual disorders.

The neck of the womb is so tender to the touch that sexual intercourse is intolerable. In some cases of insuperable aversion to the act, which you will meet with in private practice, you will find that this condition of the cervix exists. Many patients with this form of cervicitis complain of burning pain within the pelvis. This pain is usually aggravated by exercise, as in standing, riding or walking. With those who are obliged to be upon their feet, the friction of

Contact.

the swollen cervix against the vaginal walls sometimes occasions extensive ulceration of its investing mucous membrane.

Nature and Cause.—This disease consists essentially in a hypertrophy of the cellular tissue of the uterine cervix. And this hypertrophy, or hyperplasia, as Dr. Thomas prefers to style it, almost never occurs excepting in those who have been pregnant. It is a post-puerperal affair. It may follow delivery at term, but is more likely to result from an arrest of development consequent upon abortion. In many cases it supervenes the artificial induction of miscarriage, the traumatic injury sustained seeming to add to the risk of its resulting as a sequel.

Post-puerperal.

It may be either the cause or the consequence of dysmenorrhœa. In "bilious climates" it is indirectly connected with hepatic disease. In this class of cases the uterus acts as a diverticulum for the blood which should circulate more actively through the portal system. The connective tissue of the cervix becomes engorged, and an excessive development of the uterine neck is the consequence. The cause acts and re-acts. You will be on the alert for this condition of things among multiparæ in malarious districts.

From bilious complication.

Diagnosis.—A few symptoms, carefully considered, will generally enable us to differentiate between this disease and cancer of the uterine neck, which is usually of the scirrhous variety. I am pretty confident that, in this case, the swelling of the cervix is not due to scirrhous deposit, because it is smooth and regular in outline and feels like a fibrous tissue. If it were cancerous, the outline would be irregular, nodulated, and bosselated, and it would feel hard and cartilaginous. Cervical metritis is almost always a sequel to pregnancy and to labor. It bears no especial relation to the climacteric. Cervical cancer is not at all infrequent in nulliparæ, and is most common at the "change of life." In the former, no matter how much the organ is swollen or displaced, it is mobile. In the latter, it may be fixed and immovable. In cervical metritis there is no evidence of a particular cachexy, while in cervical cancer such a dyscrasia is, sooner or later, manifest. In cervicitis there is no tendency to deep-seated ulceration, with destruction of

From uterine cancer.

tissue and hæmorrhage; in cancer, such a tendency is very marked.

But, even with the greatest care, it is not always possible to distinguish between these two diseases, more especially in the non-ulcerated state of uterine cancer. I have several times resorted to an expedient that has helped me to settle the diagnosis between them. You will do no harm by trying it. It is simply to use the cotton tampon saturated with pure glycerine, just as it was employed in this case. If the enlargement is due to plain, uncomplicated cervicitis, the depletion by means of the glycerine will soon lessen the size of the uterine cervix very perceptibly. If, however, the swollen state of the cervix arises from cancerous infiltration, or from an interstitial fibroid, the glycerine will not sensibly diminish its bulk. If this simple test had been applied in the case before us, my unknown predecessor would not have decided this to be a case of uterine cancer; for now the cervix is nearly normal both in size and texture.

A new diagnostic test.

The increased depth of the womb, the liability to hæmorrhage, to endometritis, to uterine displacements, and to coincident peritonitis, which belong to chronic corporeal metritis, and not to corporeal cervicitis, will serve to separate these two diseases. In some cases they succeed each other, and again they co-exist.

Diagnosis from corporeal metritis.

Prognosis.—This disease may continue indefinitely. Its course and termination will depend upon the nature and severity of the disorders with which it is complicated. It may decline at the climacteric, or possibly develop into a more serious form of organic disease. In a reflex manner it may cause the gravest lesions of the heart, the lungs, or of the nervous centers. Frequent abortions render it more chronic and intractable. If the patient is ill in other respects and incapacitated from exercise, the cure is more doubtful.

Treatment.—It is quite as important to prescribe the proper posture for this class of patients as it is in case of acute cervical metritis.* Keep them in a horizontal or reclining posture, and off their feet, at the month especially. Shopping, visiting, party-going are as injurious as a

Postural treatment.

* See page 277.

journey by rail, or an excursion on horseback. Such a patient should let her sewing-machine rest, and her servants take care of themselves.

General indications.

If there is obstructive dysmenorrhœa, remove the cause and relieve the consequent engorgement of the cervix. If she has intermenstrual dysmenorrhœa, cure it. If the flow is too scanty, try and prompt it to be more free. If the rectum is paralyzed, or the bowels are badly constipated, she may be relieved when these conditions are set aside. She should be especially careful not to do anything before, during or directly after the flow that can by any possibility complicate the case and increase the cervical hypertrophy.

If there are "bilious" symptoms remember that they are likely to afford the most prominent and cardinal indications for the remedy or remedies. Podophyllin, mercurius, chamomilla, bryonia, nux vomica, china, natrum mur., nitric or nitro-muriatic acid, or some similar remedy, may be specifically called for.

Bell., lach. and apis.

Other remedies that I have found especially useful are belladonna, lachesis and apis mellifica. Some of the best cures that I have ever made have been performed with these three remedies in this class of cases.

Local adjuvants.

Locally the same treatment as already recommended for the acute form of this disease is equally suited to the chronic variety.* The cotton tampon saturated with glycerine can do no possible harm, will not interfere with the action of internal remedies, and may do a positive good. After the first application it can be prepared, introduced and removed by the nurse or the patient herself. I generally recommend that it shall be used two or three times per week, according to circumstances.

*See page 278.

LECTURE XXXIV.

VASCULAR TUMOR OF THE MEATUS URINARIUS.

GENTLEMEN:

The refined and cultivated physician is sometimes at a loss to know when it is best to propose, and to insist upon the necessity for a physical examination of the female generative organs. He will not pander to the vulgar habit of resorting to this measure almost indiscriminately; while, for the sake of his patient's welfare, as well as of his own reputation as a skillful diagnostician and practitioner, he must not postpone it too long, neither neglect it entirely. So important is this matter that a physician's reputation is sometimes made or ruined by the rumor that he is in the habit of using the speculum on the slightest pretext, or that he is opposed to its employment altogether.

I am led to these reflections in consequence of the examination which I have just made of a case in the ante-room. This case had been attended by two physicians, one of whom pretended to have made a proper "examination" of the patient, while she refused to allow the other to do so. Both were wrong in their conclusions, and, consequently, neither of them did the patient any good.

Case.—Mrs. T——, 30 years of age, the mother of two children, the youngest of which is four years old, has been in poor health for twelve months. One year ago she got her feet wet while menstruating. She has not been well since. Prior to that date her menstruation had always been regular; but since that sudden check of the flow, the periods have returned every three weeks. There is no pain, but from time to time the flow is becoming more scanty.

Soon after the taking cold she began to have trouble in passing water. The inclination to urinate was very frequent, and sometimes quite irresistible. It was aggravated by being much upon the feet. Anxiety of mind, sudden good or bad news, and excitement of any kind would induce a paroxysm. At first, but only for a short time, the urine was copious and colorless, but for many months it has been perfectly natural in quantity and quality. The only exception to this rule is that it has, once or twice, been a very little bloody.

The only real pain experienced is after the flow of urine, or rather, while the last drops are running away. This induces a burning, stinging pain, which is peculiar, and "very dreadful," to her. Walking is painful, and, for some reason which she can not explain, intercourse occasions the most excruciating suffering.

The first physician who treated her for this difficulty made an examination with the speculum, and after analyzing all the symptoms that were gathered, pronounced her to be suffering from "disease of the kidneys." After some months of treatment with no especial reference either to the menstrual or the urethral difficulties, she changed her physician for one of more intelligence and experience.

Her second physician prescribed for her for a time, and then requested permission to make an examination with the speculum. But it was denied, and he continued to treat her for "disease of the womb."

The physical examination just made discloses a vascular tumor which is nearly the size of my thumb-nail, at and within the mouth of the urethra. It is very tender to the touch, and of a cherry-red color. The urethra around and beyond it is tumefied and evidently somewhat inflamed. The womb is *in situ*, and the os uteri has a healthy appearance.

These vascular tumors, which are not at all infrequent, are very troublesome and often give rise to much suffering. They are located just at the mouth of the urethra, and within its canal, being attached thereto by a pedicle, like a polypus. They consist of a hypertrophy of the mucous papillæ, and are very vascular. Sometimes the tumor is lobulated; more rarely there are two instead of one. The pedicle may be so slender as to break very readily when you seize the growth with a pair of small forceps; or it may be firm and unyielding.

Nature and location.

The symptoms accompanying such a case have already been detailed in this report. Painful and frequent micturition, especially after exercise upon the feet; pain upon walking, intolerance of coitus, and the most peculiar and exquisite suffering with the passage of the last drops of urine, are almost pathognomonic. These symptoms may con-

Symptoms.

tinue until the patient is very weak and irritable. But the diagnosis can not be made with certainty except by a physical examination of the parts involved. Indeed this examination must be *visual*, for unless you see the tumor, you can not be certain of its existence.

Necessity for physical examination.

The question recurs upon the necessity for such an examination. This woman, who lives within a stone's throw of the hospital, has suffered for twelve months when she might have been relieved in as many minutes. But two things were in the way of her getting well so speedily. The first was the ignorance of the doctor who examined her with a uterine speculum, and reported that she had "disease of the kidneys." How this instrument could aid in the diagnosis of renal disease, and what particular affection of the kidneys she was thought to have, I do not know.

Obstacles to recovery in this case.

The second obstacle was her own shrinking sensitiveness, which would not permit the other physician (who was competent) to do as he thought best. And so she has failed to obtain the hoped-for relief.

Rule regulating a resort to physical exploration.

How shall you act in similar cases? The best rule that I can suggest is that you wait a reasonable length of time, providing the symptoms are not very urgent. Give the appropriate remedies meanwhile, and place the patient under such hygienic regulations as will favor her recovery. But if the symptoms do not yield as they should, or if they show a decided tendency to relapse, the inference will be that there is a local cause which perpetuates the mischief, and prevents a radical cure by internal means, alone. Under such circumstances a few sensible and cogent reasons addressed to the patient, will satisfy her of the necessity of a local examination, and obtain her consent thereto. You can explain the case by saying that the persistence of the symptoms and their liability to return when they have been relieved, leads you to conclude that they do not afford a reliable criterion of the nature of her disease. And, above all things, assure her beforehand that you will on no account proceed to operative interference, until the case is fully understood by both parties.

This plan is as appropriate in a case in which the symptoms

are connected with urination, where the quality of the urine is unaltered, as it is in case of chronic and inveterate uterine disease. For you may be morally certain that when you have given cantharis, mercurius, aconite, apis mel., cannabis, hyoscyamus, and kindred remedies, under appropriate indications, and relief has not followed, that the case needs a local examination, and perhaps topical treatment also.

Especially requisite in diseases of the female urethra.

Treatment.—Excision is the remedy. You may seize the growth with a pair of delicate forceps, and snip it off with a pair of sharp scissors, or the bistoury. Or ligation, or astringents and cauterization may answer; but they are more slow and painful. The stump, or point of attachment, may be touched with the per-chloride of iron, or with a stick of the nitrate of silver, in case of hæmorrhage. In order to prevent the subsequent growth of the tumor it may be necessary to repeat the application of the caustic after a few days.

Excision.

The after treatment consists in keeping her in the horizontal posture for twenty-four hours or more, in order to avoid consecutive inflammation. If there are any signs of urethritis, it should then be treated as if the case were an idiopathic one.*

After-treatment.

LATERO-FLEXION OF THE UTERUS.

Case.—Mrs. ——, aged 51, of nervo-bilious temperament, was admitted to the hospital one month ago. She has been suffering more or less for ten years with uterine difficulties. At 40 years of age she was treated locally for ulceration of the os uteri, and cured. She has had three children, the last of which is 16 years old. She passed the climacteric eight months ago without accident, and attributes her present troubles to having to ascend and descend three flights of stairs at her boarding place last winter.

She complains of pain in the back and a sense of dragging down in the pelvis, profuse vaginal leucorrhœa, and a burning pain in the right inguinal region. The last symptom, however, is not constant. She can not lie upon her left side. The right leg is at times numb and almost paralyzed. The bowels are tolerably regular, the appetite is not very good, the urine is normal.

Physical examination reveals a right latero-flexion of the womb,

*See page 181.

the body of the organ being apparently adherent to the right wall of the pelvic cavity. This deviation of the uterus was corrected by means of the sound, which, together with a few doses of nux vomica 3rd, promptly relieved the paralytic feeling in the right limb. The patient was ordered to lie on the left or opposite side, and upon the back exclusively. Subsequently she took the citrate of iron and strychnine in the third decimal trituration, a dose every three hours.

Cases of latero-flexion are comparatively rare. Nonat met with it in but one out of 339 examples of uterine displacement. As in other flexions of the organ the cervix is but slightly, if at all displaced, while the body is more or less curved upon its neck. The pain and distress are usually referred to one side or the other of the pelvis. The womb inclines more frequently to the right than to the left side, probably because in a majority of cases it has taken that direction during pregnancy. In some of these cases it is possible that the involution of the womb after delivery may be less complete in the right or dependent part of the organ, and that, consequently, its increased weight may cause it to topple over in that direction. Occasionally it is said to follow as a sequel of chronic metritis, and also of constipation with paralysis and a stuffed condition of the rectum. It may occur in a woman who, being confined to her couch, persists in lying day and night, always, upon one side of the body. Or it may be displaced laterally by direct pressure from uterine and ovarian tumors, peri-uterine deposits and pelvic abscess.

Relative frequency of.

Causes.

The symptoms are not distinctive. Most patients complain of burning pains in the iliac or the inguinal regions, which pains are severe and protracted, and extend more or less into the corresponding hip and thigh in proportion as the nerves are pressed upon mechanically, and the free distribution of the nervous currents is interfered with. Inability to lie on the opposite or sound side is suggestive, although not by any means pathognomonic of this particular variety of uterine deviation.

Symptoms.

It is only by the introduction of the sound that we can be quite positive in our diagnosis. If, after being passed as far as the internal os uteri, the point shall enter the organ and then travel towards the right or left acetabulum, the concavity of the instrument looking to the corresponding limb of the patient, it is safe to conclude that she has a lateral deviation of the womb. If the direction of the sound is changed when she turns over and lies for a little on the opposite side, the displacement is not a very serious affair.

Physical signs.

I have now passed the sound to the fundus uteri. You will observe that the roughened surface of the handle, which corresponds to the tip of the instrument, and its anterior curve, looks towards the right thigh of the patient. And although, as I have told you, the sound is of little use as a means of repositing the organ, still in these cases of lateral displacement, and with proper precautions, it may be of service in this way. While she is lying upon the opposite side therefore, so that gravity may assist us, we gradually turn the sound, and the uterus along with it, until its pelvic curve or concavity looks towards the symphysis pubis.

Passing the sound.

Now the organ is *in situ*, and the sound has served the double purpose of acquainting us with the precise nature of the displacement, and of furnishing us with a means for its reduction.

Repositing the organ.

The treatment of such a case as this is very simple. The first indication, after having put the organ in place again, is to select a proper posture for the patient. Manifestly she should lie on the opposite side, in order to keep the womb from gravitating into its unnatural position. This woman had right latero-flexion, in which the fundus uteri had toppled over against the right side of the pelvis. She must therefore lie upon her left side, if she wants to get well of this difficulty. There will be no harm in her turning upon the back occasionally, but she should not permit herself to lie upon the right side for months to come.

Postural treatment.

This will be a difficult prescription to take. For the first few days especially, it will require some moral courage to carry out those instructions faithfully. She will probably have pain in both hips, aching and unrest in consequence. She may lose her appetite, pass sleepless nights, and, altogether, feel worse for a time than when she came

Need of courage.

to the hospital. But ultimately her sufferings will be relieved, and she will be glad of her good resolution.

These cases are more readily and radically cured than what is known as latero-version, a condition in which the uterus is directly across the vagina, with the fundus at one acetabulum, and the cervix uteri at the other.

Contingent diseases.

If the uterus has been flexed laterally for a considerable time, it may be so bound down by unnatural adhesions that its reposition will be followed by more or less of peritoneal inflammation. Again it will be followed by a species of sciatica, which is persistent and troublesome. For the former, such remedies as rhus toxicodendron, belladonna, or bryonia, may be required. For the latter, I know of nothing to compare with colocynth.

SPINAL IRRITATION, WITH AMENORRHŒA, VICARIOUS VOMITING AND CONVULSIONS.

I was consulted in the following case by my friend, Dr. Wm. D. Foster, of Hannibal, Mo. The notes thereof were furnished by the patient, who is a most estimable and intelligent person:

Case.—My parents were born in Vermont, and up to within a short period before their death, were very healthy and robust. With my mother the "turn of life" came at 53. This caused a severe illness, which developed into insanity, and finally terminated in death from heart disease. My father lived to be 68, and died of dropsy of the heart. I was born in Cleveland, Ohio, and, when my mother died, was 14 years of age. While visiting Chicago the same season, I had a severe illness, of which I remember nothing, excepting that I had a very sore mouth. Previous to this illness, I had always been very well, except that when I was about seven years old I was vaccinated, and it made me very sick. I lost the use of my left arm for some time; had swellings in the arm-pit and upon the arm, which had to be lanced.

In the spring of 1862, the corner of a falling door struck me between the shoulders, and left me insensible for a day or two. Upon recovery I could not see out of my right eye. It did not pain me much until I began to recover my sight, which was several months after the accident. Often since that time I have been troubled with very severe pains in that eye. At these times the pupil enlarges, and I can not see out of it.

Soon after my illness in Chicago I realized that there was something wrong with my spine. The physicians predicted that I would outgrow it. The pains in the back were almost constant, but were very much aggravated whenever there were signs of torpidity of the liver, which generally occurred two or three times a year. Sometimes I would be prostrated with these attacks for from two to four weeks.

In 1864, I was troubled with the passage of gall-stones. Every few days I would suddenly be prostrated with dreadful pains in my side, which would last for several hours. These attacks developed into such a derangement of the stomach that it would not retain food. The pain finally became constant, and I was seriously ill for about six weeks; was confined to the bed, my back and head troubling me greatly. Prior to this, the worst pains in my back were between the shoulders, extending upwards to the head, and so severe as often to make me delirious for a few hours.

In 1865, I had several abscesses, which were thought to have been caused by my having fallen down stairs. These abscesses are now believed to have formed in the left ovary. I had no more of them until about a year ago, but within a year have had several, all of which have been on the right instead of the left side. They have discharged through the vagina.

I always had more or less headache during my "periods." For the last five years have had considerable pain in the small of my back, and in the womb itself. In the winter of 1867, I think it was, I was laid up for several weeks with lameness in the small of the back, could not move without help, and for some time there was no action of the bladder, the urine being retained. From that time until now I have suffered from scanty and irregular menstruation. The flow finally stopped entirely, and I suffered each month with pain, violent crampings, etc.

I was married in 1860, at the age of 21; always menstruated properly until the time aforesaid, excepting about four months in the year 1859, when, for some unknown reason, my courses stopped. I did not, however, suffer much on account of it. My back always pains me somewhat, but when the different organs named are in a proper condition, I suffer no serious inconvenience from it.

This statement shows, in very graphic outline, the chief points of interest in this case. But there are additional symptoms which our patient could not catalogue.

Vicarious hæmatemesis.

For two years past, whenever the menses have been arrested, scanty, or tardy in their appearance, she has had vomiting of blood. This hæmatemesis never comes excepting at the month, is not very copious, nor is it accompanied or followed by any evidences of inflammation or of other organic disease of the stomach.

She is also subject to periodical attacks of severe pain in the back and head, which end in spasms, delirium, and finally in clonic spasms of the muscles of the back, with opisthotonos and fearful convulsions of all the voluntary muscles. Concerning these paroxysms, which are even more painful to her friends than to herself, the Doctor says; "I have observed that the cramps, delirium, dilatation of the right pupil, pains in the spine, etc., invariably come on when there is any difficulty with the liver. The menstrual approach excites the same train of symptoms. So also does any mental trouble, disappointment, or other cause of serious mental excitement.

Convulsions.

The causes of.

"The sensitiveness of the spine is most marked in the lower cervical and upper dorsal regions. The spine, however, is somewhat sensitive throughout. She frequently falls to the floor; but, when she has any premonition, usually gets to a chair or lounge, and saves herself. These spells usually follow the more severe symptoms of spinal irritation. She has never been pregnant."

Prodromata.

The patient came to this city, and was under my care for several weeks. Her case was interesting and intricate, for several theories of her disease suggested themselves. Her illnesss might be said to have dated from her vaccination; or to have been caused by the traumatic injury of the spine from the falling door, and from falling down stairs (spinal irritation); to the hepatic complication; the menstrual irregularity and suffering; or to the epileptiform nature of the paroxysms. But the history of the case led us to infer that these causes had acted conjointly, or rather consecutively, to produce so complicated a set of symptoms.

Theories concerning the nature of the disease.

My friend, the Doctor, had faithfully applied the most appropriate remedies for the relief of the individual and collective symptoms, but without any real or lasting benefit. In this treatment he had persisted for more than two years. The menstrual derangement being marked and prominent, we concluded that it must be an important factor in the case. In his letter, the Doctor said:

Fidelity in the use of remedies.

"The non-appearance of the menses and the scant flow have been invariably owing to the spasmodic closure of the uterine cervix. Whenever I have succeeded in passing a tent within the internal os uteri, the flow proceeded properly. But the introduction of that instrument was a proceeding in which I think there were more failures than successes. By the use of Atlee's dilator, however, I could accomplish the purpose with much greater certainty."

Cause of the menstrual disorder.

Dilatation was therefore persevered with so as, if possible, to overcome the spasmodic closure of the cervix and to secure a free and easy flow of the menses. If this end were obtained, it was thought the result would be to bring relief to the nervous centers that were surcharged with blood—the patient being very fleshy and of full habit. But this means failed because of the persistent inclination to spasm of the uterine neck. For almost as soon as the tent, or Priestly's dilator, had been removed, the cervix would shut so tightly that it would be next to impossible to pass the sound.

Failure of dilatation.

We accordingly determined upon incision. The Doctor came to town and assisted me in the operation. I performed the bilateral section with a Simpson's hysterotome, but did not cut the wall of the cervix entirely through, as recommended by Sims, and practiced by my friend Comstock. The hæmorrhage, which was not severe, was arrested by a cervical tampon that had been saturated with the tincture of the per-chloride of iron. The patient was kept in bed for one week only, the cervix being dilated every alternate day with Priestly's dilator, to prevent atresia of its canal.

The operation of incision of the cervix.

She soon returned home, and with the occasional passage of the sound, and of the dilator (which are introduced without difficulty since the operation of incision), she menstruates more regularly and copiously than she has done for a long time. Thus far she has had no more vomiting of blood. In other respects, also, her health is somewhat improved. The convulsive paroxysms are less frequent than they were. Their character and severity, however, are unchanged. The cervical and dorsal pains continue. The dilatation of the pupil and the temporary amaurosis are relatively infrequent of late, but

Subsequent history.

when they are present they have the same characters as before. This patient is therefore still under treatment.

Practical points.

Now, gentlemen, I have brought this case to your notice for the sake of illustrating three very important points, viz.: (1.) That in your daily experience as practitioners, you will discover that the diseases of women are often more complicated than you had supposed they could be; (2) that Uterine Surgery, and Uterine Therapeutics are by no means perfect and infallible; and (3) that, in this as in some other departments of our art, rapid and brilliant cures are the exception and not the rule.

A fallacious idea.

If clinical teachers were always faithful to their trust, and if those who report their experience in our societies and journals always told the plain, unvarnished truth, such cardinal facts need not be mentioned in this connection. But it is not so. Students are often led to believe that nosological distinctions are real, and that diseases run an uncomplicated and unvarying course. If they have little knowledge of human nature and of human frailties, and especially if they have seen but little of the "practice," they are decidedly impressed with this idea. But the illusion vanishes when they are brought face to face with disease. And I have sometimes thought that they are more likely to be undeceived in this respect in treating the diseases that are peculiar to women, than in their experience with any other class of ailments. This is a case in point.

Dogmatic surgery and medicine.

It is so easy to dictate and dogmatize in these matters that one might prescribe a manual operation, or an internal remedy for such a patient, and insist that either of them should effect a cure. But you will find that these very complicated cases are not so easily disposed of. A certain operation, or a single remedy, may need to be modified or changed repeatedly, perhaps, before the cure is effected, if indeed it ever is. The incision of the cervix uteri in this case was of real service. It is a great point gained to have secured the regularity and freedom of the menstrual flow, and more than all, to have put a period to the hæmatemesis before any manifest organic disease of the stomach had supervened. But the operation has not cured the woman at all. And it would be wrong for me to report her as well again, when she is not.

There are those who will tell you that this or that remedy, in a particular potency, would undoubtedly have cured her. But such an opinion is presumptuous. We can accomplish much with our remedies. When fitly chosen they are wonderfully efficacious. Every year their curative scope is widened, and their clinical range more accurately defined. But, although we can accomplish more than our predecessors ever did, and with means that they deemed too insignificant to be of any practical use, we should not claim that our skill and success are unbounded. If we are unreasonably confident we defeat our purpose and disgrace our calling.

Do not claim too much.

The health of woman is exposed to so many vicissitudes, and she is the victim of so many interior sources of mischief, that you will always do well to qualify your prognosis and your promises to cure her, even of the simplest ailment. Especially should you forbear from engaging to restore her rapidly to a good state of health, in case of any disorder of menstruation or of the nervous system. I once heard a physician claim that a single dose of sepia had entirely cured one of his patients of a long-standing and serious dysmenorrhœa. It had cut short her suffering and relieved her like magic. This last result we were prepared to credit; but, when he went on to say that the prescription had been made only a fortnight before, and that the menstrual cycle had not yet returned, every experienced person present knew just what to think of the rapid and radical cure which, in all probability, had *not* been effected.

Qualify your promises.

Case.

VULVO-VAGINITIS. — PRURIGENOUS VULVITIS.

Case. — Mrs. T——, aged 45, English, married and the mother of eight children, was admitted to the hospital yesterday. She has never had a miscarriage. Three years ago she was troubled with a sudden arrest of the menses, which continued for eight months. They finally came on again spontaneously, and in the usual quantity, but the flow was subsequently attended with considerable pain. The climacteric was passed without any untoward symptoms one year ago.

During the period of arrest of the catamenia, this patient was treated for ulceration of the womb, which, she says, was accompanied by considerable discharge. At one time she remembers a sudden flow of "matter" which, she thinks, amounted in all to nearly or quite a tea-cup full. This discharge came suddenly "like the waters." There has been no trouble in micturition. The bowels have been constipated, and she has been annoyed with internal hæmorrhoids which occasionally bleed.

At present she complains of intense itching of the genitals, and says that pimples sometimes form on the labia and then burst. There is heat in the vagina, especially after exercise, and occasionally a slight, but never a copious, leucorrhœa.

She also has considerable pain in the right leg, which extends from the right iliac region in front, around and over the hip, and down the limb to the inner malleolus and the inside of the foot. This pain is not affected by changes of weather, but is aggravated by motion. The right knee-joint is enlarged, as in chronic synovitis.

On physical examination the uterus was found in position, and of normal size. Examination with the speculum revealed the mucous membrane lining the vagina and reflected over the vaginal portion of the cervix to be studded with a papulous eruption resembling prurigo. The same eruption extends over the vulva and the adjacent integuments.

This, gentlemen, is one of the old-fashioned women, whose maternal record is in every respect a creditable one. She has borne eight children, and has never suffered a miscarriage. If it were possible, I would take occasion to name all the physical and moral exemptions that she has enjoyed in consequence. Not the least among them is that she has escaped any serious illness at the climacteric.

An exceptional case.

Three years ago, at the age of 42, she had suppression of the menses for eight months. Meanwhile she received treatment for ulceration of the womb, but whether she ever had that disease, we do not know. It is very probable that her physician mistook the suppression for a sign of ulceration, and proceeded to cauterize her with a view to restore the catamenial flow. It is equally probable that the menstrual arrest was due to a physiological and not to a morbific cause, or in other words, that it was a sign of the approach of the "change of life;" for, as I have already said, such intermissions in the performance of this function are by no

Intermittent menstruation before the change.

means rare in women who have reached their fortieth year, and in whom the period for its entire cessation can not be very distant.

Defective ovulation.

The probable cause for such a temporary arrest, and which is apt to be overlooked, is a failure in the ripening of the ovule, and in the dehiscence of the Graäfian follicle. By-and-by the function of ovulation is resumed and the menstrual flow re-appears.

The sudden discharge.

The muco-purulent discharge of which she speaks may have been due to a vicarious accumulation and retention within the uterine cavity, which finally found vent with the suddenness of a rupture of the bag of waters. She could not have had an abscess without previous local pain and suffering, and general constitutional symptoms, of which she makes no mention.

Constipation is the rule in similar cases, and a woman at 45, who has had eight children, can hardly have escaped hæmorrhoids. Concerning the latter I have questioned her carefully, and find that they are not inveterate.

Symptoms.

This prurigenous eruption is always accompanied by a loss of rest and sleep, constant irritation and distress. It is very apt to become chronic. The heat of the parts, and the torment sometimes occasioned by walking, sitting, intercourse, and physical exercise of every kind, are almost insupportable. If the characteristic peculiarities of the eruption have not been destroyed by the scratching and rubbing of the parts to which the poor victim is compelled to resort, the papulæ resemble those of prurigo when it is seated on other parts of the body, as, for example, the neck, shoulders, back and outer surfaces of the extremities. So much of it as is located upon the cutaneous surface of the labia, the perineum, and even about the anus, may be colorless and invisible, but if the parts have been wounded by friction, you may perhaps find little black scabs scattered here and there. Sometimes, as in this case, there are occasional vesicles and wheals, which are readily discharged.

The eruption.

On the mucous side of the raphé and within the vagina, however, the color of the eruption differs from that of the surface upon which the papulæ are located. This is especially true in the case of elderly women in whom there is no diffuse vaginitis, and whose vaginal mucous membrane has not recently been discolored either by pregnancy or menstruation. But, in younger persons, in whom the opposite condition of this membrane prevails, there would be very little difference in hue between them.

The color of.

The causes of this peculiar affection are really unknown. It has been ascribed to various infractions of the rules of hygiene, such as the eating of unwholesome food, and the lack of proper clothing, cleanliness and exercise, to sexual excesses, to the change of life, and to the non-elimination by the proper emunctories of certain impurities from the blood. It may alternate with chronic skin disease.

Causes.

There is a form of granular vaginitis from which pregnant women sometimes suffer that should not be confounded with this. In it the eruption, or rather the pin-head pimples, consists of myriads of little granulations which give rise to pain, heat, and sometimes to considerable discharge. It is self-limited, is not accompanied by vulvar prurigo, and terminates with delivery.

Diagnosis from granular vaginitis.

Prurigenous vulvitis, of which this is an example, can be distinguished from the follicular variety by the fact that in the latter the lesion is limited to the follicles which are found upon the vulva, and just within the ostium vaginæ. These follicles become inflamed and finally discharge a purulent or muco-purulent secretion which, in many cases, may be seen exuding from the mouths of the separate follicles. But these diseases often co-exist. Follicular vulvitis is also incident to gestation, and may occur as a contingent or sequel of the eruptive fevers, and of diphtheria. More frequently, however, it is due to a very depraved and vitiated habit. Sometimes it is a sequel of gonorrhœal inflammation.

From follicular vulvitis.

This form of vulvo-vaginitis not being purulent as it would be if the eruption were eczematous, or herpetic, or if the inflammation were more diffuse and deep-seated, the amount of the leucorrhœal discharge is not in proportion with the local suffering. Mrs. T. has but little flow of this kind. Where, however, the eruption and the inflammation extend within the cervix uteri, and possibly into the uterine cav-

The leucorrhœa.

ity, as there is good reason for believing that they sometimes do, the quantity of mucus and of pus secreted may be very large. In middle-aged and more vigorous subjects the presence of these little papulæ (as in case of other vegetative growths within the vulva), may excite a very troublesome leucorrhœa. If the discharge that is poured out is thin and serous in character, it is very apt to dry upon the parts and then to crack and break into little scales which cause an intolerable pruritus. Some of these patients will tell you that they have no leucorrhœa, when in fact they are deceived and the discharge is disposed of in this way. In rare instances the eruption invades the urethra and occasions a very persistent and troublesome form of urethritis.

A practical inference concerning uterine displacements.

The entire exemption of our patient from urinary troubles, such as strangury and the like, affords an indirect proof that she has not suffered from any variety of uterine deviation. For this reason I felt almost confident that her womb was *in situ* before passing the sound. You remember that the attachments between the neck of the uterus and the bladder are such that it is next to impossible to displace the former without pressing upon, or changing the position of, the latter. And when a woman tells you that she is not subject to, and has not suffered from, vesical troubles of any kind, you may be reasonably assured that her womb is where it should be. But you are not to conclude that because she has strangury, dysuria, etc., therefore her womb is displaced; for these symptoms may arise from other and very different causes.

Prognosis.

The prognosis is generally favorable, but the time required for the cure will vary according to circumstances. Such cases recover more readily in winter than in summer, in cool than in warm climates, and in young than in old patients. Scrofulous persons, and those who are predisposed to aphthous conditions, or to chronic cutaneous eruptions of whatever kind, get well very slowly. The syphilitic taint may retard the cure. If it follows the climacteric very closely, or co-exists, as in the case before us, with rheumatism, we shall not be warranted in promising very speedy and permanent relief.

Treatment.—As affording direct relief, and being capable of making life tolerable, the topical treatment is very important. The proper palliatives have already been mentioned when speaking of pruritus of the vulva.* Cleanliness, frequent bathing with cool or tepid water, and the application of a bland demulcent, as bran-water, glycerine, almond oil with or without chloroform, or of the muriate of hydrastin with glycerine, will answer an excellent purpose. Cloths or compresses anointed or saturated with one of these may be applied to the vulva; or the cotton tampon may be the vehicle for introducing the same into the vagina.

Topical treatment.

The diet should be plain and unstimulating, the exercise moderate, and coitus positively forbidden.

The internal remedies should be suited more especially to the character of the eruption, the patient's peculiar dyscrasia, and the relation of the disease to child-bearing and the climacteric. Among the remedies that may be required in different cases are rhus tox., sepia, sulphur, arsenicum, calcarea carb., conium, hydrastis, croton tig., carbo veg., mercurius, natrum mur., kali carb., creasotum, thuja and the mineral acids.

Constitutional treatment.

Taking the peculiar eruption, and the incidental rheumatic symptoms as a guide, I shall select the rhus tox. as the remedy for this patient. She will take of the 3d attenuation a dose every three hours. This frequent repetition is justified in her case by the severity of her rheumatism. She will also have the glycerine and hydrastin applied locally morning and evening.

INFANTILE LEUCORRHŒA.

There is a form of vulvo-vaginitis to which little girls are liable, and of which I may speak in this connection. The mucous membrane reflected over the vulva becomes so inflamed, heated and irritated, that the child has no rest, but is constantly tempted to relieve itself by rubbing the parts, which only increases the trouble and extends the inflammation. Sometimes the first symptom complained of is pain on passing water, which also creates a sense of scalding and itching. This is accompanied by dryness, redness, and heat of the inflamed surfaces. Soon, however, the parts become moist from the exu-

Symptoms.

* See page 159.

dation of a thin, colorless mucus which, as the case progresses, becomes of a thick and creamy consistence.

The leucorrhœal flow.

The amount and quality of the leucorrhœal discharge varies with the constitutional taint, as well as with the duration of the disease. In scrofulous children, more especially if they have been allowed improper food and have not been kept in a cleanly, healthful condition, the leucorrhœal flow may be either very copious, or perhaps ichorous and corrosive. In bad cases of this kind there is not only inflammation, but ulceration also of the vaginal mucous membrane. When these patches of ulceration are present, they may be seen by stretching the labia apart. More rarely they are found in the upper portion of the vagina.

Causes.

The causes of this form of vaginitis in children are numerous. Sometimes the urine has such acrid properties as by its flow over the vaginal surface to induce this disease. Simple catarrhal urethritis may develop into vulvo-vaginitis. Or it may arise idiopathically from exposure to cold, or a sudden check of perspiration. Sometimes it takes the form of an epidemic, and prevails in winter along with a more or less severe influenza. I have known it to alternate with a severe and troublesome coryza. It may attack several children in the same family or neighborhood. Irritation of the rectum, and sometimes of the colon, may induce it. In some instances it is due to the presence of worms that have escaped at the anus, and crawled within the vaginal orifice, where, by their presence, they excite a great degree of itching and irritation. And sometimes there is no doubt that it has been caused by a mischievous rubbing and irritation of the parts by nurses and servants who have had the children in charge.

Treatment.

The proper treatment for cases of infantile leucorrhœa is first, if possible, to remove the cause. It is very important to avoid exposure to cold and wet, and to order a proper and digestible diet. Cleanliness, bathing and drying the parts carefully afterwards, either with a very soft towel, or better still, with an application of finely pulverized starch, or lycopodium powder, as in case of infants to prevent intertrigo, are very useful.

If the complaint is related to influenza, the internal remedies will be the same as are suited to the epidemic catarrhal inflammation, no matter where it is located. If it occurs in scrofulous children, the remedies which suggest themselves, and which are most useful, are calcarea carb., hepar sulph., and mercurius. A majority of cases may be cured with pulsatilla, or calcarea carb.

Local and general.

If the passage of the urine occasions great suffering, give cantharis, and have cloths that have been dipped in warm water applied over the vulva. If there is ulceration, or aphthous inflammation, add hydrastin or calendula to the water. If ascarides have created the mischief, order lard to be smeared about the anus, or a decoction of garlic, or an injection of olive oil to be thrown into the bowel, and give the child teucrium.

It is important that children who have this affection should not be allowed to sleep in the same bed, or to be washed with the same towels as those who are healthy. For although the disease is not always easy of communication, yet it might happen that it would spread through a whole family of little ones, and occasion much suffering and anxiety. It is a pleasure to be able to assure the mother or nurse that, with proper time and care, this disease may be readily and certainly cured.

Isolation.

INDEX.

A.

D.

E.

F.

G.

I.

P.

T.